Medical Terminology

A Student-Centered Approach, Second Edition

Marie A. Moisio, MA, RHIA
formerly of Northern Michigan University, Marquette, Michigan

Elmer W. Moisio, PhD, RN
formerly of Northern Michigan University, Marquette, Michigan

DISCARD

Australia Canada Mexico Singapore Spain United Kingdom United States

DELMAR
™
THOMSON LEARNING

Medical Terminology: A Student-Centered Approach, Second Edition
Marie A. Moisio and Elmer W. Moisio

Vice President, Health Care Business Unit:
William Brottmiller

Director of Learning Solutions:
Matthew Kane

Acquisitions Editor:
Matthew Seeley

Editorial Assistant:
Megan Tarquinio

Product Manager:
Debra Myette-Flis

Marketing Director:
Jennifer McAvey

Marketing Manager:
Michele C. McTighe

Marketing Coordinator:
Chelsey Iaqunita

Production Director:
Carolyn Miller

Content Project Manager:
Thomas Heffernan

Technology Product Manager:
Carolyn Fox

Senior Art Director:
Jack Pendleton

Library of Congress Cataloging-in-Publication Data
Moisio, Marie A.
  Medical terminology : a student-centered approach / Marie A. Moisio and Elmer W. Moisio. -- 2nd ed.
    p. ; cm.
  Includes index.
  ISBN-13: 978-1-4018-9750-5
  ISBN-10: 1-4018-9750-9
  1. Medicine--Terminology--Problems, exercises, etc. I. Moisio, Elmer W. II. Title.
  [DNLM: 1. Terminology--Problems and Exercises. W 18.2 M714m 2008]
  R123.M595 2008
  610.1'4--dc22

                                         2007011934

NOTICE TO THE READER

Contents

Preface

Introduction

Medical terminology is the language of the health care industry. Successful functioning of health care workers in any position related to the industry requires a working knowledge of this language. *Medical Terminology: A Student-Centered Approach, Second Edition* provides basic information about the structures and functions of each body system and numerous reinforcement exercises designed to assist the student in mastering the meaning and spelling of literally thousands of medical terms.

The text is designed for use by educational programs in the areas of medical assisting, medical transcription, medical coding, health insurance billing, nursing, surgical technician, health unit coordinating, and other health related professions. It can also be used for in-service training and professional development.

Objectives

The primary objective of this text is to provide students with a clear, concise understanding of commonly used medical terms by:

- Introducing students to the foundations of medical terminology
- Presenting techniques for breaking complex medical terms into roots, prefixes, and suffixes
- Providing a variety of reinforcement exercises to enable students to learn to spell, define, and use medical terms

Features of the Text

This text has many features designed to encourage student success in learning medical terminology.

- Learning objectives identify expectations for each chapter.
- Numerous reinforcement exercises following each major chapter topic were field-tested by medical terminology students.
- A CD-ROM with exercises, pronunciations, and games is available to supplement the reinforcement exercises.
- Medical reports provide an opportunity to learn medical terms in context.
- End-of-chapter reviews include objective and subjective measures of student comprehension.
- Term pronunciation lists at the end of each chapter correlate to the terms recorded on the CD-ROM.
- Challenge exercises encourage students to use the Internet for further study.
- Appendices include word elements and abbreviations.

Changes to the Second Edition

Based on instructor recommendations, the second edition was reorganized from 20 chapters to 16 chapters.

- Chapter 1 Medical Terminology Building Blocks includes roots, prefixes, suffixes, combining and pronunciation rules, and instructions for analyzing medical terms. This chapter is a combination of the previous Chapter 1 and Chapter 2 Prefixes and Suffixes.
- Chapter 4 Skeletal System now includes material related to joints, which was removed Chapter 6 Muscular System
- Chapter 13 Female Reproductive System includes both reproductive and obstetric terminology. This chapter is a combination of the previous Chapter 14 Female Reproductive System and Chapter 15 Obstetrics.
- Chapter 15 Sensory System: Vision and Hearing includes medical terminology of the eye and ear. This chapter is a combination of the previous Chapter 17 Sensory System: The Eye and Chapter 18 Sensory System: The Ear.
- Chapter 16 Specialty Terminology is a new chapter that includes terminology related to oncology, pharmacology, and surgical terminology. Anesthesia terminology in this chapter includes sedation and conscious sedation.

Other major changes include:

- Several disease photographs added to help learners visualize medical conditions
- New medical reports added to chapters 4, 9, 15, and 16
- Blood group content added to Chapter 7
- Bariatric surgery content added to Chapter 9
- Information related to human papilloma virus (HPV) infections is included with other sexually transmitted infection material in Chapter 12
- Descriptions of various biopsies was added to Chapter 16
- Answers to chapter exercises were moved to the Instructor's Manual on the Electronic Classroom Manager CD-ROM.
- A StudyWARE™ CD-ROM offering additional practice through quizzes, activities and animations.

Comprehensive Teaching and Learning Resources

Medical Terminology: A Student-Centered Approach, Second Edition StudyWARE™

The StudyWARE™ CD-ROM offers an exciting way to gain additional practice in working with medical terms. The quizzes and activities help you remember even the most difficult terms. See "How to Use *Medical Terminology: A Student-Centered Approach*, Second Edition StudyWARE™ on page xi for details.

The Electronic Classroom Manager

The Electronic Classroom Manager is a robust, computerized tool for your instructional needs! A must have for all instructors, this comprehensive and convenient CD-ROM contains:

- **The Instructor's Manual** is designed to help you with lesson preparation and performance assessment. It includes:
  - Fifteen-and Ten-Week Course Schedules
  - Generic Lecture Plans
  - Suggested Classroom Activities
  - Chapter Quizzes with Answer Keys
  - Final Exam with Answer Keys
  - Case Reports
  - Answers to review exercises in the text

- **Exam View®Computerized Testbank** contains 980 questions. You can use these questions, and add your own questions to create review materials or tests.
- **PowerPoint® Presentations** designed to aid you in planning your class presentations. If a learner misses a class, a print-out of the slides for a lecture makes a helpful review page.

Electronic Classroom Manager, ISBN 1-4018-9752-5

WebTUTOR™

Designed to compliment the book, WebTUTOR™ is a content rich, web-based teaching and learning aid that reinforces and clarifies complex concepts. The WebCT™ and Blackboard™ platforms also provide rich communication tools to instructors and students, including a course calendar, chat, email, and threaded discussions.

WebTUTOR™ on WebCT™, ISBN 1 4018-9755-X
Text Bundled with WebTUTOR™ on WebCT™, ISBN 1-4283-9366-8
WebTUTOR™ on Blackboard™, ISBN 1-4018-9756 8
Text Bundled with WebTUTOR™ on Blackboard™, ISBN 1-4283-9368-4

Delmar Learning's Medical Terminology Audio Library

This extensive audio library of medical terminology includes four Audio CDs with over 3,700 terms pronounced, and a software CD-ROM. The CD-ROM presents terms organized by body systems, medical specialty, and general medical term categories. The user can search for a specific term by typing in the term or key words, or click on a category to view an alphabetical list of all terms within the category. Hear the correct pronunciation of one term or listen to each term on the list pronounced automatically. Definitions can be viewed after hearing the pronunciation of terms.

Institutional Version ISBN: 1-4018-3223-7
Individual Version ISBN: 1-4018-3222-9

Flashcards

The flashcards provide practice for more than 800 medical terms, with phonetic pronunciations and definitions provided.

ISBN: 1-4283-4122-6

Acknowledgments

Reviewers

A special thank-you is extended to the following reviewers who provided suggestions for improvement throughout the development of this text. Their experience and knowledge served as a valuable resource for the authors.

Constance L. Allen, MS Anatomy & Physiology
Professor of Biology
Edison College
Ft. Myers, Florida

Debra Biddle, MS, RTR
Instructor
Portland Community College
Portland, Oregon

Karen Feltner, RHIT, CCS
Program Director
Health Information Technology
Roane State Community College
Harriman, Tennessee

Deborah Newton, BS, MA, PhD
Program Director
Montana State University College of Technology
Great Falls, Montana

Frederika de Yampert, MSN, RN
Associate Professor
Nursing Department
ChairFinlandia University
Hancock, Michigan

Marie A. Moisio and Elmer W. Moisio

How to Use *Medical Terminology: A Student-Centered Approach, Second Edition* StudyWARE™

The StudyWARE™ software helps you learn terms and concepts in *Medical Terminology: A Student-Centered Approach, Second Edition*. As you study each chapter in the text, be sure to explore the activities in the corresponding chapter in the software. Use StudyWARE™ as your own private tutor to help you learn the material in your *Medical Terminology: A Student-Centered Approach, Second Edition* textbook.

Getting started is easy. Install the software by inserting the CD-ROM into your computer's CD-ROM drive and following the on-screen instructions. When you open the software, enter your first and last name so the software can store your quiz results. Then choose a chapter from the menu to take a quiz or explore one of the activities.

MENUS:

You can access the menus from wherever you are in the program. The menus include Quizzes, Activities, and Scores.

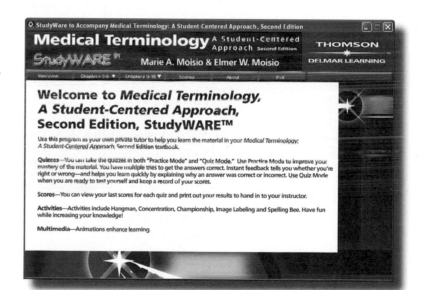

QUIZZES:

Quizzes include multiple choice and fill-in-the-blank questions. You can take the quizzes in both Practice Mode and Quiz Mode. Use Practice Mode to improve your mastery of the material. You have multiple tries to get the answer correct. Instant feedback tells you whether you're right or wrong—and helps you learn quickly by explaining why an answer was correct or incorrect. Use Quiz Mode when you are ready to test yourself and keep a record of your scores. In Quiz Mode, you have one try to get the answers right, but you can take each quiz as many times as you want.

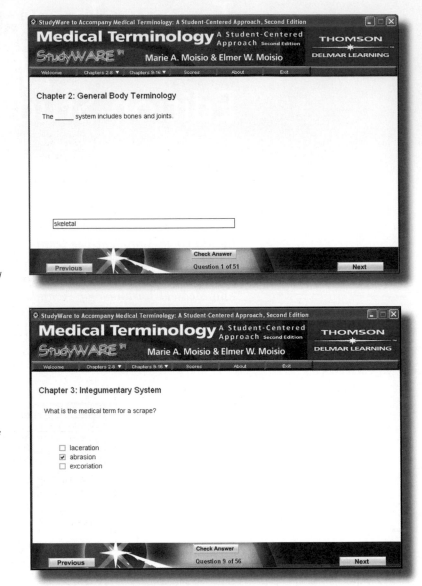

SCORES:

You can view your last scores for each quiz and print your results to hand in to your instructor.

Reports for Student 1

Date Taken	Quiz Name	Score	
5/30/2007 (3:20 p.m.)	Chapter 11: Endocrine System	34	View Details

Title	StudyWare to Accompany Medical Terminology: A Student-Cent
Quiz	Chapter 11: Endocrine System
Name	Student 1

Date   5/30/2007
Time   3:20 p.m.
Score   34%

Question Type	Question	Result	Correct Answer	Your Answer
Multiple Choice	Which hormone is responsible for decreasing blood glucose levels?	✓	insulin	insulin
Multiple Choice	Select the term for male physical traits found in women.	✗	virilism	hirsutism
True/False	Progesterone stimulates placental growth and development.	✓	True	True

ACTIVITIES:

Activities include concentration, hangman, image labeling, Spelling Bee, and a Jeopardy!-style Championship game. Have fun while increasing your knowledge!

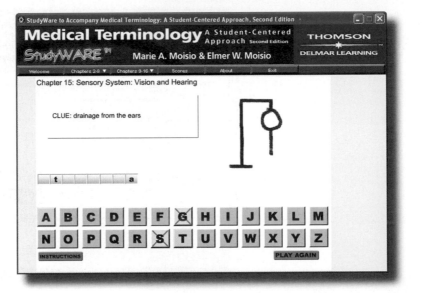

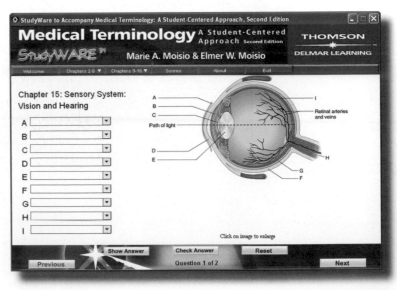

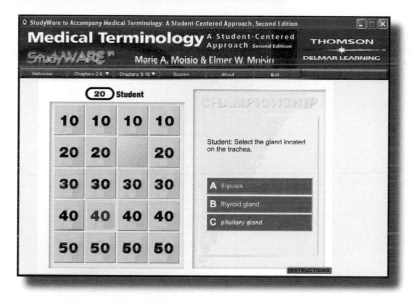

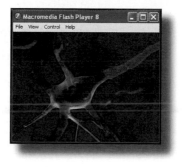

ANIMATIONS:
Animations help you
visualize concepts.

Chapter 1
Building Blocks of Medical Terminology

OBJECTIVES

At the completion of this chapter, the student should be able to:
1. Briefly define roots, prefixes, suffixes, combining forms, and combining vowels.
2. Analyze medical terms by identifying the root, prefix, and suffix.
3. Combine roots and suffixes accurately.
4. Build medical terms using roots, prefixes, suffixes, and combining vowels.

OVERVIEW

Learning medical terminology is very much like learning a foreign language. You begin by studying the rules of the language, progress to learning words, move on to putting the words together to form sentences, and finally, develop the ability to communicate using the language.

It is virtually impossible to "memorize" a language, but you can, and must, memorize the rules and word parts associated with the language. For example, in Spanish the word parts *-a* (pronounced "ah") and *-ita* (pronounced "eetah") represent the female gender. Señor*a* is an adult or married woman and señor*ita* is a young or unmarried woman. One rule of the Spanish language states that *el* precedes a singular male noun and *la* precedes a singular female noun (*los* and *las* are used for plural male and female nouns, respectively). Therefore, the correct way to write *the young girl* in Spanish is *la señorita.*

Most medical terms are derived from Greek and Latin. Fortunately, you do not need to learn those languages to understand medical terminology. The Greek and Latin bases for medical terms are included in all medical dictionaries. As you look up the definitions for medical terms, you will notice that the Greek and Latin foundations are included in the definitions.

Medical terminology is the language of the health care industry. To use this language, you must memorize the word parts and rules. Many medical words, like English words, are made up of three basic parts: roots, prefixes, and suffixes. Various combinations of these components determine the meaning of the words.

In the English language, the root word *cycle* takes on a new meaning when combined with the prefixes *bi-, tri-,* and *uni-.* Bicycles, tricycles, or unicycles are vehicles with wheels and pedals that require "person-power" to move. Combining the root word *cycle* with another root, *motor,* results in the term *motorcycle.* A motorcycle is a vehicle with wheels and pedals that is powered by a motor or engine. If you know the meaning of the roots, prefixes, and suffixes, you are able to understand the word.

This chapter introduces roots, prefixes, and suffixes as they apply to medical terminology. Rules for combining the word parts, also called **word elements**, are presented as well.

Roots

A **root** is the foundation of a medical term. Medical terms usually have at least one root. Roots usually identify a part of the body or a color and always keep the same meaning. Prefixes and suffixes change the meaning of words that have the same root. Some of the more common body part roots are as follows:

- arthr = joint
- cardi = heart
- derm or dermat = skin
- gastr = stomach

All medical term roots have a **combining form** that is created when a root is combined with a vowel. The vowel, called the **combining vowel**, is usually an *o* and occasionally an *i* or *e*. The combining vowel is used to join word elements and helps ease the pronunciation of medical terms. The combining form of a root is written with a slash followed by the combining vowel. Review the following examples of combining forms:

- arthr**/o** = joint
- cardi**/o** = heart
- dermat**/o** = skin
- gastr**/o** = stomach

The combining form of a root is used when joining roots with roots or combining roots with suffixes that begin with a consonant. In this text, word roots are introduced with the appropriate body system. For example, *cardi/o* means "heart" and is included with other word roots in the cardiovascular system chapter; *gastr/o* means "stomach" and is included with other word roots in the digestive system chapter.

Roots that identify color are found throughout each body system chapter. The combining form of these roots are listed here:

- cyan/o = blue; bluish
- eosin/o = rosy red; rosy
- erythr/o = red
- leuk/o = white
- melan/o = black
- xanth/o = yellow

Prefixes

A **prefix** is a word element or part that is added to the beginning of the word root. All medical terms do not have a prefix. In a list of word parts, prefixes are easily identified because they are written with a hyphen after the prefix. Many prefixes associated with medical terms keep their English meaning. For example, pre- (before), post- (after), and anti- (against) are commonly used medical terminology prefixes that retain the English meaning. Review the following examples of prefixes:

- ante- = before; forward
- hemi- = half
- multi- = many
- neo- = new
- sub- = under; below

Prefixes are added to a word root without additional vowels or combining forms. Commonly used prefixes are presented later in this chapter. You must memorize these prefixes so that you can apply their meaning to the medical terms presented in the body system chapters.

Suffixes

A **suffix** is a word element or part that is added to the end of the word root. All medical terms must have a suffix to complete the term, except in those rare instances when the root can stand alone as a word. In a list of word parts, suffixes are easy to recognize because they are written with a hyphen preceding the suffix.

As with prefixes, suffixes change the meaning of the medical term. In addition, suffixes indicate whether a medical term is a noun or an adjective. Remember that a noun identifies a person, place, animal, or thing and an adjective is a word that describes a noun. Review the following examples of adjective suffixes:

- -ac; -al; -ar; -ary = pertaining to; like
- -ic; -iac = pertaining to
- -oid = like; resembling

Adjective suffixes have the same meaning both for English words and for medical terms. For example, circul**ar** driveway means that your driveway is like a circle; a theatric**al** event means that the event pertains to the theater; an andr**oid** is an object that resembles a human. A few noun suffixes and their meanings are presented here:

- -ectomy (ek-toh-mee) = surgical removal; excision
- -itis (igh-tis) = inflammation of
- -megaly (meg-ah-lee) = enlargement
- -pathy (path-ee) = disease

Commonly used suffixes are also presented later in this chapter. You must memorize these suffixes so that you can apply their meaning to the medical terms presented in the body system chapters.

EXERCISE I

Fill in the blanks.

1. Word parts that make up medical terms are also called
   _____ .

2. A/An ___root___ is the foundation of a medical term.

3. _Combining vowels_ are added to the end of word roots.

4. A/An ___Prefix___ is added to the beginning of a word root.

5. Most medical terms have a/an ___Prefix___ and a/an
   ___Suffix___

6. The _____ is used to join word elements and help the pronunciation of medical terms.

7. A/An _____ is created when a root is combined with a vowel, usually *o* or sometimes an *i* or *e*.

8. Suffixes indicate whether a medical term is a/an _____ or a/an _____

EXERCISE 2

Write the meaning of the listed word elements.

1. arthr/o _____ *joint*
2. gastr/o _____ *stomach*
3. ante- _____ *before or forward*
4. multi- _____ *many*
5. -oid _____ *like or resembling*
6. -ic _____ *pertaining to*
7. -megaly _____ *large*
8. -pathy _____ *disease*

Combining Roots, Prefixes, and Suffixes

Combining roots, prefixes, and suffixes is the basic way to create medical terms. A few rules apply to this process. Review the following rules and examples and complete the exercises.

1. *When combining more than one root in a medical term, the combining form of the root is usually used between the roots.*
   Example: **cardi**o**gastric** (**kar**-dee-oh-**GASS**-trik) = pertaining to the heart and stomach.
   Note that the combining form *cardi/o* is used to join the roots *cardi* and *gastr*.
2. *When combining a root with a suffix that begins with a consonant (any letter other than a, e, i, o, u, and y), the combining form of the root must be used to connect the suffix and root.*
   Example: **gastr**o**megaly** (gass-troh-**MEG**-ah-lee) = enlarged stomach or enlargement of the stomach.
   The root *gastr* means stomach, and the suffix *-megaly* means enlarged. Note how using the combining form gastr/o aids in the pronunciation of this term. Imagine how difficult it would be to say gastrmegaly!
3. *When combining a root with a suffix that begins with a vowel, the combining form is not used.*
   Example: **gastrectomy** (gass-**TREK**-toh-mee) = surgical removal of the stomach. Because the suffix *-ectomy*, which means surgical removal, begins with a vowel, the root *gastr* is used to create the medical term. Pronunciation is much smoother without the combining vowel.
4. *There will always be some exceptions to these rules.* For example, when combining word roots and one of the roots begins with a vowel, the combining vowel is retained.
   Example: **gastr**o**enterology** (**gass**-troh-en-ter-**ALL**-oh-jee) = the study of the stomach and intestines, which are the major organs of the digestive system. The root *gastr* means stomach and the root *enter* means intestine. To ease pronunciation of this term, the combining vowel *o* is retained with the root *gastr*.

Pronunciation Rules

Pronouncing medical terms seems difficult at times because medical terms are often very long. A comprehensive medical dictionary is a valuable tool for learning the pronunciation and meaning of medical terms. You should have this type of dictionary available at all times while you are learning this "language." In addition, there are several rules that provide guidance for term pronunciation. These rules are presented here. Note that in this text, pronunciations are written phonetically (by sound) with the primary accented syllable presented in bold, uppercase letters. Secondary accented syllables are presented in bold, lowercase letters.

1. *Medical terms with two syllables are usually accented on the first syllable.*
   Example: gastric = **GASS**-trik; pertaining to the stomach
2. *Medical terms with more than two syllables are usually accented on the third to last or next to last syllable.*
   Example A: gastritis = gass-**TRY**-tis = inflammation of the stomach
   Example B: gastromegaly = gass-troh-**MEG**-ah-lee = enlarged stomach
   Example A illustrates the next to last syllable accent rule. Example B illustrates the third to last syllable accent rule.
3. *The vowel in the accented syllable is pronounced with the long vowel sound when the syllable ends with the vowel.*
   Example: gastritis = gass-**TRY**-tis. The accented syllable *tri* is pronounced with the long *i* sound.
4. *The vowel in the accented syllable is pronounced with the short vowel sound when the syllable ends with a consonant.*
   Example: cardiomegaly = **kar**-dee-oh-**MEG**-ah-lee. The accented syllable *meg* is pronounced with the short *e* sound.
5. *There will always be exceptions to these rules.*

Singular and Plural Words

In the English language, singular words are often made plural by adding *s* or *es* to the word, for example, tree (singular), trees (plural); and box (singular), boxes (plural). Because medical terms are often derived from Latin, the plural forms of many medical terms follow Latin rules. You are already familiar with these rules and may not even be aware of it. For example, the word *data* is actually the plural form of the word *datum*; *alumnus* is the singular form of *alumni*. Table 1-1 lists several singular medical terms with examples of the plural forms. Note that the word ending changes to form the plural.

TABLE 1-1   SINGULAR AND PLURAL ENDINGS

Singular Ending	Plural Ending	Singular Example	Plural Example
-a	-ae	papill*a* (pah-**PILL**-ah) a small nipple-shaped projection	papill*ae* (pah-**PILL**-ay)
-en	-ina	lum*en* (**LOO**-men) cavity or channel of an organ or structure	lum*ina* (**LOO**-min-ah)
-ex; -ix	-ices	ap*ex* (**AY**-pecks) top, end, or tip of a structure	ap*ices* (**AY**-pih-seez)

(continues)

TABLE 1-1 SINGULAR AND PLURAL ENDINGS (continued)

Singular Ending	Plural Ending	Singular Example	Plural Example
-ies	-ietes	paries (**PAIR**-ee-ess) wall of an organ or cavity	parietes (pah-**RIGH**-ih-teez)
-is	-es	diagnosis (digh-ag-**NOH**-sis) name of a disease or condition	diagnoses (digh-ag-**NOH**-seez)
-is	-ides	epididymis (**ep**-ih-**DID**-ih-miss) coiled duct of the testicle	epdididymides (**ep**-ih-did-ih-**MY**-deez)
-nx	-nges	larynx (**LAIR**-inx) voice organ of the throat	larynges (lah-**RIN**-jeez)
-on	-a	ganglion (**GANG**-lee-on) knot or knotlike mass	ganglia (**GANG**-lee-ah)
-um	-a	atrium (**AY**-tree-um) upper chamber of the heart	atria (**AY**-tree-ah)
-us	-i	bronchus (**BRONG**-kus) air passage of the respiratory system	bronchi (**BRONG**-kigh)
-us	-era	viscus (**VISS**-kuss) internal organ	viscera (**VISS**-eh-rah)
-us	-ora	corpus (**KOR**-pus) body	corpora (**KOR**-por-ah; kor-**POR**-ah)

EXERCISE 3

Correctly combine each root with the suffix to form a medical term. You must decide whether or not to use the combining form.

EXAMPLE:	ROOT	SUFFIX	TERM
	arthr/o	-megaly	arthromegaly

	ROOT	SUFFIX	TERM
1.	arthr/o	-itis	arthritis
2.	arthr/o	-ectomy	arthrectomy
3.	arthr/o	-pathy	arthropathy
4.	dermat/o	-itis	dermatitis
5.	dermat/o	-pathy	dermatopathy
6.	gastr/o	-ic	gastric
7.	gastr/o	-ectomy	gastroectomymegaly
8.	gastr/o	-megaly	gastromegaly
9.	cardi/o	-megaly	cardiomegaly
10.	cardi/o	-pathy	cardiopathy

EXERCISE 4

Based on the meaning of the roots and suffixes, write a definition for each term you created in Exercise 3.

1. arthritis — inflamation or infection of a joint
2. arthroectomy — surgical removal of a joint
3. arthropathy — the study of disease of a joint
4. dermatitis — inflamation or infection of the skin
5. _____
6. Pertaining to the stomach
7. Surgical removal of the stomach
8. Inflammation of the stomach
9. enlargement of the heart
10. disease of the heart

EXERCISE 5

Write the plural form for the following singular terms.

1. ampulla   ampullae
2. fornix   formices
3. foramen   foramina
4. ovum   ova
5. phalanx   phalanices
6. testis   testices
7. thrombus   thrombery

Analyzing Medical Terms

Once you have mastered the meanings of roots, prefixes, and suffixes, you are able to analyze a medical term and arrive at a basic definition of the term. For example, *arthr/o* means joint and *itis* means inflammation; *arthritis* is briefly defined as inflammation of a joint.

To analyze a medical term, identify the root(s), prefix, and suffix. Most medical terms have a root and a suffix, but might not have a prefix. Once you have identified the word elements, recall the meaning of each element. When you write the brief definition, define the suffix first, the prefix second, and the root last. Many, but not all, medical terms can be analyzed and briefly defined with this technique. The best place to find the complete definition of any medical term is, of course, in a medical dictionary.

Practice analyzing medical terms by completing the following exercise. Table 1-2 lists the meanings of the roots, prefixes, and suffixes for the medical terms included in the exercise.

TABLE 1-2 ROOTS, PREFIXES, SUFFIXES, AND MEANINGS

Root	Meaning	Prefix	Meaning	Suffix	Meaning
arthr/o	joint	endo-	within	-algia	pain
cardi/o	heart	epi-	above, upon	-ic	pertaining to
derm/o; dermat/o	skin	hemi-	half	-itis	inflammation
gastr/o	stomach	hypo-	below, deficient	-megaly	enlarged
hepat/o	liver	peri-	around	-pathy	disease
oste/o	bone	poly-	many	-plasty	repair

EXERCISE 6

Analyze each medical term. Write a brief definition for the term based on the meaning of each word part.

EXAMPLE: hemigastrectomy
ROOT: gastr = stomach
PREFIX: hemi = half
SUFFIX: ectomy = surgical removal
DEFINITION: surgical removal of half the stomach

1. arthralgia
   ROOT: _arthr_ =
   PREFIX: _____
   SUFFIX: _algia_ –
   DEFINITION: _Pain in a joint_

2. endocarditis
   ROOT: _cardi_ (around the
   PREFIX: _endo_
   SUFFIX: _itis_
   DEFINITION: _____

3. hemigastroplasty
   ROOT: _gastro_
   PREFIX: _hemi_
   SUFFIX: _plasty_
   DEFINITION: _disease, repair, small_

4. hepatomegaly
   ROOT: _hepato_
   PREFIX: _____
   SUFFIX: _megaly_
   DEFINITION: _enlargement of the liver_

5. hypogastric

ROOT: _gast_

PREFIX: _hypo - below_

SUFFIX: _ic_

DEFINITION: _Pertaining to below the stomach_

6. osteoarthritis

ROOT: _Osteo, arthr_

PREFIX: _____

SUFFIX: _itis_

DEFINITION: _inflammation of the bone and joint_

7. osteopathy

ROOT: _Osteo_

PREFIX: _____

SUFFIX: _Pathy_

DEFINITION: _disease of the bone_

8. pericarditis

ROOT: _Card_

PREFIX: _Peri_

SUFFIX: _itis_

DEFINITION: _inflammation around heart_

9. polyarthritis

ROOT: _arthr_

PREFIX: _Poly_

SUFFIX: _itis_

DEFINITION: _inflammation or infection in joints_

10. hepatitis

ROOT: _hepat_

PREFIX: _____

SUFFIX: _itis_

DEFINITION: _inflammation of the liver_

Building Medical Terms

A working knowledge of roots, prefixes, and suffixes allows you to analyze and define many medical terms. That same knowledge can also help you build medical terms from a definition. It is important to remember that not all terms can be created from a definition. Many medical terms are not built from prefixes or suffixes, and there are many instances when the basic definition based on prefixes and suffixes does not provide a full or completely accurate definition. For example, in this chapter, the definition of gastrectomy, based solely on the meaning of the root and suffix, is surgical removal or excision of the stomach. In practice, the term *gastrectomy* commonly means surgical excision of *part* of the stomach. However, analyzing, defining, and building medical terms with roots, prefixes, and suffixes provides an excellent foundation for developing a working knowledge of medical terminology.

Practice building medical terms by completing the following exercise. Refer to Table 1-2 for a list of the roots, prefixes, and suffixes included in the exercise.

EXERCISE 7

Read each definition. Write the name of the body part, the combining form for the root, the suffix, and the prefix on the lines provided. Using the rules for word building, write a medical term for each definition.

EXAMPLE:

DEFINITION:	inflammation of joints
BODY PART:	joints
ROOT:	arthr/o
SUFFIX:	-itis
PREFIX:	none
MEDICAL TERM:	arthritis

1. DEFINITION: disease of the heart

   BODY PART: *Heart*

   ROOT: *Cardio*

   SUFFIX: *Pathy*

   PREFIX: _____

   MEDICAL TERM: *Cardiopathy*

2. DEFINITION: surgical repair of the liver

   BODY PART: *Liver*

   ROOT: *Hepato*

   SUFFIX: _____

   PREFIX: *Plasty*

   MEDICAL TERM: *hepatoplasty*

3. DEFINITION: stomach pain

   BODY PART: *Stomach*

   ROOT: *gastro*

   SUFFIX: *algia*

   PREFIX: _____

   MEDICAL TERM: *gastralgia*

4. DEFINITION: skinlike; resembling skin
   BODY PART: _Skin_
   ROOT: _dermato_
   SUFFIX: _Oid_
   PREFIX: _____
   MEDICAL TERM: _dermatoid_

5. DEFINITION: pertaining to the area around the heart
   BODY PART: _heart_
   ROOT: _Cardio_
   SUFFIX: _Peri_
   PREFIX: _Pei_
   MEDICAL TERM: _Pericardic_

6. DEFINITION: inflammation of bone
   BODY PART: _bone_
   ROOT: _Osteo_
   SUFFIX: _itis_
   PREFIX: _____
   MEDICAL TERM: _Ostitis_

7. DEFINITION: surgical repair of the skin
   BODY PART: _Skin_
   ROOT: _dermato_
   SUFFIX: _Plasty_
   PREFIX: _____
   MEDICAL TERM: _dermoplasty_

8. DEFINITION: pain in many joints
   BODY PART: _Joints_
   ROOT: _arthro_
   SUFFIX: _algia_
   PREFIX: _Poly_
   MEDICAL TERM: _Polyarthralgia_

9. DEFINITION: under the liver
   BODY PART: _liver_
   ROOT: _hepato_
   SUFFIX: _____
   PREFIX: _Sub_
   MEDICAL TERM: _Sub hepato_

Prefixes

Prefixes and their meanings should be memorized early in your study of medical terminology. In this section, commonly used prefixes are presented and defined. Exercises focus on mastering the meaning of each prefix. Memorization is often boring. To make learning the prefixes less so, it is helpful to use gamelike formats. For example: Create flashcards with the prefix or suffix on one side and its meaning on the other. Place the cards on a smooth surface, prefix/suffix side up, and with several other students see how many cards each of you can "capture" by giving the correct meaning for the prefix or suffix. Ask a friend or partner to help you complete various flashcard drills. Think of words you already know that include the prefixes given in this section.

Prefixes can be divided into four categories: general, negative, numeric, and problem or disease prefixes. Each category of prefixes is presented individually.

General Prefixes

General prefixes make up the largest number of prefixes presented in this text and often refer to size, shape, direction, and location. The first set of general prefixes is listed in Table 1-3. Note that the table includes the meaning of the prefix and an example of a medical term containing the prefix. Some examples include an everyday word with the prefix. Learn this group of prefixes and complete the exercises.

TABLE I-3 GENERAL PREFIXES

Prefix	Meaning	Examples
ab-	away from	**ab**normal = away from being normal **ab**duct (ab-**DUCT**) = to move away from the body
ad-	to; toward	**ad**dendum = in addition to; added to **ad**duct (ad-**DUCT**) = to move to or toward the body
ante-	before	**ante**room = a room or area before a larger room or area **ante**febrile (an-tee-**FEE**-brill) = before a fever
astr-	star	**astr**ology = study of the stars **astr**ocyte (**ASS**-troh-sight) = star-shaped cell
auto-	self	**auto**biography = story written by yourself about your life **auto**graft (**AH**-toh-graft) = surgical transplant of one's own tissue
brady-	slow	**brady**cardia (bray-dih-**KAR**-dee-ah) = slow heart rate
ect-	outside; outer	**ect**oderm (**EKT**-oh-derm) = outermost layer of the skin
en-	within; in	**en**trails = organs within or inside a human or animal **en**tropia (en-**TROH**-pee-ah) = turning in of the eyes
endo-	within; inner	**endo**cardium (en-doh-**KAR**-dee-um) = within the heart; inner lining of the heart
epi-	above; upon	**epi**gastric (ep-ih-**GAS**-trik) = above the stomach
ex-	out; outer	**ex**it = to go out; passage/doorway used to go out **ex**icision (ek-**SIH**-zhun) = taking out; cutting away
hemi-	half	**hemi**sphere = half of a sphere **hemi**plegia (**heh**-mih-**PLEE**-jee-ah) = paralysis of one side (half) of the body
infra-	below; inferior	**infra**orbital (in-frah-**OR**-bih-tal) = below the eye socket

(continues)

TABLE 1-3   GENERAL PREFIXES (continued)

Prefix	Meaning	Examples
inter-	between; among	**inter**mission = time period between events or periods of activity **inter**cellular (**in**-ter-**SELL**-yoo-lar) = between the cells
intra-	within	**intra**state = existing or occurring within a state **intra**cellular (**in**-trah-**SELL**-yoo-lar) = within the cells
iso-	same; equal	**iso**metric (eye-soh-**MET**-rik) = having the same length or dimension

EXERCISE 8

Read each sentence. Write the prefix and its definition for each italicized medical term. Using your medical dictionary, write a brief definition of the term.

EXAMPLE: *Macroglossia* is associated with a specific type of birth defect.
PREFIX: macro- = large   DEFINITION: hypertrophied or large tongue

1. *Autoimmune* diseases are difficult to treat.
   PREFIX: _Auto_____   DEFINITION: _Self_____

2. The *endocardium* includes the heart valves.
   PREFIX: _endo_____   DEFINITION: _within or in_____

3. *Abduction* is the opposite of adduction.
   PREFIX: _ab_____   DEFINITION: _away from_____

4. *Adduction* is the opposite of abduction.
   PREFIX: _Ad_____   DEFINITION: _to, toward_____

5. An *intradermal* injection is often used to administer a TB test.
   PREFIX: _intra_____   DEFINITION: _within_____

6. *Bradykinesia* might be a side effect of some medications.
   PREFIX: _Brady_____   DEFINITION: _Slow_____

7. An *ectopic* pregnancy often occurs in the fallopian tubes.
   PREFIX: _ect_____   DEFINITION: _outside,   out_____

8. An *astrocyte* is a specific cell of the nervous system.
   PREFIX: _star_____   DEFINITION: _____

9. The brain is divided into a right and left *hemisphere*.
   PREFIX: _____   DEFINITION: _____

10. *Epigastric* pain caused a restless evening for the patient.
    PREFIX: _____   DEFINITION: _____

EXERCISE 9

Match the prefix in Column 1 with the meaning in Column 2.

COLUMN 1	COLUMN 2
_____ 1. ab-	a. above; upon
_____ 2. ante-	b. away from
_____ 3. astr-	c. before
_____ 4. auto-	d. below; inferior
_____ 5. brady-	e. between
_____ 6. ect-	f. within; in
_____ 7. epi-	g. same; equal
_____ 8. infra-	h. self
_____ 9. inter-	i. slow
_____ 10. intra-	j. star
_____ 11. iso-	k. outside; out

EXERCISE 10

Write the prefix for each meaning.

1. above; upon   _____
2. away from   _____
3. before   _____
4. below; inferior   _____
5. between   _____
6. half   _____
7. out; outer   _____
8. outside; outer   _____
9. same; equal   _____
10. self   _____
11. slow   _____
12. star   _____

The last set of general prefixes is listed in Table 1-4. Note that the table includes the meaning of the prefix and an example of a medical term containing the prefix. Some examples also include an everyday word with the prefix. Learn this group of prefixes and complete the exercises.

TABLE 1-4 GENERAL PREFIXES

Prefix	Meaning	Examples
macro-	large	**macro**cyte (**MAK**-roh-sight) = abnormally large red blood cell
meta-	change; after; beyond	**meta**plasia (met-ah-**PLAY**-zee-ah) = change from one type of growth to another
micro-	small	**micro**cyte (**MY**-kroh-sight) = abnormally small red blood cell
multi-	many	**multi**lobular (mull-tigh-**LOB**-yoo-lar) = having many lobes
neo-	new	**neo**plasm (**NEE**-oh-plazm) = new growth
pan-	all	**pan**carditis (**pan**-kar-**DIGH**-tiss) = inflammation of the entire heart
para-	near; beside	**para**nasal (**pair**-ah-**NAY**-sal) = near or beside the nose
peri-	around; surrounding	**peri**meter = boundary surrounding a specific location **peri**cardium (**pair**-ih-**KAR**-dee-um) = membrane around the heart
poly-	many	**poly**arthritis (**pall**-ee-ar-**THRIGH**-tiss) = inflammation of many joints
post-	after	**post**partum (post-**PAR**-tum) = after giving birth
pre-	before; in front of	**pre**natal (pre-**NAY**-tal) = before giving birth
retro-	behind; backward	**retro**spect = looking back at past events **retro**grade (**REH**-troh-grayd) = moving backward
semi-	half	**semi**lunar (sem-eye-**LOO**-nar) = half-moon shaped
sub-	below; under	**sub**hepatic (**sub**-heh-**PAT**-ik) = below or under the liver
super-	above; over; excess	**super**ior (soo-**PEER**-ee-or) = above or toward a higher place
supra-	above; on top of	**supra**spinal (**soo**-prah-**SPIGH**-nal) = above the spine
sym-	with; association	**sym**pathy = having an association with another's feelings **sym**biosis (sim-bee-**OH**-siss) = living with or in close association
syn-	together; with; union	**syn**chronize = to move or operate together or in unison **syn**ergistic (sin-er-**JISS**-tik) = related to working together
tachy-	fast	**tachy**cardia (**tak**-ih-**KAR**-dee-ah) = fast heart rate

EXERCISE 11

Read each sentence. Write the prefix and its definition for each italicized medical term. Using your medical dictionary, write a brief definition of the term.

1. A caterpillar experiences *metamorphosis* to become a butterfly.

  PREFIX: _____ DEFINITION: _____

2. The laboratory technician uses a *microscope* to examine tissue samples.

  PREFIX: _____ DEFINITION: _____

3. Some heart valves are *semilunar* in shape.

PREFIX: _____ DEFINITION: _____

4. *Tachycardia* might cause the patient to feel dizzy.

PREFIX: _____ DEFINITION: _____

5. *Substernal* chest pain is a sign of "heartburn."

PREFIX: _____ DEFINITION: _____

6. A *neoplasm* can be cancerous or noncancerous.

PREFIX: _____ DEFINITION: _____

7. The adrenal glands are also known as the *suprarenal* glands.

PREFIX: _____ DEFINITION: _____

8. Humans are *multicelluar* organisms.

PREFIX: _____ DEFINITION: _____

9. *Retroflexion* prevents an organ from functioning properly.

PREFIX: _____ DEFINITION: _____

10. The patient's *postoperative* course was uneventful.

PREFIX: _____ DEFINITION: _____

EXERCISE 12

Match the prefix in Column 1 with the meaning in Column 2.

COLUMN 1	COLUMN 2
_____ 1. pan-	a. above; over; excess
_____ 2. para-	b. after
_____ 3. peri-	c. all
_____ 4. poly-	d. around; surrounding
_____ 5. post-	e. before; in front of
_____ 6. pre-	f. change
_____ 7. meta-	g. many
_____ 8. super-	h. near; beside
_____ 9. sym-	i. together; with; union
_____ 10. syn-	j. with; association

EXERCISE 13

Write the prefix for each meaning.

1. above; on top of _____

2. above; over; excess _____

3. behind; backward _____

4. change _____

5. fast _____

6. half   _____

7. large   _____

8. near; beside   _____

9. new   _____

10. together; with; union   _____

Negative, Numeric, and Disease Prefixes

Negative and numeric prefixes are self-explanatory. **Problem or disease prefixes** provide some information about an abnormal structure or function. Learn this group of prefixes, listed in Table 1-5, and complete the exercises.

TABLE 1-5   NEGATIVE, NUMERIC, AND DISEASE AND PROBLEM PREFIXES

NEGATIVE PREFIXES

Prefix	Meaning	Example
a; an; ana	no; not; without	**an**archy = without laws or government **an**algesia (**an**-al-**JEE**-zee-ah) = without pain; no sensation of pain
anti-	against	**anti**fungal (an-tigh-**FUNG**-al) = against fungus
contra-	against; opposite	**contra**ception (con-trah-**SEP**-shun) = against conception
non-	not	**non**functioning = does not function

NUMERIC PREFIXES

Prefix	Meaning	Example
bi-	two; double; both	**bi**lateral (bigh-**LAT**-er-al) = both sides; two sides
centi-	hundred; hundredth	**centi**meter (**SEN**-tih-me-ter) − one hundredth of a meter
dec-	ten	**dec**aliter (**DEK**-ah-lee-ter) = ten liters
milli-	one thousandth	**milli**liter (**MILL**-ih-**lee**-ter) = one thousandth of a liter
quadr-	four	**quadr**iplegia (**kwod**-rih-**PLEE**-jee-ah) = paralysis of all four limbs
tri-	three	**tri**cuspid (trigh-**KUSS**-pid) = having three flaps
uni-	one	**uni**lateral (yoo-nih-**LAT**-er-al) = one side

DISEASE and PROBLEM PREFIXES

Prefix	Meaning	Example
carcin-	cancerous	**carcin**oma (kar-sin-**OH**-mah) = cancerous tumor
dys-	difficult; painful	**dys**uria (dis-**YOO**-ree-ah) = painful urination
hyper-	above; excessive	**hyper**thyroidism (**high**-per-**THIGH**-royd-izm) = excessive thyroid activity
hypo	deficient; below	**hypo**thyroidism (**high**-poh-**THIGH**-royd-izm) = deficient thyroid activity
mal-	bad; poor; abnormal	**mal**absorption (mal-ab−**SORP**-shun) = abnorma absorption

EXERCISE 14

Read each sentence. Write the prefix and its definition for each italicized medical term. Using your medical dictionary, write a brief definition of the term.

1. The *bicuspid* valve in the heart is also called the mitral valve.

   PREFIX: _____ DEFINITION: _____

2. *Antibiotic* medications are an effective treatment for some diseases.

   PREFIX: _____ DEFINITION: _____

3. *Hypertension* can be successfully treated and controlled.

   PREFIX: _____ DEFINITION: _____

4. Squamous cell *carcinoma* might involve the cervix.

   PREFIX: _____ DEFINITION: _____

5. *Hypothyroidism* often responds to medication therapy.

   PREFIX: _____ DEFINITION: _____

6. A stroke sometimes results in *dysphagia*.

   PREFIX: _____ DEFINITION: _____

7. Some procedures are done with local *anesthesia*.

   PREFIX: _____ DEFINITION: _____

8. Some birth defects are characterized by *malformation* of an organ or limb.

   PREFIX: _____ DEFINITION: _____

9. Most medications have at least one *contraindication*.

   PREFIX: _____ DEFINITION: _____

10. After taking fertility medications, Helen gave birth to *quadruplets*.

    PREFIX: _____ DEFINITION: _____

EXERCISE 15

Write the prefix for each definition.

1. above; excessive _____

2. against _____

3. against; opposite _____

4. bad; poor; abnormal _____

5. cancerous _____

6. deficient; below _____

7. difficult; painful _____

8. hundred; hundredth _____

9. no; not; without _____

10. not _____

11. one _____

12. one thousandth _____

13. ten   _____

14. three   _____

15. two; double; both   _____

Suffixes

Suffixes are added to the end of a word root and, as with prefixes, change the meaning of the medical term. In addition to identifying a medical term as a noun or an adjective, a suffix indicates if the term is related to a diagnosis, abnormal condition, or procedure. Several suffixes also are used to describe general medical processes and functions.

General Suffixes

General suffixes are used to describe general medical processes and functions and are the largest number of suffixes presented in this text. Review the suffixes and meanings in Table 1-6 and complete the exercises.

TABLE 1-6   GENERAL SUFFIXES

Suffix	Meaning	Example
-ac; -al; -ar; -ary	pertaining to	cardiovascular (**kar**-dee-oh-**VASS**-kyoo-lar) = pertaining to the heart and vessels
-crine	to secrete	endocrine (**EN**-doh-krin) = to secrete within, into
-crit	to separate	hematocrit (hee-**MAT**-oh-krit) = to separate blood
-cyte	cell	leukocyte (**LOO**-koh-sight) = white cell; white blood cell
-gen; -genesis; -genic	producing, forming	spermatogenesis (sper-**mat**-oh-**JEN**-eh-siss) = producing sperm
-globin; -globulin	protein	hemoglobin (**HEE**-mah-gloh-bin) = blood protein
-gram	record	venogram (**VEE**-noh-gram) = record of the veins
-graph	instrument for recording	cardiograph (**KAR**-dee-oh-graf) = instrument that records heart activity
-graphy	process of recording	cardiography (kar-dee-**AH**-grah-fee) = recording the activity of, or a picture of the heart
-iac; ic	pertaining to	cardiac (**KAR**-dee-ak) = pertaining to the heart
-oid	resembling; like	ovoid (**OH**-voyd) = resembling an oval or an egg
-(o)logist	specialist	dermatologist (**der**-mah-**TALL**-oh-jist) = skin specialist
-(o)logy	study of	dermatology (**der**-mah-**TALL**-oh-jee) = study of the skin
-ous	pertaining to	mucous (**MEW**-kuss) = pertaining to mucus
-pepsia	digestion	dyspepsia (diss-**PEP**-see-ah) = difficult or painful digestion

(continues)

TABLE 1-6 GENERAL SUFFIXES (continued)

Suffix	Meaning	Example
-phagia	eating; swallowing	**a**phagia (ah-**FAY**-jee-ah) = lack of the ability to swallow
-phonia	voice; sound	**a**phonia (ah-**FOH**-nee-ah) = lack of the ability to produce sound; lack of voice

EXERCISE 16

Read each sentence. Write the suffix and its definition for each italicized medical term. Using your medical dictionary, write a brief definition of the term.

1. *Endocrine* glands do not have ducts.

   SUFFIX: _____ DEFINITION: _____

2. Many bacteria are *pathogenic*.

   SUFFIX: _____ DEFINITION: _____

3. *Gammaglobulins* are found in circulating blood.

   SUFFIX: _____ DEFINITION: _____

4. After reviewing the *renogram*, Dr. Jones noted the patient had an enlarged kidney.

   SUFFIX: _____ DEFINITION: _____

5. The *echograph* is an important diagnostic tool.

   SUFFIX: _____ DEFINITION: _____

6. *Echocardiography* is a noninvasive method for inspecting the heart.

   SUFFIX: _____ DEFINITION: _____

7. Mark's family physician referred him to a *urologist*.

   SUFFIX: _____ DEFINITION: _____

8. *Aphonia* might be the result of a stroke.

   SUFFIX: _____ DEFINITION: _____

9. *Radiology* is one of several medical specialties.

   SUFFIX: _____ DEFINITION: _____

10. *Erythrocytes* are one of the major components of blood.

    SUFFIX: _____ DEFINITION: _____

EXERCISE 17

Match the suffix in Column 1 with the meaning in Column 2.

COLUMN 1	COLUMN 2
_____ 1 -crine	a. cell
_____ 2. -crit	b. digestion
_____ 3. -cyte	c. eating; swallowing

_____ 4. -genesis; -genic   d. record; picture

_____ 5. -globin; -globulin   e. pertaining to

_____ 6. -gram   f. process of recording

_____ 7. -graphy   g. protein

_____ 8. -(o)logist   h. secrete

_____ 9. -ous   i. specialist

_____ 10. -pepsia   j. separate

_____ 11. -phagia   k. voice; sound

_____ 12. -phonia   l. producing

Review the general suffixes and meanings in Table 1-7 and complete the exercises.

TABLE 1-7   GENERAL SUFFIXES

Suffix	Meaning	Example
-phoresis	carrying; transmission	electro**phoresis** (ee-lek-troh-for-**EE**-siss) = carrying or transmission of an electrical charge
-phoria	feeling; mental state	dys**phoria** (diss-**FOR**-ee-ah) = bad feeling
-pnea	breathing	dys**pnea** (disp-**NEE**-ah) = difficult breathing
-poiesis	formation	erythro**poiesis** (air-**rith**-roh-poy-**EE**-siss) = formation of red blood cells
-scope	instrument for viewing	micro**scope** (**MY**-kroh-scope) = instrument for viewing small objects
-scopy	process of viewing	arthro**scopy** (ar-**THROSS**-koh-pee) = viewing joint(s)
-somnia	sleep	in**somnia** (in-**SOM**-nee-ah) = inability to sleep
-stasis	control; stop	hemo**stasis** (hee-moh-**STAY**-siss) = stopping blood flow
-therapy	treatment	chemo**therapy** (kee-moh-**THAIR**-ah-pee) = treatment using drugs
-thorax	chest; pleural cavity	hemo**thorax** (hee-moh-**THOR**-acks) = blood in the chest or pleural cavity
-tocia	labor; birth	dys**tocia** (diss-**TOH**-see-ah) = abnormal labor
-tresia	opening	a**tresia** (ah-**TREE**-see-ah) = lack of a normal opening
-trophy	growth; development	dys**trophy** (**DISS**-troh-fee) = abnormal or bad growth
-tropin	nourish; develop; stimulate	somato**tropin** (soh-mat-oh-**TROH**-pin) = stimulates body growth
-version	to turn	retro**version** (**reh**-troh-**VER**-zhun) = to turn backward

EXERCISE 18

Read each sentence. Write the suffix and its definition for each italicized medical term. Using your medical dictionary, write a brief definition of the term.

1. Dr. Jefferson used an *otoscope* during Marilyn's annual physical.

   SUFFIX: _____ DEFINITION: _____

2. *Hematopoiesis* takes place in the bone marrow.

   SUFFIX: _____ DEFINITION: _____

3. *Cardioversion* is used to correct heart rhythm problems.

   SUFFIX: _____ DEFINITION: _____

4. Disuse *atrophy* is caused by prolonged confinement to bed.

   SUFFIX: _____ DEFINITION: _____

5. After experiencing a *pneumothorax*, the patient's lung collapsed.

   SUFFIX: _____ DEFINITION: _____

6. *Orthopnea* is sometimes associated with congestive heart failure.

   SUFFIX: _____ DEFINITION: _____

7. After winning the lottery, Robert experienced *euphoria*.

   SUFFIX: _____ DEFINITION: _____

8. *Endoscopy* is an important diagnostic technique.

   SUFFIX: _____ DEFINITION: _____

9. *Cryotherapy* is often used to treat skin problems.

   SUFFIX: _____ DEFINITION: _____

EXERCISE 19

Match the suffix in Column 1 with the meaning in Column 2.

COLUMN 1	COLUMN 2
_____ 1. -phoresis	a. breathing
_____ 2. -phoria	b. carrying; transmission
_____ 3. -pnea	c. control; stop
_____ 4. -poiesis	d. feeling; mental state
_____ 5. -scopy	e. formation
_____ 6. -somnia	f. labor; birth
_____ 7. -stasis	g. nourish; develop
_____ 8. -therapy	h. opening
_____ 9. -tocia	i. process of viewing
_____ 10. -tresia	j. sleep
_____ 11. -tropin	k. treatment

EXERCISE 20

Write the meaning for each suffix.

1. to secrete _____

2. separate _____

3. producing; forming _____

4. cell _____

5. process of recording _____

6. study of _____

7. specialist _____

8. eating; swallowing _____

9. formation _____

10. sleep _____

11. to turn _____

12. development; growth _____

13. like; resembling _____

14. chest; pleural cavity _____

Disease and Abnormal Condition Suffixes

Disease and **abnormal condition suffixes** are used to describe what is wrong with a given body part. Review the suffixes and meanings in Table 1-8 and complete the exercises.

TABLE 1-8 DISEASE AND ABNORMAL CONDITION SUFFIXES

Suffix	Meaning	Example
-algia	pain	arthr**algia** (ar-**THRAL**-jee-ah) = joint pain
-cele	hernia; herniation	recto**cele** (**REK**-toh-seel) = herniation into the rectum
-cytosis	condition of cells	leuko**cytosis** (**loo**-koh-sigh-**TOH**-siss) = condition of white blood cells (abnormal increase)
-dynia	pain	gastro**dynia** (**gass**-troh-**DIN**-ee-ah) = pain in the stomach
-emesis	vomiting	hemat**emesis** (hee-mah-**TEM**-eh-siss) = vomiting blood
-emia	blood condition	an**emia** (ah-**NEE**-mee-ah) = lack of quantity or quality of blood
-ia; iasis	abnormal condition	lith**iasis** (lih-**THIGH**-ah-siss) = abnormal presence of stones
-itis	inflammation	gingiv**itis** (jin-jih-**VIGH**-tiss) = inflammation of the gums
-lysis; -lytic	break down; destruction	hemo**lysis** (hee-**MALL**-oh-siss) = destruction of blood or red blood cells

(continues)

TABLE 1-8   DISEASE AND ABNORMAL CONDITION SUFFIXES (continued)

Suffix	Meaning	Example
-malacia	softening	osteo**malacia** (**oss**-tee-oh-mah-**LAY**-she-ah) = softening of bone
-megaly	enlargement	cardio**megaly** (**kar**-dee-oh-**MEG**-ah-lee) = enlarged heart
-oma	tumor	aden**oma** (ad-en-**OH**-mah) = tumor of the gland
-osis	abnormal condition	dermat**osis** (der-mah-**TOH**-siss) = skin condition

EXERCISE 21

Read each sentence. Write the suffix and its definition for each italicized medical term. Using your medical dictionary, write a brief definition of the term.

1. Exposure to UV rays is the leading cause of *melanoma*.

    SUFFIX: _____   DEFINITION: _____

2. *Spherocytosis* is often seen in some types of anemia.

    SUFFIX: _____   DEFINITION: _____

3. *Bacteremia* is treated with antibiotics.

    SUFFIX: _____   DEFINITION: _____

4. Health care workers are at risk for *hepatitis*.

    SUFFIX: _____   DEFINITION: _____

5. Inadequate nutrition might contribute to *chondromalacia*.

    SUFFIX: _____   DEFINITION: _____

6. *Halitosis* can be a symptom of dental problems.

    SUFFIX: _____   DEFINITION: _____

7. Muscle spasms of the head and neck may cause *cephalalgia*.

    SUFFIX: _____   DEFINITION: _____

8. A *cystocele* might require surgical intervention.

    SUFFIX: _____   DEFINITION: _____

9. *Nephromegaly* might be visualized with an x-ray.

    SUFFIX: _____   DEFINITION: _____

10. After exercising for several hours, Rhonda experienced *myodynia*.

    SUFFIX: _____   DEFINITION: _____

EXERCISE 22

Write the suffix for each meaning.

1. blood condition   _____

2. break down; destruction   _____

3. abnormal condition   _____

4. enlargement; enlarged   _____

5. hernia; herniation   _____

6. inflammation   _____

7. pain   _____

8. softening   _____

9. tumor   _____

10. vomiting   _____

Review the disease and abnormal condition suffixes and meanings in Table 1-9 and complete the exercises.

TABLE 1-9   DISEASE AND ABNORMAL CONDITION SUFFIXES

Suffix	Meaning	Example
-paresis	slight paralysis	hemi**paresis** (**hem**-ee-pah-**REE**-siss) = slight paralysis of one side of the body
-pathy	disease	neuro**pathy** (noo-**ROP**-ah-thee) = disease of nerves
-penia	decreased number	leukocyto**penia** (**loo**-koh-sigh-toh-**PEE**-nee-ah) = decreased number of white cells (white blood cells)
-phobia	abnormal fear	arachno**phobia** (ah-**rak**-noh-**FOH**-bee-ah) = abnormal fear of spiders
-plegia	paralysis	quadra**plegia** (kwad-rah-**PLEE**-gee-ah) = paralysis of all four limbs
-ptosis	drooping; sagging; prolapse	nephro**ptosis** (**neff**-rop-**TOH**-siss) = drooping kidney
-ptysis	spitting up	hemo**ptysis** (hee-**MOP**-tih-siss) = spitting up blood
-(r)rhage; (r)rhagia	bursting forth of blood	hemo**rrhage** (**HEM**-oh-rij) = bursting forth of blood
-(r)rhea	flow; discharge	rhino**rrhea** (**righ**-noh-**REE**-ah) = discharge from the nose; runny nose
-(r)rhexis	rupture	utero**rrhexis** (yoo-ter-oh-**RECKS**-iss) = rupture of the uterus
-sclerosis	hardening	arterio**sclerosis** (ar-**teer**-ee-oh-sclair-**ROH**-siss) = hardening of the arteries
-spasm	contraction; twitching	cardio**spasm** (**KAR**-dee-oh-spasm) = twitching of the heart muscle
-stenosis	narrowing; tightening	arterio**stenosis** (ar-teer-ree-oh-sten-OH-siss) = narrowing of an artery

EXERCISE 23

Read each sentence. Write the suffix and its definition for each italicized medical term. Using your medical dictionary, write a brief definition of the term.

1. Sara's infection caused her to experience *hemiparesis*.

   SUFFIX: _____   DEFINITION: _____

2. Elizabeth hoped the physician could find the cause of her *menorrhagia*.

   SUFFIX: _____   DEFINITION: _____

3. *Splenorrhexis* might lead to blood in the abdominal cavity.

   SUFFIX: _____   DEFINITION: _____

4. *Neutropenia* is often a side effect of chemotherapy.

   SUFFIX: _____   DEFINITION: _____

5. An acrobat with *acrophobia* might find it difficult to perform.

   SUFFIX: _____   DEFINITION: _____

6. *Nephroptosis* might require surgical intervention.

   SUFFIX: _____   DEFINITION: _____

7. *Atherosclerosis* is associated with heart disease.

   SUFFIX: _____   DEFINITION: _____

8. After the accident, Marilyn was diagnosed with *hemiplegia*.

   SUFFIX: _____   DEFINITION: _____

9. *Neuropathy* is a complication of diabetes.

   SUFFIX: _____   DEFINITION: _____

10. *Otorrhea* is sometimes present with an ear infection.

    SUFFIX: _____   DEFINITION: _____

EXERCISE 24

Match the suffixes in Column 1 with the meanings in Column 2.

COLUMN 1	COLUMN 2
_____ 1. -malacia	a. abnormal condition
_____ 2. -megaly	b. abnormal fear
_____ 3. -osis	c. bursting forth of blood
_____ 4. -paresis	d. contraction; twitching
_____ 5. -pathy	e. drooping; sagging; prolapse
_____ 6. -phobia	f. disease
_____ 7. -plegia	g. enlargement; enlarged
_____ 8. -ptosis	h. flow; discharge
_____ 9. -ptysis	i. hardening
_____ 10. -(r)rhage	j. narrowing; tightening
_____ 11. -(r)rhea	k. paralysis

_____ 12. -sclerosis   l. slight paralysis

_____ 13. -spasm   m. softening

_____ 14. -stenosis   n. spitting up

EXERCISE 25

Write the suffix for each meaning.

1. bursting forth of blood   _____

2. decreased number   _____

3. drooping; sagging   _____

4. hernia   _____

5. inflammation   _____

6. mass; tumor   _____

7. pain   _____

8. rupture   _____

9. slight paralysis   _____

10. vomiting   _____

Treatment and Procedure Suffixes

Treatment and **procedure suffixes** describe a variety of medical interventions such as the removal or repair of a body part or an organ. Review the suffixes and meanings in Table 1-10 and complete the exercises.

TABLE 1-10 TREATMENT AND PROCEDURE SUFFIXES

Suffix	Meaning	Example
-centesis	surgical puncture	thora**centesis** (**thor**-ah-sen-**TEE**-siss) = surgical puncture into the chest or thoracic cavity
-desis	binding together	arthro**desis** (ar-throh-**DEE**-siss) = binding together of joints
-ectasia; -ectasis	stretching; dilatation	gast**rectasia** (**gass**-trek-**TAY**-zee-ah) = stretching or dilatation of the stomach
-ectomy	surgical removal; excision	gast**rectomy** (gass-**TREK**-toh-mee) = surgical removal of all or part of the stomach
-(o)stomy	create a new opening	colo**stomy** (koh-**LOSS**-toh-mee) = create a new opening for the colon
-(o)tomy	incision into	laparo**tomy** (**lap**-ah-**ROT**-oh mee) = incision into the abdominal wall
-pexy	surgical fixation	utero**pexy** (**yoo**-ter-oh-**PEK**-see) = surgical fixation of the uterus
-plasty	surgical repair	rhino**plasty** (**RIGH**-noh-plass-tee) = surgical repair of the nose

(continues)

TABLE 1-10 TREATMENT AND PROCEDURE SUFFIXES (continued)

Suffix	Meaning	Example
-(r)rhaphy	suture	hernior**rhaphy** (**her**-nee-**OR**-ah-fee) = suturing a hernia
-tripsy	crushing; friction	litho**tripsy** (**LITH**-oh-trip-see) = crushing of stones

EXERCISE 26

Read each sentence. Write the suffix and its definition for each italicized medical term. Using your medical dictionary, write a brief definition of the term.

1. Erik underwent an *arthrocentesis* to remove the fluid around his knee.

   SUFFIX: _____ DEFINITION: _____

2. Mark sustained internal injuries and underwent a *splenectomy*.

   SUFFIX: _____ DEFINITION: _____

3. An *ileostomy* is often associated with ulcerative colitis.

   SUFFIX: _____ DEFINITION: _____

4. *Septoplasty* might be the treatment of choice for a broken nose.

   SUFFIX: _____ DEFINITION: _____

5. A *tracheotomy* was performed to allow the patient to breathe.

   SUFFIX: _____ DEFINITION: _____

6. After the birth of her seven children, Mrs. Wilde was scheduled for a *colporrhaphy*.

   SUFFIX: _____ DEFINITION: _____

7. An *orchidopexy* was scheduled to correct Roger's problem.

   SUFFIX: _____ DEFINITION: _____

8. Following *esophagectasia*, Victoria was able to swallow with ease.

   SUFFIX: _____ DEFINITION: _____

EXERCISE 27

Match the suffixes in Column 1 with the meanings in Column 2.

COLUMN 1	COLUMN 2
_____ 1. -centesis	a. binding together
_____ 2. -desis	b. create a new opening
_____ 3. -ectasia; ectasis	c. crushing; friction
_____ 4. -ectomy	d. drooping; sagging; prolapse
_____ 5. -(o)stomy	e. incision into
_____ 6. -(o)tomy	f. opening
_____ 7. -pexy	g. rupture
_____ 8. -plasty	h. spitting up

_____ 9. -ptosis   i. stretching; dilatation

_____ 10. -ptysis   j. surgical fixation

_____ 11. -(r)rhaphy   k. surgical removal; excision

_____ 12. -(r)rhexis   l. surgical repair

_____ 13. -tresia   m. surgical puncture

_____ 14. -tripsy   n. suture

SUMMARY

Prefixes and suffixes are word parts that are added to the beginning and end of word roots. These word parts change the meaning of a medical term. Prefixes can signify colors and numbers as well as indicate a negative meaning for a medical term. Suffixes identify a medical term as a noun or an adjective. There are general, disease, and procedure suffixes.

It is important to memorize the commonly used prefixes and suffixes because these word parts are found in the majority of medical terms. Additional prefixes and suffixes will be presented in the body system chapters, along with the word roots associated with each body system.

CHAPTER REVIEW

EXERCISE 28

Read the medical report. The italicized medical terms are listed after the report. Write the prefixes, suffixes, and the meanings for each term. Using your medical dictionary, look up the definition for each term.

PATIENT NAME: MATTSON, SARA
PHYSICIAN NAME: Erik Gervais, MD

BRIEF HISTORY
The patient is a 28-year-old female who presents with gradual onset of right upper quadrant pain, vomiting and (1) _diarrhea_. She was recently (2) _postpartum_ and had a postpartum tubal ligation.

PHYSICAL EXAMINATION
Exam today revealed that she was (3) _afebrile_. She exhibited (4) _tachycardia_ and massive (5) _hepatomegaly_. Pelvic exam revealed no cervical motion tenderness.

HOSPITAL COURSE
The patient was admitted for workup of her hepatomegaly. She was given (6) _intravenous_ fluids for her dehydration and was started on iron for her (7) _anemia_. A liver biopsy revealed several (8) _hepatic_ lesions and the tissue resembled neutrophils. (9) _Laparoscopy_ was scheduled, a larger sample was taken, and a frozen section was sent to the lab. The final (10) _pathology_ report confirmed (11) _adenocarcinoma_. (12) _Oncology_ was then consulted and a chemotherapy regime was recommended. Further lab and x-ray reports revealed (13) _hypoalbuminemia_ and (14) _bilateral_ pleural effusion, respectively. Pain control at home will be accomplished with a (15) _subcutaneous_ morphine pump.

MEDICAL TERM	PREFIX AND MEANING	SUFFIX AND MEANING
1. diarrhea	_____	_____
2. postpartum	_____	_____
3. afebrile	_____	_____
4. tachycardia	_____	_____
5. hepatomegaly	_____	_____
6. intravenous	_____	_____
7. anemia	_____	_____
8. hepatic	_____	_____
9. laparoscopy	_____	_____
10. pathology	_____	_____
11. adenocarcinoma	_____	_____
12. oncology	_____	_____
13. hypoalbuminemia	_____	_____
14. bilateral	_____	_____
15. subcutaneous	_____	_____

EXERCISE 30

Write the plural form for the singular word endings listed here.

1. a   _____
2. ex   _____
3. is   _____
4. on   _____
5. um   _____
6. us   _____
7. nx   _____

EXERCISE 31

Write a short answer for each of the following questions.

1. What is the purpose of a combining vowel?

_____

2. When is it necessary to use a combining vowel?

_____

3. How do you know which syllable should be accented when pronouncing medical terms?

_____

Chapter 2
General Body Terminology

OBJECTIVES	At the completion of this chapter, the student should be able to:

1. Identify, define, and spell word roots associated with the body structure and organization.
2. Label the five body cavities presented in this chapter.
3. Spell correctly the medical terms related to body structure and organization.
4. Describe the basic components of the 13 body systems.
5. Define the three body planes.
6. Label and define the nine body regions and four body quadrants.
7. Analyze body structure and organization terms by defining the roots, prefixes, and suffixes of these terms.

OVERVIEW

General body terminology includes terms related to structural organization and body cavities, planes, regions, quadrants, and direction. These terms apply to the body as a whole and provide a foundation for understanding the medical terminology related to individual body systems.

General Body Terminology Word Roots

To understand and use general body terminology, it is necessary to acquire a thorough knowledge of the associated word roots. Word roots in Table 2-1 are listed with the combining vowel. Review the word roots and complete the exercises that follow.

TABLE 2-1   BODY TERMINOLOGY WORD ROOTS

Word Root/Combining Form	Meaning
abdomin/o; lapar/o; ceil/o	abdomen
adip/o; lip/o	fat; fatty
anter/o	front
chondr/o	cartilage
crani/o	skull
cyt/o	cell
dors/o	back
gastr/o	stomach
hist/o	tissue

(continues)

TABLE 2-1   BODY TERMINOLOGY WORD ROOTS (continued)

Word Root/Combining Form	Meaning
inguin/o	groin
later/o	side; away from the midline
lumb/o	loin
medi/o	middle
nucle/o	nucleus
pelv/i	pelvis
poster/o	back
proxim/o	near
spin/o	spine
thorac/o	chest
umbilic/o	navel
ventr/o	front side; belly
viscer/o	internal organs

EXERCISE 1

Write the meaning of each word root.

1. cyt/o   _____

2. abdomin/o   _____

3. hist/o   _____

4. later/o   _____

5. ventr/o   _____

6. thorac/o   _____

7. pelv/i   _____

8. chondr/o   _____

9. gastr/o   _____

10. lapar/o   _____

EXERCISE 2

Write the word root with its meaning and a brief definition for each term.

EXAMPLE: laparotomy
ROOT: lapar/o = abdomen   Definition: incision into the abdomen

1. abdominal

   ROOT: _____   DEFINITION: _____

2. cytology

   ROOT: _____   DEFINITION: _____

3. umbilical

   ROOT: _____ DEFINITION: _____

4. posterior

   ROOT: _____ DEFINITION: _____

5. anterior

   ROOT: _____ DEFINITION: _____

6. histology

   ROOT: _____ DEFINITION: _____

7. ventral

   ROOT: _____ DEFINITION: _____

8. proximal

   ROOT: _____ DEFINITION: _____

9. adipose

   ROOT: _____ DEFINITION: _____

10. spinal

    ROOT: _____ DEFINITION: _____

11. cranial

    ROOT: _____ DEFINITION: _____

EXERCISE 3

Write the correct word root(s) for the following definitions.

1. abdomen   _____ _____

2. front   _____

3. internal organs _____

4. navel   _____

5. back   _____

6. front side   _____

7. side   _____

8. near   _____

9. nucleus   _____

10. tissue   _____

11. cartilage   _____

12. stomach   _____

13. loin   _____

14. groin   _____

Structural Organization Terms

Structures of the body are organized into four general categories: cells, tissues, organs, and systems. The categories are described as follows:

- **Cells** are the foundation for all parts of the body.
- **Tissues** are composed of similar cells that come together to perform a common or specialized function. For example, muscle tissue is made up of several types of cells, including muscle cells.
- **Organs** are made up of different types of tissue arranged together to perform a specific function. For example, the heart is an organ with several types of tissue.
- **Systems** include different organs that work together to perform the various functions of the body as a whole. For example, the cardiovascular system consists of the heart, arteries, and veins.

Cells

The human body is made up of literally trillions of cells that vary in size and shape depending on their function. The study of cells is called **cytology** (sigh-**TALL**-oh-jee). Figure 2-1 illustrates a human cell and some of its structures.

Cells are surrounded by a (1) **cell membrane**, which is the cell's outer covering. The membrane allows materials to pass in and out of the cell so that the cell can receive nutrients and release waste products. The cell's structures are housed in a gel-like substance called (2) **cytoplasm** (**SIGH**-toh-plazm). The (3) **nucleus** (**NOO**-klee-us) controls cellular functions and is made up of threadlike strands called **chromosomes** (**KROH**-moh-sohms). Chromosomes control the growth, repair, and reproduction functions of the body. Chromosomes contain **deoxyribonucleic** (dee-**ocks**-ee-**righ**-boh-noo-**KLAY**-ic) **acid** (**DNA**), which transmits genetic information. The chromosomes also have thousands of segments called **genes**, which are responsible for all hereditary characteristics.

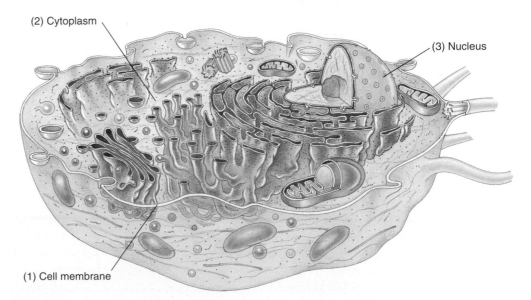

(2) Cytoplasm

(3) Nucleus

(1) Cell membrane

Figure 2-1 Human cell

Tissues

Tissues are groups of cells working together to perform a specific function. There are four main types of body tissue: **connective**, **epithelial** (ep-ih-**THEEL**-ee-al), **muscle**, and **nervous**. The study of tissue is called **histology**.

Connective Tissue

Connective tissue functions as the name implies: to connect or support other body tissue or structures. Connective tissue can be liquid, **adipose** (**ADD**-ih-pohs), fibrous, or solid. Table 2-2 lists examples of each type of tissue.

TABLE 2-2 TYPES OF CONNECTIVE TISSUE

Connective Tissue	Example(s)
liquid	blood; lymph
adipose	fat
fibrous	tendons; ligaments
cartilage	nose; rings of the trachea
solid	bone

Epithelial Tissue

Epithelial tissue provides a covering for body organs. It also lines body vessels, cavities, glands, and organs. The skin is an example of epithelial tissue. The lining of the heart, called the **endocardium** (**en** doh-**KAR**-dee-um), is another example of epithelial tissue.

Muscle Tissue

Muscle tissue functions to produce movement in all parts of the body. Some movement, such as walking, is normally under our control, while other movement, such as the movement of food through the small intestines, is not. There are three types of muscle tissue: skeletal, smooth, and cardiac. Table 2-3 lists each type of muscle tissue and a brief description.

TABLE 2-3 TYPES OF MUSCLE TISSUE

Muscle Tissue	Description
skeletal	attached to bone; moves the skeleton; voluntary muscle
smooth	located in the walls of hollow organs such as the stomach and intestines; produces movement in those organs; involuntary muscle
cardiac	makes up the muscular layer of the heart

Nervous Tissue

Nervous tissue transmits information throughout the body that allows us to move, think, taste, see, and experience all functions associated with being alive. From blinking the eyes to solving the most complex mathematical equation, nervous tissue is ready to activate the body parts necessary to complete these activities.

Organs

Organs are groups of tissues working together to perform a specific function. Examples of various organs include the heart, stomach, eyes, and skin. The internal organs of the body are known as the **viscera** (**VISS**-er-ah) or **visceral** organs.

Systems

Systems are groups of organs working together to perform the many functions of the body as a whole. Each body system is discussed in the remaining chapters. Table 2-4 lists the body systems and related organs as described in this text.

TABLE 2-4 BODY SYSTEMS AND ORGANS

Body System	Organs
integumentary	skin; hair; nails; glands
skeletal	bones; joints
muscular	muscles; cartilage; ligaments; tendons
cardiovascular	heart; arteries; veins
blood/lymph	blood; blood cells; lymph; lymph cells; lymph glands
respiratory	lungs; trachea; bronchi
digestive	mouth; throat; esophagus; stomach; small and large intestines; rectum; liver; gallbladder; and pancreas
urinary	kidneys; ureters; urethra; bladder
endocrine	glands; hormones
male reproductive	testes; vas deferens; penis; accessory organs
female reproductive	ovaries; uterus; vagina; fallopian tubes; accessory organs
nervous	nerves; brain; spinal cord
sensory	eyes; ears

EXERCISE 4

Write the term for each definition.

1. foundation for all parts of the body   _____

2. organs working together to perform a function   _____

3. cells working together to perform a function   _____

4. tissues working together to perform a function   _____

5. internal organs   _____

6. covering and lining for glands and organs   _____

7. supports and binds other body tissue   _____

8. transmits impulses   _____

9. produces movement   _____

EXERCISE 5

Match the term in Column 1 with the definition in Column 2.

COLUMN 1

_____ 1. chromosome

_____ 2. cytology

_____ 3. cytoplasm

_____ 4. histology

_____ 5. integumentary system

_____ 6. nucleus

_____ 7. proximal

_____ 8. sensory system

_____ 9. ventral

_____ 10. viscera

COLUMN 2

a. eyes; ears

b. study of tissue

c. internal organs

d. pertaining to something near

e. pertaining to the front side

f. contains genes and DNA

g. skin; hair; nails; glands

h. gel-like substance within a cell

i. controls cellular functions

j. study of cells

EXERCISE 6

Write the name of the body system that includes the listed organs.

1. bones; joints _____

2. muscles; tendons; cartilage _____

3. lungs; trachea; bronchi _____

4. kidneys; ureters; urethra; bladder _____

5. glands; hormones _____

6. heart; arteries; veins _____

7. mouth; stomach; large and small intestines _____

8. brain; spinal cord _____

9. testes; vas deferens _____

10. ovaries; uterus _____

Body Cavities

Body cavities are hollow spaces that contain an orderly arrangement of internal organs. The main body cavities are (1) the **ventral cavity**, located on the front side of the body, and (2) the **dorsal cavity**, located on the backside of the body. Each main body cavity is further subdivided and named for its specific location. Figure 2-2 illustrates the location and name of the main cavities and their subdivisions. Refer to Figure 2-2 as you read about the body cavities.

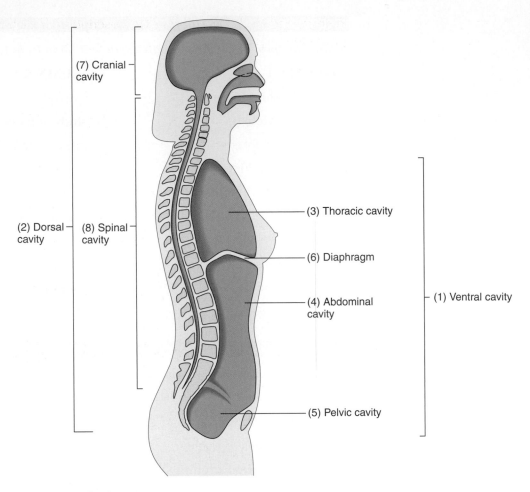

Figure 2-2 Body cavities

Ventral Cavity

The ventral cavity is divided into the (3) **thoracic** (thoh-**RASS**-ik) **cavity**, the (4) **abdominal cavity**, and the (5) **pelvic cavity**. The thoracic cavity, which is also called the chest cavity, houses the lungs, heart, aorta, esophagus, and the trachea. The (6) **diaphragm** (**DIGH**-ah-fram), the muscle that helps us breathe, separates the thoracic cavity from the abdominal cavity.

The abdominal cavity houses the liver, gallbladder, spleen, stomach, pancreas, intestines, and kidneys. There is no specific structure that separates the abdominal cavity from the pelvic cavity. The pelvic cavity houses the urinary bladder and reproductive organs. The abdominal cavity and pelvic cavity are often called the abdominopelvic cavity.

Dorsal Cavity

The dorsal cavity is divided into the (7) **cranial cavity** and the (8) **spinal cavity**. The cranial cavity houses the brain, and the spinal cavity houses the spinal cord.

Body Regions and Quadrants

Body regions are imaginary sections of the abdominopelvic cavity that are located between the diaphragm and pelvis. Physicians use these regions to identify the location of abdominal organs and describe the location of pain. There are nine body regions.

Refer to Figure 2-3 as you read the description of each region. The descriptions are presented in Table 2-5.

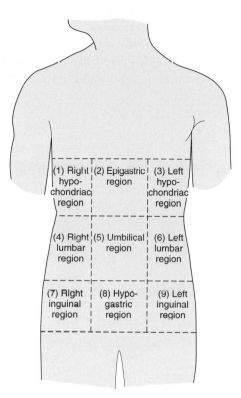

Figure 2-3   Body regions

TABLE 2-5   BODY REGIONS

Region	Name and Description
1	**Right hypochondriac (high-poh-KON-dree-ak) region**. Located beneath the cartilage of the lower ribs in the upper-right section of the abdomen.
2	**Epigastric (ep-ee-GASS-trik) region**. Located above the stomach and navel, between the right and left hypochondriac regions.
3	**Left hypochondriac region**. Located beneath the cartilage of the lower ribs in the upper-left section of the abdomen.
4	**Right lumbar region**. Located in the midportion of the abdomen directly below the right hypochondriac region.
5	**Umbilical region**. Located in the midsection of the abdomen at the level of the umbilicus or navel.
6	**Left lumbar region**. Located in the midportion of the abdomen directly below the left hypochondriac region.
7	**Right inguinal (ING-gwih-nal) region**. Located in the lower-right portion of the abdomen, directly below the right lumbar region. Also called the **right iliac region**.
8	**Hypogastric region**. Located in the lower midsection of the abdomen, directly below the umbilical region.
9	**Left inguinal region**. Located in the lower-right portion of the abdomen, directly below the left lumbar region. Also called the **left iliac region**.

Body quadrants are four imaginary sections of the abdomen that, like the nine body regions, provide a reference point for locating abdominal organs and pain. The quadrants are named based on their relationship to the umbilicus or navel. Figure 2-4 illustrates the body quadrants. The (1) **right upper quadrant (RUQ)** and (2) **left upper quadrant (LUQ)** are positioned above and to the right and left of the umbilicus. The (3) **right lower quadrant (RLQ)** and (4) **left lower quadrant (LLQ)** are positioned below and to the right and left of the umbilicus.

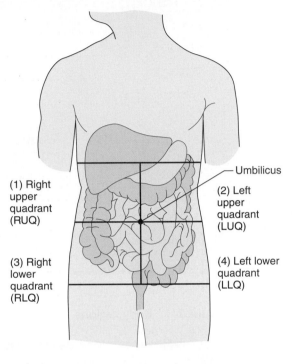

Figure 2-4 Body quadrants

EXERCISE 7

Analyze the listed body region terms. Identify and define the root, prefix, and suffix for each term. Write the definition for each term.

EXAMPLE:	hemigastrectomy
ROOT:	gastr = stomach
PREFIX:	hemi- = half
SUFFIX:	-ectomy = surgical removal, excision
DEFINITION:	surgical removal of all or part of the stomach

1. hypochondriac

    ROOT: _____

    PREFIX: _____

    SUFFIX: _____

    DEFINITION: _____

2. inguinal

   ROOT: _____

   PREFIX: _____

   SUFFIX: _____

   DEFINITION: _____

3. epigastric

   ROOT: _____

   PREFIX: _____

   SUFFIX: _____

   DEFINITION: _____

4. hypogastric

   ROOT: _____

   PREFIX: _____

   SUFFIX: _____

   DEFINITION: _____

5. umbilical

   ROOT: _____

   PREFIX: _____

   SUFFIX: _____

   DEFINITION: _____

EXERCISE 8

Write the name of the body cavities shown in Figure 2-5 on the spaces provided.

   1. _____

   2. _____

   3. _____

   4. _____

   5. _____

   6. _____

   7. _____

   8. _____

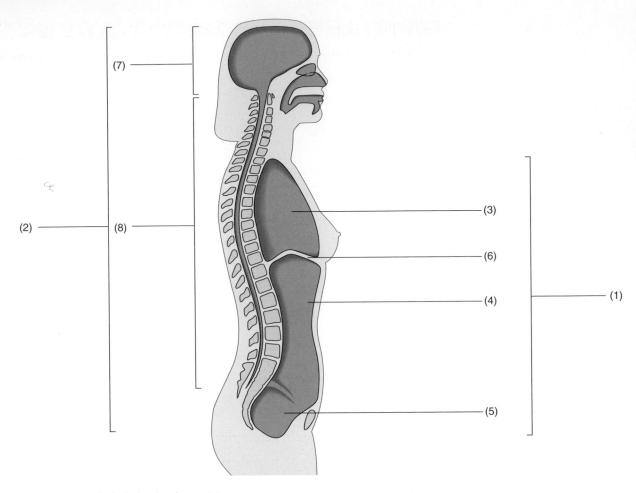

Figure 2-5 Label the body cavities

EXERCISE 9

Write out the following abbreviations.

1. RUQ _____

2. LLQ _____

3. LUQ _____

4. RLQ _____

EXERCISE 10

Place the abbreviations listed in Exercise 9 in the correct location on Figure 2-6.

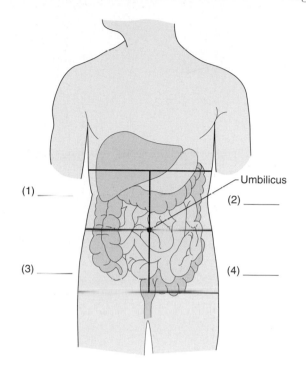

Figure 2-6   Label the body quadrants

EXERCISE 11

Write the names of the body regions shown in Figure 2-7 on the spaces provided.

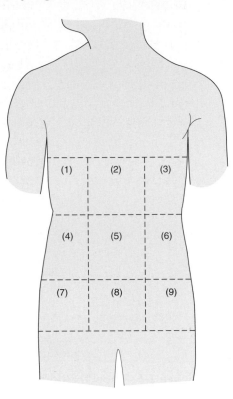

Figure 2-7 Label the body regions

1. _____

2. _____

3. _____

4. _____

5. _____

6. _____

7. _____

8. _____

9. _____

Body Planes

Body planes are imaginary slices, or cuts, that divide the body into right and left, front and back, and upper and lower segments. These slices pass through the body in a specific direction. Table 2-6 lists and describes commonly used body planes. Refer to Figure 2-8 as you review the descriptions of the body planes.

TABLE 2-6   BODY PLANES

Body Plane	Description
(1) midsagittal plane (mid-**SAJ**-ih-tal)	divides the body, starting with the head and continuing through the pelvic region, into right and left halves or sides
sagittal plane (**SAJ**-ih-tal)	parallel to the midsagittal plane; divides the body into right and left portions or segments
(2) frontal plane	divides the body, starting with the head and continuing through the legs and feet, into front and back portions or segments; also called the coronal (koh-**ROH**-nal) plane
(3) transverse plane	divides the body into upper and lower portions or segments; also called the horizontal plane

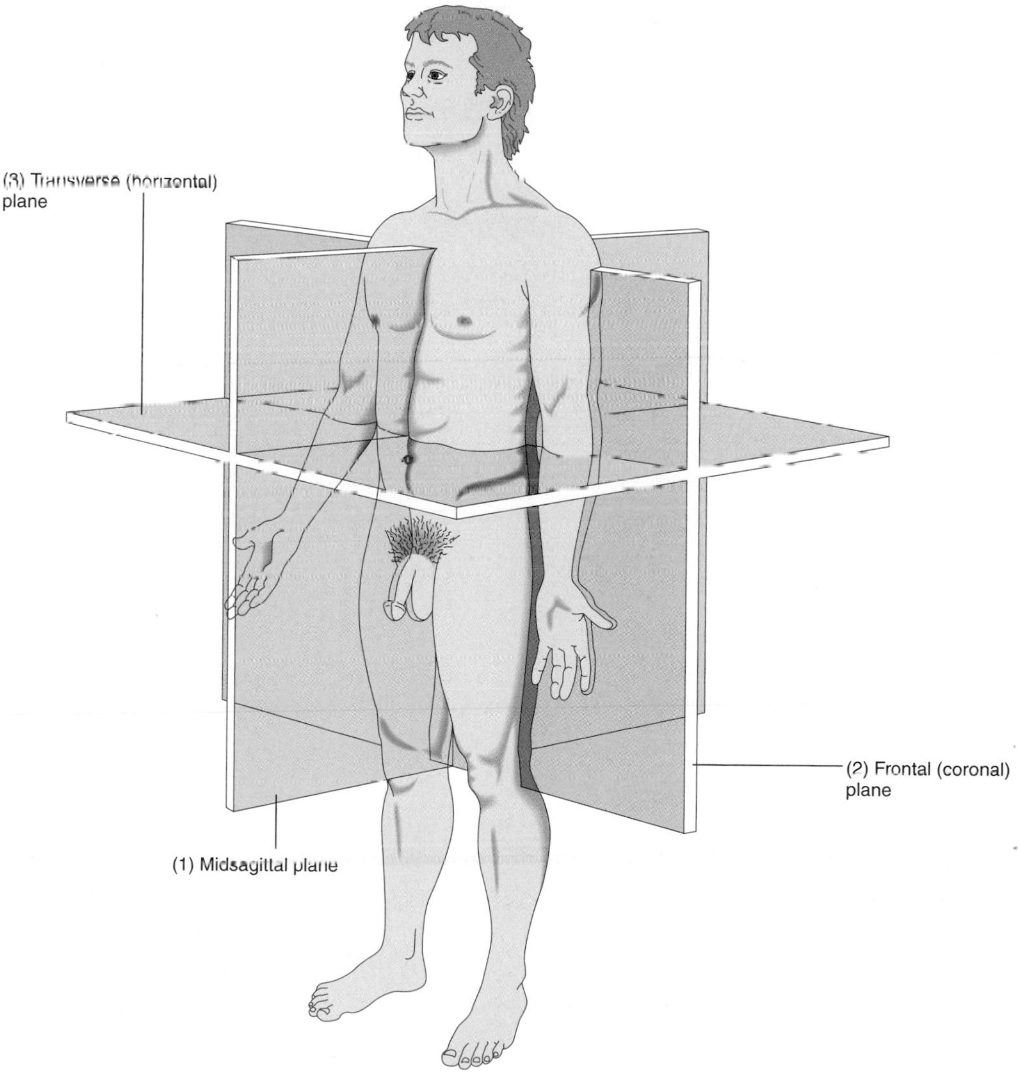

(3) Transverse (horizontal) plane

(2) Frontal (coronal) plane

(1) Midsagittal plane

Figure 2-8   Body planes

Body Direction Terms

Body direction terms are literally the north, south, east, and west of medical terminology. These terms provide health-care professionals with a vocabulary that readily describes the location of another body part, an incision, a problem, diagnosis, or disease and other information related to the human body.

Body direction terms are described in terms of a standard reference position of the body as a whole. This standard reference position is called the **anatomical position**. In the anatomical position, the body is viewed as erect, with the arms at the sides, palms of the hands facing forward, and the head and feet also facing forward. Directional terms keep the same meaning as long as the individual is standing or lying down, face up.

Commonly used directional terms, with pronunciations and meanings, are listed in Table 2-7. Review the pronunciation and meaning of each term and complete the exercises.

TABLE 2-7 DIRECTIONAL TERMS

Term with Pronunciation	Definition
anterior (an-**TEE**-ree-or)	toward the front; pertaining to the front
anteroposterior (AP) (**an**-ter-oh-poss-**TEE**-ree-or)	from the front to the back; pertaining to the front and the back
caudal (**KAWD**-al)	pertaining to the tail; downward
cranial (**KRAY**-nee-al)	toward the head; pertaining to the head
cephalad (**SEFF**-ah-lad)	toward the head; pertaining to the head
deep	away from the surface
distal (**DISS**-tal)	away from the trunk of the body; farthest from the point of origin of a body part (Figure 2-9)

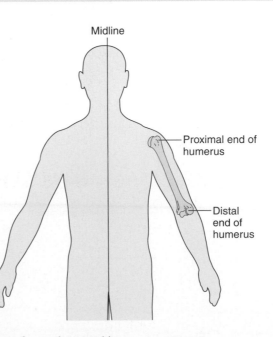

Midline

Proximal end of humerus

Distal end of humerus

Figure 2-9 Distal (away from the trunk)

(continues)

TABLE 2-7   DIRECTIONAL TERMS (continued)

Term with Pronunciation	Definition
dorsal (**DOR**-sal)	toward the back; pertaining to the back
inferior (in-**FEER**-ee-or)	below; downward toward the tail or feet
lateral (**LAT**-er-al)	to the side; away from the midline of the body
medial (**MEE**-dee-al)	toward the midline of the body; pertaining to the middle
posterior (poss-**TEE**-ree-or)	toward the back; pertaining to the back of the body
posteroanterior (PA) (**poss**-ter-oh-an-**TEE**-ree-or)	from the back to the front; pertaining to the back and front
prone (PROHN)	face down; lying on the abdomen
proximal (**PROCKS**-ih-mal)	toward the trunk of the body; nearest to the point of origin of a body part (see Figure 2-9)
superficial (soo-per-**FISH**-al)	near the surface; pertaining to the surface
superior (soo-**PEE**-ree-or)	above; upward; toward the head
supine (soo-**PINE**)	face up; lying on the back
ventral (**VEN**-tral)	toward the front; pertaining to the front side

EXERCISE 12

Fill in the blanks.

1. The _____ plane divides the body into right and left segments.

2. Horizontal plane is another name for the _____ plane.

3. Coronal plane is also known as the _____ plane.

4. The _____ plane divides the body into right and left halves.

5. A/An _____ wound is near the surface of the body.

6. The _____ position is best for examining the abdomen.

7. The knees are located in a/an _____ position from the ankles.

EXERCISE 13

Match the term in Column 1 with the definition in Column 2.

COLUMN 1

_____ 1. anterior

_____ 2. caudal

_____ 3. distal

_____ 4. lateral

_____ 5. medial

_____ 6. posterior

COLUMN 2

a. toward the tail

b. upper and lower segments

c. face up

d. toward the front

e. farthest away from

f. nearest to

_____ 7. proximal   g. toward the side

_____ 8. supine   h. toward the back

_____ 9. midsagittal plane   i. toward the midline

_____ 10. transverse plane   j. equal right and left segments

EXERCISE 14

Write the directional term that has the opposite meaning of each listed directional term.

EXAMPLE:	DIRECTIONAL TERM	OPPOSITE MEANING DIRECTIONAL TERM
	deep	superficial

DIRECTIONAL TERM	**OPPOSITE MEANING DIRECTIONAL TERM**
1. anterior	_____
2. anteroposterior	_____
3. caudal	_____
4. distal	_____
5. lateral	_____
6. prone	_____
7. superficial	_____
8. superior	_____
9. ventral	_____

SUMMARY

General body terminology includes words associated with the organization of the body from cells to body systems; the names of the major body cavities, planes, and organ systems; and the regions and quadrants of the chest and abdomen. The roots and terms presented in this chapter provide a foundation for understanding the medical terminology of the individual body systems.

CHAPTER REVIEW

The Chapter Review can be used as a self-test. Go through each exercise and answer as many questions as you can without referring to previous exercises or earlier discussions within this chapter. Check your answers and fill in any blanks. Practice writing the terms that are misspelled.

EXERCISE 15

Write the meaning of each abbreviation.

1. RLQ   _____

2. LLQ   _____

3. RUQ   _____

4. LUQ   _____

5. AP   _____

6. PA   _____

EXERCISE 16

Select the best answer to each statement.

1. Select the type of tissue that supports other body structures.
   a. connective
   b. muscle
   c. nervous
   d. adipose

2. Which tissue transmits information throughout the body?
   a. adipose
   b. nervous
   c. muscle
   d. connective

3. Choose the tissue that is responsible for body movement.
   a. connective
   b. nervous
   c. adipose
   d. muscle

4. Which tissue is composed of fat?
   a. muscle
   b. nervous
   c. adipose
   d. connective

5. Select the term that means internal body organs.
   a. systems
   b. viscera
   c. ventral
   d. abdominus

6. Which body cavity is **not** a division of the ventral cavity?
   a. thoracic cavity
   b. pelvic cavity
   c. abdominal cavity
   d. cranial cavity

7. Select the group of organs located in the thoracic cavity.
   a. heart, aorta, diaphragm
   b. lungs, esophagus, spleen
   c. lungs, heart, trachea
   d. esophagus, trachea, liver

8. Choose the group of organs located in the pelvic cavity.
   a. kidneys, uterus, ovaries
   b. uterus, ovaries, vas deferens
   c. kidneys, ureters, urinary bladder
   d. urinary bladder, ovaries, spleen

9. Which group of organs is located in the abdominal cavity?
   a. esophagus, liver, stomach
   b. intestines, stomach, urinary bladder
   c. stomach, trachea, spleen
   d. liver, gallbladder, kidneys

10. Select the body cavity that houses the brain.
    a. cranial cavity
    b. dorsal cavity
    c. thoracic cavity
    d. ventral cavity

EXERCISE 17

Match the body system in Column 1 with the components in Column 2.

COLUMN 1	**COLUMN 2**
_____ 1. blood/lymph	a. bones, joints
_____ 2. cardiovascular	b. blood, blood cells, lymph glands
_____ 3. digestive	c. cartilage, ligaments, tendons
_____ 4. endocrine	d. eyes, ears
_____ 5. female reproductive	e. glands, hormones
_____ 6. integumentary	f. heart, arteries, veins
_____ 7. male reproductive	g. kidneys, ureters, bladder
_____ 8. muscular	h. lungs, trachea, bronchi
_____ 9. nervous	i. mouth, stomach, intestines
_____ 10. respiratory	j. nerves, brain, spinal cord
_____ 11. sensory	k. ovaries, uterus, vagina
_____ 12. skeletal	l. skin, hair, nails
_____ 13. urinary	m. testes, vas deferens, penis

EXERCISE 18

Write a brief definition for each term.

1. cell _____
2. tissue _____
3. organ _____
4. system _____
5. cytology _____

6. sagittal plane   _____

7. transverse plane   _____

8. supine   _____

9. prone   _____

10. distal   _____

EXERCISE 19

Fill in the blanks.

1. The _____ controls all cellular functions.

2. _____ tissue covers organs and lines vessels.

3. Tendons and ligaments are examples of _____ tissue.

4. The _____ region of the body is at the level of the navel.

5. The _____ region of the body is located above the stomach.

6. A gel-like substance called _____ houses the cell's structures.

7. _____ muscle is attached to bones.

8. The _____ region of the body is located below the stomach and navel.

9. _____ is defined as the study of tissue.

10. _____ muscle produces movement in hollow organs.

Chapter 3
Integumentary System

At the completion of this chapter, the student should be able to:

1. Identify, define, and spell word roots associated with the integumentary system.
2. Label the basic structures of the integumentary system.
3. Discuss the functions of the integumentary system.
4. Provide the correct spelling of integumentary terms, given the definition of the term.
5. Analyze integumentary terms by defining the roots, prefixes, and suffixes of these terms.
6. Identify, define, and spell disease, disorder, and procedure terms related to the integumentary system.

OVERVIEW

The integumentary system is made up of the skin, hair, nails, and glands. The structures of the integumentary system function together for the following purposes: (1) to provide a protective covering for the entire body; (2) to produce sweat, which cools the body, and oil, which lubricates the body; and (3) to receive sensory information associated with pain, temperature, pressure, and touch. Each integumentary system structure and its unique characteristics are presented individually.

Integumentary System Word Roots

To understand and use integumentary system medical terms, it is necessary to acquire a thorough knowledge of the associated word roots. Integumentary system word roots are listed with the combining vowel. Review the word roots in Table 3-1 and complete the exercises that follow.

TABLE 3-1   INTEGUMENTARY SYSTEM WORD ROOTS

Word Root/Combining Form	Meaning
cut/o; cutane/o	skin
derm/o; dermat/o	skin
hidr/o	sweat
kerat/o	horny tissue; hard
melan/o	black
myc/o	fungus
onych/o; ungu/o	nail
pachy/o	thick

(continues)

TABLE 3-1 INTEGUMENTARY SYSTEM WORD ROOTS (continued)

Word Root/Combining Form	Meaning
pil/o	hair
rhytid/o	wrinkles
seb/o	sebum
squam/o	scale
sud/o; sudor/o	sweat
trich/o	hair
xer/o	dry

EXERCISE I

Write the definitions of the following word roots.

1. melan/o _____
2. trich/o _____
3. onych/o _____
4. cutane/o _____
5. sud/o; sudor/o _____
6. hidr/o _____
7. xer/o _____
8. myc/o _____
9. pachy/o _____
10. rhytid/o _____

EXERCISE 2

Write the word root and meaning for each of the listed medical terms.

EXAMPLE: cutaneous
ROOT: cutan   MEANING: skin

1. dermatitis

   ROOT: _____ MEANING: _____

2. keratosis

   ROOT: _____ MEANING: _____

3. melanocyte

   ROOT: _____ MEANING: _____

4. rhytidoplasty

   ROOT: _____ MEANING: _____

5. squamous

   ROOT: _____ MEANING: _____

6. sebum

   ROOT: _____ MEANING: _____

The hair shaft is actually dead tissue and does not have nerve endings or a blood supply, which is why it does not hurt when your hair is cut. Figure 3-2 illustrates the major structures of hair.

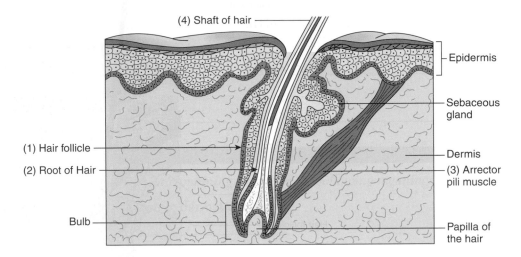

Figure 3-2 Structures of hair

Fingernails and toenails are also made up of keratin and originate in the epidermis. Although both hair and nails contain keratin, nails are arranged as flat, hard, plate-like coverings located at the ends of toes and fingers. Nails consist of the (1) **nail plate,** also called the nail body; the (2) **lunula (LOO**-noo-lah), a pale or white half-moon shaped area at the base of the nail plate; and the (3) **cuticle,** a narrow band of epidermal skin at the base and sides of the nail plate. Figure 3-3 highlights nail structures.

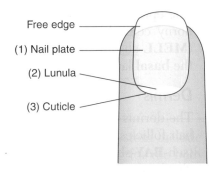

Figure 3-3 Structures of nails

EXERCISE 4

Match the structures in Column 1 with the definitions in Column 2.

COLUMN 1	COLUMN 2
_____ 1. arrector pili	a. secretes sebum
_____ 2. cuticle	b. "living" skin tissue
_____ 3. dermis	c. produces sweat
_____ 4. epidermis	d. flat, plate-like coverings
_____ 5. follicle	e. outermost skin layer

_____ 6. hair

_____ 7. lunula

_____ 8. melanin

_____ 9. nail

_____ 10. sebaceous gland

_____ 11. sweat gland

f. contains hair root

g. provides skin color

h. meshwork of cells with protein

i. area at the base of the nail

j. band of skin around the nail plate

k. provides support to the hair follicle

EXERCISE 5

Write the name of the skin structures shown in Figure 3-4 on the spaces provided.

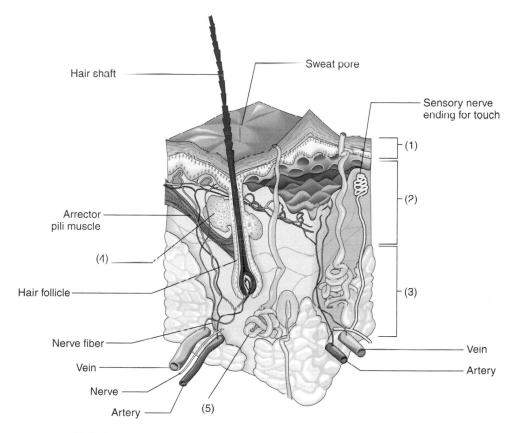

Hair shaft

Sweat pore

Sensory nerve ending for touch

(1)

(2)

Arrector pili muscle

(4)

Hair follicle

(3)

Nerve fiber

Vein

Nerve

Artery

(5)

Vein

Artery

Figure 3-4 Label the structures of the skin

1. _____

2. _____

3. _____

4. _____

5. _____

6. Joe made an appointment to have a *boil* removed.

   MEDICAL TERM: _____

7. Henry's *scratch* became infected.

   MEDICAL TERM: _____

8. After sliding across the basketball floor, Jenny had a large *scrape* on her arm.

   MEDICAL TERM: _____

9. Rachel's *scar* required surgical intervention.

   MEDICAL TERM: _____

EXERCISE 10

Using your medical dictionary, write a brief definition for the italicized medical terms.

1. The *ecchymosis* on Julia's forearm did not prevent her from playing volleyball.

   DEFINITION: _____

2. Many over-the-counter lotions claim they can relieve *erythema*.

   DEFINITION: _____

3. Standing on your feet for prolonged periods may cause *edema*.

   DEFINITION: _____

4. Marlena's dermatologist prescribed a new medication for her *eczema*.

   DEFINITION: _____

5. *Actinic keratosis* is related to excessive sunlight exposure.

   DEFINITION: _____

6. Jim's *herpes zoster* affected his trunk and back.

   DEFINITION: _____

7. *Acne* can affect an individual at any age.

   DEFINITION: _____

8. When Lisa was diagnosed with *impetigo* she avoided contact with her fellow students.

   DEFINITION: _____

EXERCISE 11

Match the medical term in Column 1 with the definition in Column 2.

COLUMN 1	COLUMN 2
_____ 1. abrasion	a. shingles
_____ 2. acne	b. cancerous tumor of the epidermis
_____ 3. albinism	c. disease of sebaceous glands and hair follicles
_____ 4. basal cell carcinoma	d. scratch
_____ 5. cicatrix	e. highly contagious superficial skin infection

_____	6. contusion	f. lack of skin pigmentation
_____	7. diaphoresis	g. scar
_____	8. eczema	h. scraping away of the skin; a scrape
_____	9. excoriation	i. excessive sweating
_____	10. herpes zoster	j. bruise
_____	11. impetigo	k. skin disorder; redness, itching, weeping, and crusting

EXERCISE 12

Review the list of medical terms and rewrite the terms that are misspelled.

1. alopecea   _____

2. abrasion   _____

3. exzema   _____

4. furuncle   _____

5. erithema   _____

6 excoriation   _____

7. diaphoresis   _____

8. impatigo   _____

9. basil cell carcinoma   _____

10. carbuncle   _____

Review the pronunciation and definition for each term in Table 3-5 and complete the exercises.

TABLE 3-5   INTEGUMENTARY SYSTEM DISEASE AND DISORDER TERMS

Term with Pronunciation	Definition
jaundice (**JAWN**-dis)	yellow discoloration of the skin
Kaposi's sarcoma (**KAP**-oh-seez sar-**KOH**-mah) sarc/o = flesh -oma = tumor	a cancerous growth that begins as soft, purple-brown papules on the feet and gradually spreads in the skin
keloid (**KEE**-loyd)	abnormally large, raised or thickened scar
laceration (lass-er-**AY**-shun)	a cut
lesion (**LEE**-zhun)	any damage to tissue caused by trauma or disease

(continues)

TABLE 4-1 SKELETAL SYSTEM WORD ROOTS (continued)

Word Root/Combining Form	Meaning
crani/o	skull
femor/o	femur; thigh bone
fibul/o	fibula; outer lower leg bone
humer/o	humerus; upper arm bone
ili/o	ilium; pelvic bone, upper section
ischi/o	ischium; pelvic bone, lower section
lamin/o	lamina; thin, flat plate or layer
lumb/o	lower back
mandibul/o	mandible; lower jaw bone
maxill/o	maxilla; upper jaw bone
metacarp/o	hand bones
metatars/o	foot bones
myel/o	bone marrow
orth/o	straight
oste/o	bone
patell/o	patella; kneecap
pelv/i	pelvis
phalang/o	finger and toe bones
pubi/o; pub/o	pubis; pelvic bone, anterior section
radi/o	radius; outer lower arm bone
scapula/o	scapula; shoulder blade
spondyl/o	vertebra
stern/o	sternum; breastbone
tars/o	ankle bones
vertebr/o	vertebra

EXERCISE 1

Write the meaning for each word root.

1. carp/o _____

2. cost/o _____

3. coccyg/o _____

4. lumb/o _____

5. metacarp/o _____

6. myel/o _____

7. orth/o _____

8. phalang/o _____

9. spondyl/o _____

10. arthr/o _____

11. articul/o _____

12. burs/o _____

EXERCISE 2

Write the word root and meaning for the following medical terms.

EXAMPLE: costochondritis
ROOT: cost/o   MEANING: rib   ROOT: chondr/o   MEANING: cartilage

1. chondritis

   ROOT: _____   MEANING: _____

2. clavicular

   ROOT: _____   MEANING: _____

3. laminectomy

   ROOT: _____   MEANING: _____

4. osteomalacia

   ROOT: _____   MEANING: _____

5. craniotomy

   ROOT: _____   MEANING: _____

6. costovertebral

   ROOT: _____   MEANING: _____

7. femorocele

   ROOT: _____   MEANING: _____

8. pelvimetry

   ROOT: _____   MEANING: _____

9. pubiotomy

   ROOT: _____   MEANING: _____

10. arthritis

    ROOT: _____   MEANING: _____

EXERCISE 3

Write the correct word root/combining forms for the following bones.

1. fibula _____

2. humerus _____

3. ilium _____

4. ischium _____

5. mandible _____

6. maxilla _____

7. metatarsal _____

8. patella _____

Bone depressions are holes or indentations that allow nerves and blood vessels to pass through or into the bones. Commonly known bone depressions include the following:

- **fissure**—groove or slit-like opening
- **foramen** (foh-RAY-men)—hole or opening in a bone
- **fossa** (FOSS-ah)—indentation in the surface of a bone
- **sinus**—air space or opening in the bones of the skull

Bone processes and depressions are noted on the bone illustrations in this chapter.

Bones of the Head, Shoulders, Chest, Arms, and Hands

The bones of the head are collectively called the **cranium**. The cranial bones protect the brain, eyes, and inner structures of the ears. The more commonly known cranial bones are presented here. Refer to Figure 4-2 as you read about the cranial bones.

The (1) **frontal bone** forms the forehead and part of the bony protection for the eyes. Just behind the frontal bone are the (2) **parietal** (pah-**RIGH**-eh-tal) **bones**, one on each side of the head. These bones form the top and upper sides of the cranium. A single (3) **occipital** (ok-**SIP**-ih-tal) **bone** forms the back of the head and the base of the skull. The (4) **temporal** (**TEM**-por-al) **bones**, one on each side of the head, form the lower sides and part of the base of the skull.

The facial bones of the cranium include the (5) **mandible**, the lower jawbone and the only cranial bone that moves; the (6) **maxilla** or upper jawbone; and the (7) **zygomatic** (**zigh**-goh-**MAT**-ik) **bones**, one on each side of the face, which form the cheekbones and the outer part of the bony protection for the eyes.

The bones of the shoulders, chest, arms, and hands are illustrated in Figure 4-3. Refer to the figure as you read about these bones.

The bones of the shoulder are the (1) **clavicle**, commonly called the collarbone, and the (2) **scapula**, commonly called the shoulder blade. A section of the scapula, the (3) **acromion** (ah-**KROH**-mee-on) **process**, joins with the clavicle to create the highest point of the shoulder.

The bones of the chest or thorax are the (4) **sternum**, commonly called the breastbone, and the (5) **ribs**. The **xiphoid** (**ZIGH**-foyd) **process** is a projection at the lower end of the sternum.

The bones of the arms are the (6) **humerus**, the upper arm bone and the lower arm bones that include the (7) **radius** (i.e., the lateral bone) and the (8) **ulna** (i.e., the medial bone). The bones of the hands are the (9) **carpals**, the wrist bones; the (10) **metacarpals**, the bones of the palm; and the (11) **phalanges**, commonly called the finger bones.

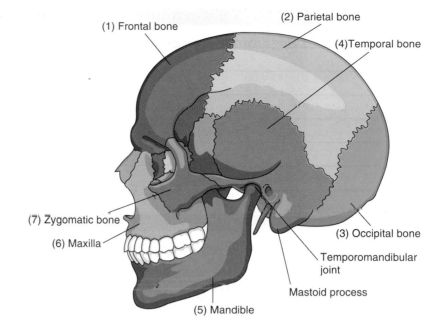

(1) Frontal bone

(2) Parietal bone

(4) Temporal bone

(7) Zygomatic bone

(6) Maxilla

(3) Occipital bone

Temporomandibular joint

Mastoid process

(5) Mandible

Figure 4-2 Bones of the face and skull

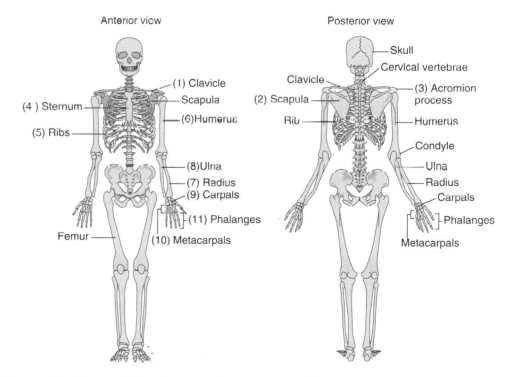

Anterior view

Posterior view

(1) Clavicle

Scapula

(4) Sternum

(6) Humerus

(5) Ribs

(8) Ulna

(7) Radius

(9) Carpals

(11) Phalanges

Femur

(10) Metacarpals

Skull

Cervical vertebrae

Clavicle

(3) Acromion process

(2) Scapula

Rib

Humerus

Condyle

Ulna

Radius

Carpals

Phalanges

Metacarpals

Figure 4-3 Bones of the thorax and upper extremities

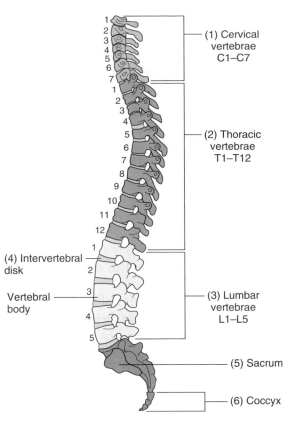

Figure 4-7 Bones of the spinal column

Joints

The area where two or more bones meet is called a **joint** or an **articulation** (ar-**tik**-yoo-**LAY**-shun). Joints are classified by the type of movement they allow. **Fibrous** (**FIGH**-brus) joints are nonmoveable and are located between the cranial bones. **Cartilaginous** (**kar**-tih-**LAJ**-in-us) joints allow limited movement. The pubic symphysis of the pelvis is an example of a cartilaginous joint. The pubic symphysis allows the pelvic bones to expand during childbirth. Figure 4-8 illustrates fibrous and cartilaginous joints.

Synovial (sin-**OH**-vee-al) joints are freely moveable. They include ball-and-socket joints that permit movement in a wide range of directions and hinge joints that move in one direction. The hip and shoulder joints are ball-and-socket joints. The elbow and knee joints are hinge joints. Synovial joints have several structures. Refer to Figure 4-9 as you read the description of the components of a synovial joint.

A synovial joint is enclosed within a **joint capsule** made up of ligaments. The (1) **synovial membrane** lines the capsule and secretes a lubricating fluid called **synovial fluid**. This fluid circulates in the (2) **synovial cavity**, the space between the bones, and allows the joint to move freely. The ends of the bones in a synovial joint are covered with (3) **articular cartilage** (ar-**TIK**-yoo-lar **KAR**-tih-laj), a protective covering for the bones. Fibrous sacs, called (4) **bursae** (**BER**-see), or bursa (singular), are filled with synovial fluid and provide a cushion for the friction points between tendons and bone. Bursae are located in the elbow, knee, and shoulder joints.

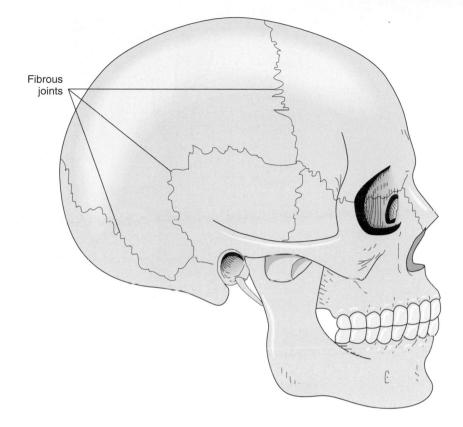

Fibrous joints

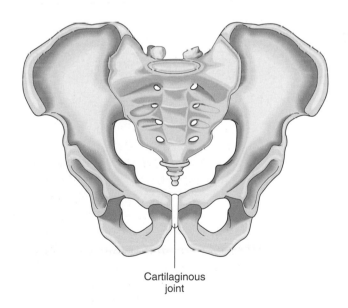

Cartilaginous joint

Figure 4-8   Fibrous and cartilaginous joints

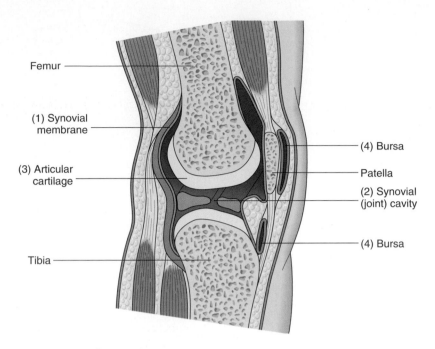

Figure 4-9 Synovial joint structures

EXERCISE 9

Using Figure 4-10 as a guide, write the medical term for the structures of the pelvic bones.

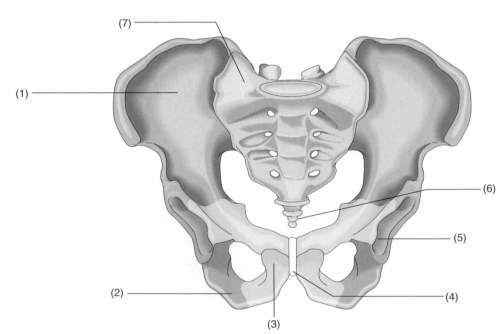

Figure 4-10 Bones of the hips and pelvis

1. _____

2. _____

3. _____

4. _____

5. _____

6. _____

7. _____

EXERCISE 10

Write the medical term for each definition.

1. ankle bone(s) _____

2. kneecap _____

3. large projection near the neck of the femur _____

4. heel _____

5. thighbone _____

6. toe bone(s) _____

7. foot bone(s) _____

8. large, rounded end of the femur _____

9. anterior segment of the pelvic bones _____

EXERCISE 11

Match the terms in Column 1 with the descriptions in Column 2.

COLUMN 1

_____ 1. cervical vertebrae

_____ 2. coccyx

_____ 3. fibula

_____ 4. intervertebral disk

_____ 5. lumbar vertebrae

_____ 6. sacrum

_____ 7. talus

_____ 8. thoracic vertebrae

_____ 9. tibia

_____ 10. vertebra

COLUMN 2

a. part of the ankle joint

b. L1–L5

c. T1–T12

d. spinal column bone

e. triangular-shaped bone

f. non–weight-bearing bone

g. larger lower leg bone

h. C1–C7

i. cushions the vertebrae

j. tailbone

EXERCISE 12

Write the joint term for each definition.

1. sac of lubricating fluid _____

2. freely moveable joint _____

3. nonmoveable joint _____

4. slightly moveable joint _____

5. lubricating fluid in a joint _____

6. lining of a joint capsule _____

7. type of joint that permits a wide range
of movement _____

8. type of joint that permits movement in one
direction _____

9. protective covering for the end of bones in a freely
moveable joint _____

10. alternate term for joint _____

Skeletal System Medical Terminology

Skeletal system medical terms are organized into three main categories: (1) general medical terms; (2) diseases and conditions; and (3) diagnostic procedure, surgery, and laboratory test terms. Roots, prefixes and suffixes listed in Table 4-3 are commonly a part of skeletal system medical terms. Review these word parts and complete the related exercises. The exercises are designed to help you learn skeletal system medical terms by recalling the meaning of the word parts.

TABLE 4-3 ROOTS, PREFIXES, AND SUFFIXES FOR SKELETAL SYSTEM TERMS

Root	Meaning	Prefix	Meaning	Suffix	Meaning
ankyl/o	stiff; immobile	sub-	below; under	-blast	immature
kyph/o	pertaining to a hump	supra-	above	-clasis	surgical fracture
				-malacia	softening
lord/o	swayback			-oma	tumor
scoli/o	crooked; bent			-osis	abnormal condition

EXERCISE 13

Write the word root, prefix, suffix, and meanings for the following medical terms. Using the meanings, write a definition for the medical term. Use a medical dictionary to check your definition.

EXAMPLE: osteoblast
ROOT: oste/o = bone   PREFIX: none   SUFFIX: -blast = immature
DEFINITION: immature bone

1. osteoma

   ROOT: _____ PREFIX: _____ SUFFIX: _____

   DEFINITION: _____

2. scoliosis

   ROOT: _____ PREFIX: _____ SUFFIX: _____

   DEFINITION: _____

3. subcostal

ROOT: _____ PREFIX: _____ SUFFIX: _____

DEFINITION: _____

4. lordosis

ROOT: _____ PREFIX: _____ SUFFIX: _____

DEFINITION: _____

5. suprapubic

ROOT: _____ PREFIX: _____ SUFFIX: _____

DEFINITION: _____

6. osteoclasis

ROOT: _____ PREFIX: _____ SUFFIX: _____

DEFINITION: _____

7. kyphosis

ROOT: _____ PREFIX: _____ SUFFIX: _____

DEFINITION: _____

8. chondromalacia

ROOT: _____ PREFIX: _____ SUFFIX: _____

DEFINITION: _____

9. ankylosis

ROOT: _____ PREFIX: _____ SUFFIX: _____

DEFINITION: _____

Skeletal System General Medical Terms

Review the pronunciation and meaning of each term in Table 4-4. Note that some terms are built from word parts and some are not. Complete the exercises for these terms.

TABLE 4-4   SKELETAL SYSTEM GENERAL MEDICAL TERMS

Term with Pronunciation	Definition
articulation (ar-**tik**-yoo-**LAY**-shun) articul/o = joint	area where two or more bones meet; a joint
chiropractor (**KIGH**-roh-prak-tor)	practitioner who uses mechanical manipulation of the spinal column as a primary treatment method
cranial (**KRAY**-nee-al) crani/o = cranium, skull -al = pertaining to	pertaining to the cranium or skull

(continues)

TABLE 4-4   SKELETAL SYSTEM GENERAL MEDICAL TERMS (continued)

Term with Pronunciation	Definition
femoral (**FEM**-or-al) femor/o = femur -al = pertaining to	pertaining to the femur
humeral (**HYOO**-mor-al) humer/o = humerus -al = pertaining to	pertaining to the humerus
intercostal (**in**-ter-**KOSS**-tal) inter- = between cost/o = ribs -al = pertaining to	pertaining to between the ribs
intervertebral (**in**-ter-**VER**-teh-bral) inter- = between vertebr/o = vertebra -al = pertaining to	pertaining to between the vertebrae
ischiopubic (**ih**-shee-oh-**PYOO**-bik) ischi/o = ischium pub/o = pubis -ic = pertaining to	pertaining to the ischium and pubis
lumbar (**LUM**-bar) lumb/o = lower back -ar = pertaining to	pertaining to the lower back
lumbosacral (**lum**-boh-**SAY**-kral) lumb/o = lower back sacr/o = sacrum -al = pertaining to	pertaining to the lower back or lumbar region and sacrum
orthopedics (**or**-thoh-**PEE**-diks) orth/o = straight ped/o = foot -ic = pertaining to	branch of medicine pertaining to the study and treatment of diseases and abnormalities of the skeletal and muscular systems
orthopedist (**or**-thoh-**PEE**-dist) orth/o = straight ped/o = foot -ist = specialist	physician who specializes in orthopedics

(continues)

TABLE 4-4 SKELETAL SYSTEM GENERAL MEDICAL TERMS (continued)

Term with Pronunciation	Definition
osteoblast (**OSS**-tee-oh-blast) oste/o = bone -blast = immature	immature bone or bone cell
osteocyte (**OSS**-tee-oh-sight) oste/o = bone -cyte = cell	mature bone cell
submandibular (**sub**-man-**DIB**-yoo-lar) sub- = below, under mandibul/o = mandible -ar = pertaining to	pertaining to under or below the mandible
submaxillary (sub-**MACKS**-ih-lair-ee) sub- = under, below maxill/o = maxilla -ary = pertaining	pertaining to under or below the maxilla
substernal (sub-**STERN**-al) sub- = under, below stern/o = sternum -al = pertaining to	pertaining to under or below the sternum
supraclavicular (**soo**-prah-klah-**VIK**-yoo-lar) supra- = above clavicul/o = clavicle -ar = pertaining to	pertaining to above the sternum and clavicle

EXERCISE 14

Analyze each term by writing the root, prefix, suffix, and combining vowel separated by vertical slashes.

EXAMPLE: subclavicular

sub	/ *clavicul*	*(none)*	/ *ar*
prefix	*root*	*combining vowel*	*suffix*

1. cranial

prefix	*root*	*combining vowel*	*suffix*

2. femoral

prefix	*root*	*combining vowel*	*suffix*

3. humeral

prefix	root	combining vowel	suffix

4. intercostal

prefix	root	combining vowel	suffix

5. intervertebral

prefix	root	combining vowel	suffix

6. ischiopubic

prefix	root	combining vowel	suffix

7. lumbosacral

prefix	root	combining vowel	suffix

8. osteocyte

prefix	root	combining vowel	suffix

9. substernal

prefix	root	combining vowel	suffix

10. supraclavicular

prefix	root	combining vowel	suffix

Skeletal System Disease and Disorder Terms

Skeletal system disease and disorder terms are presented in alphabetical order in Table 4-5. All fractures are listed under the main term *fracture*. Review the pronunciation and definition for each term and complete the exercises.

TABLE 4-5 SKELETAL SYSTEM DISEASE AND DISORDER TERMS

Term with Pronunciation	Definition
ankylosing spondylitis (**ang**-kih-**LOH**-sing **spon**-dih-**LIGH**-tiss) ankyl/o = stiff spondyl/o = spinal column -itis = inflammation	inflammation of one or more vertebrae characterized by joint stiffness or immobility; rheumatoid arthritis of the spine
ankylosis (ang-kih-**LOH**-sis) ankyl/o = stiff -osis = condition	immobility of a joint
arthralgia (ar-**THRAL**-jee-ah) arthr/o = joint -algia = pain	joint pain

TABLE 4-5 SKELETAL SYSTEM DISEASE AND DISORDER TERMS (continued)

Term with Pronunciation	Definition
arthritis (ar-**THRIGH**-tis) arthr/o = joint -itis = inflammation	inflammation of a joint
arthrochondritis (**ar**-throh-kon-**DRIGH**-tis) arthr/o = joint chondr/o = joint -itis = inflammation	inflammation of an articular cartilage
Baker's cyst	accumulation of synovial fluid in the knee joint
bunion	inflammation and enlargement of the bursa of the joint of the great (big) too; also known as hallux valgus
bursitis (ber-**SIGH**-tis)	inflammation of the bursa
chondromalacia (**kon**-droh-mah-**LAY**-she-ah) chondr/o = cartilage -malacia = softening	softening of cartilage
crepitation (**crep**-ih-**TAY**-shun) during joint movement	crackling or clicking sound present
dislocation (**diss**-loh-**KAY**-shun)	temporary displacement of a bone from its joint
fracture (Figure 4-11 illustrates five types of fractures.)	sudden breaking of a bone; broken bone

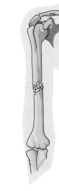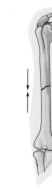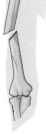

Closed (simple complete) fracture   Comminuted fracture   Greenstick fracture   Impacted fracture   Open (compound) fracture

Figure 4-11 Types of fractures

fracture, closed	break in a bone without interrupting the skin; simple or complete fracture

(continues)

TABLE 4-5 SKELETAL SYSTEM DISEASE AND DISORDER TERMS (continued)

Term with Pronunciation	Definition
fracture, Colles'	fracture of the distal end of the radius, just above the wrist
fracture, comminuted	fracture in which the bone is broken or splintered into pieces
fracture, greenstick	fracture in which the bone is partially bent and partially broken; incomplete fracture
fracture, impacted	fracture in which the bone is broken and wedged into the interior of another bone
fracture, open	fracture in which the bone is broken and bone fragments protrude through the skin; compound fracture

EXERCISE 15

Analyze each term. Identify and define the root(s), prefix, and suffix. Use your medical dictionary and write a brief definition.

1. chondromalacia

    ROOT: _____ PREFIX: _____ SUFFIX: _____

    DEFINITION: _____

2. ankylosing spondylitis

    ROOT: _____ PREFIX: _____ SUFFIX: _____

    ROOT: _____ PREFIX: _____ SUFFIX: _____

    DEFINITION: _____

3. arthralgia

    ROOT: _____ PREFIX: _____ SUFFIX: _____

    DEFINITION: _____

4. arthritis

    ROOT: _____ PREFIX: _____ SUFFIX: _____

    DEFINITION: _____

5. arthrochondritis

    ROOT: _____ PREFIX: _____ SUFFIX: _____

    ROOT: _____ PREFIX: _____ SUFFIX: _____

    DEFINITION: _____

6. bursitis

    ROOT: _____ PREFIX: _____ SUFFIX: _____

    DEFINITION: _____

EXERCISE 16

Identify each type of fracture shown in Figure 4-12.

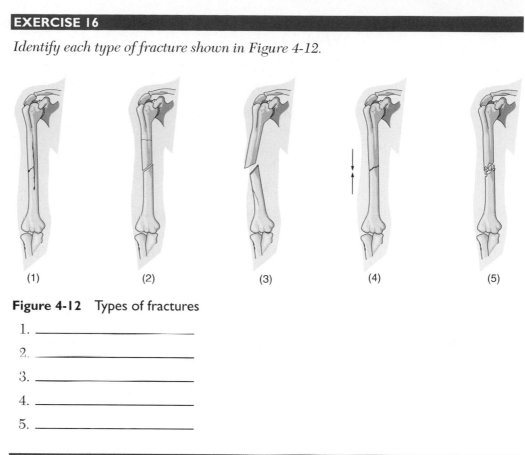

(1)   (2)   (3)   (4)   (5)

Figure 4-12   Types of fractures

1. _____
2. _____
3. _____
4. _____
5. _____

EXERCISE 16

Replace the italicized phrase with the correct medical term.

1. Rodney fell off his skateboard and sustained a *broken radius just above his wrist.*

   _____

2. Angelo experienced pain when he walked because of the *accumulation of synovial fluid in the knee joint* in his left leg.

   _____

3. Ling was scheduled for surgery to remove the *inflamed and enlarged joint bursa of her great toe* of her right foot.

   _____

4. A *crackling sound during joint movement* may indicate a fracture of the joint bones.

   _____

5. During gymnastic practice, Quo needed medical attention for the *temporary displacement* of his shoulder joint.

   _____

6. Dion was hospitalized for a *partially bent and partially broken bone.*

   _____

Review the pronunciation and definition for each term in Table 4-6 and complete the exercises.

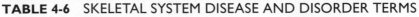

TABLE 4-6 SKELETAL SYSTEM DISEASE AND DISORDER TERMS

Term with Pronunciation	Definition
gout	acute arthritis characterized by inflammation of the first joint of the great toe
herniated disk (**HER**-nee-ay-ted disk)	rupture of the intervertebral disk, which protrudes between the vertebra and puts pressure on the spinal nerve root; commonly called a *slipped disk*
kyphosis (kigh-**FOH**-sis) kyph/o = pertaining to a hump -osis = abnormal condition	outward curvature of the upper sections of the spinal column; humpback (Figure 4-13)

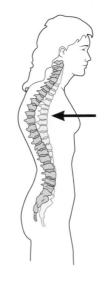

Figure 4-13 Kyphosis

lordosis (lor-**DOH**-sis) lord/o = swayback -osis = abnormal condition	forward curvature of the lower sections, usually the lumbar section, of the spinal column; swayback (Figure 4-14)
myeloma (**my**-eh-**LOH**-mah) myel/o = bone marrow -oma = tumor	tumor originating from the bone marrow
osteitis (**oss**-tee- **EYE**-tis) oste/o = bone -itis = inflammation	inflammation of the bone

(continues)

TABLE 4-6   SKELETAL SYSTEM DISEASE AND DISORDER TERMS (continued)

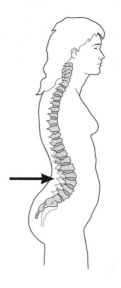

Figure 4-14   Lordosis

Term with Pronunciation	Definition
osteochondritis (**oss**-tee-oh-kon-**DRIGH**-tis) oste/o = bone chondr/o = cartilage -itis = inflammation	inflammation of bone and cartilage
osteofibroma (**oss**-tee-oh-fih-**BROH**-mah) oste/o = bone fibr/o = fibrous tissue -oma = tumor	tumor of bony and fibrous tissue
osteomalacia (**oss**-tee-oh-mah-**LAY**-she-ah) oste/o = bone -malacia = softening	softening of the bone
osteomyelitis (**oss**-tee-oh-my-eh-**LIGH**-tis) oste/o = bone myel/o = bone marrow -itis = inflammation	inflammation of the bone and bone marrow
osteoporosis (**oss**-tee-oh-poh-**ROH**-sis) oste/o = bone -porosis = porous condition	decreased bone density or loss of bone mass

(continues)

TABLE 4-6 SKELETAL SYSTEM DISEASE AND DISORDER TERMS (continued)

Term with Pronunciation	Definition
osteosarcoma (**oss**-tee-oh-sar-**KOH**-mah) oste/o = bone sarc/o = flesh -oma = tumor	malignant tumor of bone
rheumatoid arthritis (RA) (**ROO**-mah-toyd ar-**THRIGH**-tis) arthr/o = joint -itis = inflammation	chronic, systemic inflammatory disease of the joints, especially the joints of the hands and feet
scoliosis (skoh-lee-**OH**-sis) scoli/o = crooked, bent -osis = abnormal condition	abnormal lateral curvature of the spine (Figure 4-15)

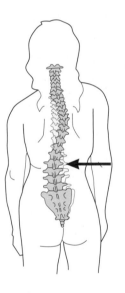

Figure 4-15 Scoliosis

spondylitis (spon-dih-**LIGH**-tiss) spondyl/o = spinal column, vertebra -itis = inflammation	inflammation of one or more vertebrae
spur	bony growth arising from the surface of the bone
subluxation (sub-luks-**AY**-shun)	incomplete dislocation of a bone from its joint
talipes (**TAL**-ih-peez)	congenital deformity characterized by an abnormal alignment of the bones of the feet; commonly called clubfoot

EXERCISE 18

Analyze each term. Identify and define the root(s), prefix, and suffix. Use your medical dictionary and write a brief definition for each term.

1. osteomalacia

   ROOT: _____ PREFIX: _____ SUFFIX: _____

   DEFINITION: _____

2. osteomyelitis

   ROOT: _____ PREFIX: _____ SUFFIX: _____

   DEFINITION: _____

3. osteoporosis

   ROOT: _____ PREFIX: _____ SUFFIX: _____

   DEFINITION: _____

4. osteosarcoma

   ROOT: _____ PREFIX: _____ SUFFIX: _____

   DEFINITION: _____

5. spondylitis

   ROOT: _____ PREFIX: _____ SUFFIX: _____

   DEFINITION: _____

6. myeloma

   ROOT: _____ PREFIX: _____ SUFFIX: _____

   DEFINITION: _____

7. osteochondritis

   ROOT: _____ PREFIX: _____ SUFFIX: _____

   DEFINITION: _____

8. osteitis

   ROOT: _____ PREFIX: _____ SUFFIX: _____

   DEFINITION: _____

9. osteofibroma

   ROOT: _____ PREFIX: _____ SUFFIX: _____

   DEFINITION: _____

EXERCISE 19

Write the medical term for each definition.

1. clubfoot   _____

2. abnormal lateral curvature of the spine   _____

3. acute arthritis and inflammation of the first joint
   of the great toe   _____

4. slipped disk   _____

5. abnormal outward curvature of the spine _____

6. incomplete dislocation of a bone from its joint _____

7. decreased bone density _____

8. abnormal forward curvature of the spine _____

9. chronic, systemic inflammatory disease of the joints _____

10. bony growth from the surface of a bone _____

Skeletal System Diagnostic, Treatment, and Surgical Terms

Review the pronunciation and definition of the diagnostic and treatment terms in Table 4-7. Complete the exercises for each set of terms.

TABLE 4-7 SKELETAL SYSTEM DIAGNOSTIC, TREATMENT, AND SURGICAL TERMS

Term with Pronunciation	Definition
arthrocentesis (**ar**-throh-sen-**TEE**-sis) arthr/o = joint -centesis = surgical puncture to withdraw fluid	surgical puncture of a joint to withdraw fluid
arthroclasis (**ar**-throh-**CLAY**-sis) arthr/o = joint -clasis = therapeutic or surgical breaking	therapeutic breaking of a joint or adhesions of a joint
arthrodesis (**ar**-throh-**DEE**-sis) arthr/o = joint -desis = surgical fixation	surgical fixation, binding, or immobilization of a joint
arthrogram (**AR**-throh-gram) arthr/o = joint -gram = picture or record of a joint	x-ray picture of a joint
arthrography (ar-**THROG**-rah-fee) arthr/o = joint -graphy = process of recording	process of obtaining a radiograph of the internal structures of a joint aided by the injection of a contrast medium
arthroplasty (**AR**-throh-**plass**-tee) arthr/o = joint -plasty = surgical repair	surgical repair of a joint
arthroscopy (ar-**THROSS**-koh-pee) arthr/o = joint -scopy = process of viewing; visualization	visualization of the internal structures of a joint using an endoscope
arthrotomy (ar-**THROT**-oh-mee) arthr/o = joint -tomy = incision into	incision into a joint
bone marrow aspiration (ass-per-**AY**-shun)	removing a sample of bone marrow using an aspiration needle
bone scan	visualization of the structure of the bone using a radioisotope

(continues)

TABLE 4-7   SKELETAL SYSTEM DIAGNOSTIC, TREATMENT, AND SURGICAL TERMS (continued)

Term with Pronunciation	Definition
bunionectomy (bun-yun-**ECK**-toh-mee) -ectomy = surgical removal	surgical removal of a bunion
bursectomy (ber-**SEK**-toh-mee) burs/o = bursa -ectomy = surgical removal	surgical removal of a bursa
bursotomy (ber-**SOT**-oh-mee) burs/o = bursa -tomy = incision into	incision into a bursa
closed reduction	process of aligning fractured bones through manual manipulation or traction
craniotomy (**kray**-nee-**OT**-oh-mee) crani/o = skull -tomy = incision into	incision into the cranium or bones of the skull
diskectomy (disk-**EK**-toh-mee) -ectomy = surgical removal	surgical removal of a herniated intervertebral disk
dual-energy x-ray absorptiometry (DEXA) (ab-**sorp**-she-**AH**-meh-tree)	noninvasive x-ray procedure that measures bone density
dual-photon absorptiometry (**FOH**-ton ab-**sorp**-she-**AH**-meh-tree)	noninvasive procedure using a small amount of radiation to measure bone density
laminectomy (lam-in-**EK**-toh-mee) lamin/o 5 lamina -ectomy 5 surgical removal	surgical removal of the posterior arch of the vertebra
open reduction	alignment of fractured bones through a surgically opened wound
open reduction and internal fixation (ORIF)	surgical alignment of fractured bones using screws, pins, wires, or nails to maintain bone alignment
osteoclasis (**oss**-tee-oh-**KLAY**-sis) oste/o 5 bone -clasis 5 surgical fracture	surgical fracture of a bone
osteoplasty (**OSS**-tee-oh-plass-tee) oste/o = bone -plasty = surgical repair	surgical repair of a bone

(continues)

TABLE 4-7 SKELETAL SYSTEM DIAGNOSTIC, TREATMENT, AND SURGICAL TERMS (continued)

Term with Pronunciation	Definition
osteotomy (**oss**-tee-**OT**-oh-mee) oste/o = bone -tomy = incision into	incision into a bone
spinal fusion	permanent joining of two or more vertebrae permanent joining of two or more vertebrae
synovectomy (**sin**-oh-**VEK**-toh-mee) -ectomy = surgical removal	surgical removal of a synovial membrane
total hip replacement (THR)	surgical replacement of the head of the femur and the acetabulum with synthetic components (Figure 4-16)

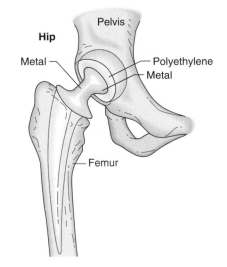

Figure 4-16 Total hip replacement

EXERCISE 20

Analyze each term. Identify and define the root, prefix, and suffix. Use your medical dictionary and write a brief definition for each term.

1. craniotomy

   ROOT: _____ PREFIX: _____ SUFFIX: _____

   DEFINITION: _____

2. diskectomy

   ROOT: _____ PREFIX: _____ SUFFIX: _____

   DEFINITION: _____

3. laminectomy

ROOT: _____   PREFIX: _____   SUFFIX: _____

DEFINITION: _____

4. osteoclasis

ROOT: _____   PREFIX: _____   SUFFIX: _____

DEFINITION: _____

5. osteoplasty

ROOT: _____   PREFIX: _____   SUFFIX: _____

DEFINITION: _____

6. osteotomy

ROOT: _____   PREFIX: _____   SUFFIX: _____

DEFINITION: _____

7. arthrocentesis

ROOT: _____   PREFIX: _____   SUFFIX: _____

DEFINITION: _____

8. arthroclasis

ROOT: _____   PREFIX: _____   SUFFIX: _____

DEFINITION: _____

9. arthrodesis

ROOT: _____   PREFIX: _____   SUFFIX: _____

DEFINITION: _____

10. arthroscopy

ROOT: _____   PREFIX: _____   SUFFIX: _____

DEFINITION: _____

11. arthrotomy

ROOT: _____   PREFIX: _____   SUFFIX: _____

DEFINITION: _____

EXERCISE 21

Write the medical term for the italicized phrase.

1. Quentin's fractured humerus was aligned via *manual manipulation*.

   _____

2. Dr. Rodriguez ordered a *bone density measurement* scan to assess the patient's osteoporosis.

   _____

3. Darrell's crushed calcaneus was repaired by *surgical alignment with pins and screws*.

   _____

4. Degenerative disk disease might be corrected by *permanent joining of vertebrae.*

_____

5. *Surgical repair of a joint* might be accomplished as an open or closed procedure.

_____

Abbreviations

Review the skeletal system abbreviations in Table 4-8. Practice writing the meaning of each abbreviation.

TABLE 4-8 ABBREVIATIONS

Abbreviation	Meaning
fx	fracture
C1–C7	cervical vertebrae, 1 through 7
DEXA	dual-energy x-ray absorptiometry
L1–L5	lumbar vertebrae, 1 through 5
ORIF	open reduction and internal fixation
T1–T12	thoracic vertebrae, 1 through 12
THR	total hip replacement

CHAPTER REVIEW

The Chapter Review can be used as a self-test. Go through each exercise and answer as many questions as you can without referring to previous exercises or earlier discussions within this chapter. Check your answers and fill in any blanks. Practice writing any terms that you might have misspelled.

EXERCISE 22

Analyze the listed medical terms by separating the root, prefix, suffix, and combining vowel with vertical slashes. Using the word part meanings, write a definition for the term. Use a medical dictionary to verify your definitions.

EXAMPLE: subclavicular

sub	*/ clavicul*	*(none)*	*/ ar*
prefix	root	combining vowel	suffix

1. intercostal

prefix	root	combining vowel	suffix

DEFINITION: _____

2. osteoblast

prefix	root	combining vowel	suffix

DEFINITION: _____

3. submandibular

prefix	root	combining vowel	suffix

DEFINITION: _____

4. supraclavicular

prefix	root	combining vowel	suffix

DEFINITION: _____

5. chondromalacia

prefix	root	combining vowel	suffix

DEFINITION: _____

6. kyphosis

prefix	root	combining vowel	suffix

DEFINITION: _____

7. myeloma

prefix	root	combining vowel	suffix

DEFINITION: _____

8. osteoporosis

prefix	root	combining vowel	suffix

DEFINITION: _____

9. craniotomy

prefix	root	combining vowel	suffix

DEFINITION: _____

10. osteoclasis

prefix	root	combining vowel	suffix

DEFINITION: _____

11. arthralgia

prefix	root	combining vowel	suffix

DEFINITION: _____

12. intervertebral

prefix	root	combining vowel	suffix

DEFINITION: _____

13. submaxillary

prefix	root	combining vowel	suffix

DEFINITION: _____

14. osteomyelitis

prefix	*root*	*combining vowel*	*suffix*

DEFINITION: _____

15. arthroscopy

prefix	*root*	*combining vowel*	*suffix*

DEFINITION: _____

16. lumbosacral

prefix	*root*	*combining vowel*	*suffix*

DEFINITION: _____

17. arthrocentesis

prefix	*root*	*combining vowel*	*suffix*

DEFINITION: _____

18. humeral

prefix	*root*	*combining vowel*	*suffix*

DEFINITION: _____

19. ischiopubic

prefix	*root*	*combining vowel*	*suffix*

DEFINITION: _____

20. laminectomy

prefix	*root*	*combining vowel*	*suffix*

DEFINITION: _____

EXERCISE 23

Fill in the blanks.

1. A/An _____ is a mature bone cell.
2. A/An _____ is a physician who specializes in disorders and treatments of the skeletal system.
3. The medical term for the sudden breaking of a bone is _____.
4. A/An _____ is commonly called a slipped disk.
5. Forward curvature of the lumbar spine is called _____.
6. The diagnosis _____ is a malignant bone tumor.
7. _____ is commonly known as clubfoot.
8. A/An _____ is an incision into the bones of the skull.

9. The medical term for surgical fracture of a bone is _____.

10. Lateral curvature of the spine is called _____.

11. _____ is also known as rheumatoid arthritis of the spine.

12. The medical term for softening of the bone is _____.

13. A(n) _____ specializes in the manipulation of the spine as a primary treatment method.

14. _____ is an incomplete dislocation of a bone from its joint.

15. Crackling and clicking sounds during joint movement is called

    _____.

16. A(n) _____ of a fracture includes surgical intervention.

17. A _____ is a bony growth on the surface of a bone.

18. Surgical fixation of a joint is called _____ .

19. A(n) _____ fracture occurs at the distal end of the radius.

20. Tennis elbow is one example of _____, an inflammation of the bursa.

EXERCISE 24

Read the following discharge note. Write the definition for each italicized medical term.

DISCHARGE NOTE
DISCHARGE DIAGNOSES: 1, (1) *Herniated nucleus pulposis*; 2. Status post anterior (2) *cervical diskectomy*
PROCEDURE(S) PERFORMED: Anterior cervical diskectomy
BRIEF HISTORY: This 27-year-old male fell twelve feet from a ladder. He complained of pain radiating to the (3) *occipital* region of the skull. Cervical x-rays were suspicious for a compression (4) *fracture* at the level of (5) *C-5*. A (6) *myelogram* and CT scan of the cervical spine confirmed a herniated nucleus pulposus at the (7) *C5-6* level.
DISPOSITION: The patient was discharged home on the third post-operative day. He will wear a cervical collar at all times and will be seen at the (8) *orthopedic* clinic in two weeks.

1. _____

2. _____

3. _____

4. _____

5. _____

6. _____

7. _____

8. _____

EXERCISE 25

Select the best answer to each statement.

1. The area where two or more bones meet is called a(n)
   a. joint capsule
   b. hinge joint
   c. articulation
   d. fibrous joint

2. Select the alternative term for a closed fracture.
   a. Colles' fracture
   b. incomplete fracture
   c. complete fracture
   d. greenstick fracture

3. Which type of fracture is characterized by splintered pieces of bone?
   a. greenstick fracture
   b. comminuted fracture
   c. impacted fracture
   d. pathological fracture

4. Select the term that best describes a fracture caused by an underlying disease.
   a. comminuted fracture
   b. greenstick fracture
   c. impacted fracture
   d. pathological fracture

5. Which term means the same as a compound fracture?
   a. impacted fracture
   b. greenstick fracture
   c. open fracture
   d. pathological fracture

6. An accumulation of synovial fluid in the knee joint is known as a(n)
   a. Baker's cyst
   b. bursal cyst
   c. synovial cyst
   d. articular cyst

7. _____ is the incomplete dislocation of a bone from its joint.
   a. Crepitation
   b. Claudication
   c. Articulation
   d. Subluxation

8. _____ is the temporary displacement of a bone from its joint.
   a. Articulation
   b. Dislocation
   c. Claudication
   d. Subluxation

9. Select the medical term for softening of the bone.
   a. osteoporosis
   b. osteofibroma
   c. osteomegaly
   d. osteomalacia

10. Choose the medical term for therapeutic breaking of joint adhesions.
    a. arthrectomy
    b. arthroplasty
    c. arthroclasis
    d. arthrocentesis

11. Which abbreviation represents a treatment for an open fracture?
    a. DEXA
    b. ORIF
    c. THR
    d. CRIF

12. Choose the diagnostic procedure that includes a radioisotope.
    a. bone scan
    b. DEXA
    c. dual-photon absorptiometry
    d. bone marrow aspiration

13. Select the phrase that is represented with the abbreviation THR.
    a. tibia and hip repair
    b. total hip radiography
    c. tarsal hinge replacement
    d. total hip replacement

14. Which type of fracture is also called an incomplete fracture?
    a. comminuted fracture
    b. open fracture
    c. greenstick fracture
    d. impacted fracture

15. Select the type of fracture characterized by a bone wedged into another bone.
    a. open fracture
    b. impacted fracture
    c. greenstick fracture
    d. comminuted fracture

16. Select the medical term that means incision into a joint.
    a. arthrectomy
    b. arthrotomy
    c. arthroplasty
    d. arthrocentesis

17. Which medical term best describes an x-ray picture of a joint?
    a. arthroscopy
    b. arthrography
    c. arthrogram
    d. arthroplasty

18. The medical term for joint immobility is
    a. arthrodesis
    b. arthroplasty
    c. arthrocentesis
    d. ankylosis

19. A physician specialist for the skeletal system is called a(n)
    a. orthopedist
    b. orthoarthropedist
    c. chiropractor
    d. osteologist

20. Which treatment is usually associated with a simple fracture?
    a. closed reduction
    b. THR
    c. DEXA
    d. open reduction

CHALLENGE EXERCISE

Search the Internet using the keyword "osteoporosis." Using the information you find, create a one-page handout that summarizes the cause, prevention, and treatment aspects of this common condition. Share the handout with your instructor and/or other students in your class.

Pronunciation Review

Review the terms from this chapter. Pronounce each term using the following phonetic pronunciations. Check off each term when you are comfortable saying it.

TERM	PRONUNCIATION
☐ ankylosing spondylitis	**ang**-kih-**LOH**-sing **spon**-dih-**LIGH**-tis
☐ ankylosis	ang-kih-**LOH**-sis
☐ arthralgia	ar-**THRAL**-jee-ah
☐ arthritis	ar-**THRIGH**-tis
☐ arthrocentesis	**ar**-throh-sen-**TEE**-sis
☐ arthrochondritis	**ar**-throh-kon-**DRIGH**-tis
☐ arthroclasis	**ar**-throh-**CLAY**-sis
☐ arthrodesis	**ar**-throh-**DEE**-sis
☐ arthrogram	**AR**-throh-gram
☐ arthrography	ar-**THROG**-rah-fee
☐ arthroplasty	**AR**-throh-**PLASS**-tee
☐ arthroscopy	ar-**THROSS**-koh-pee
☐ arthrotomy	ar-**THROT**-toh-mee
☐ articulation	ar-**tik**-yoo-**LAY**-shun
☐ Baker's cyst	Baker's cyst

☐ bone marrow aspiration   bone marrow **ass**-per-**AY**-shun
☐ bunion   **BUN**-yun
☐ bunionectomy   bun-yun-**ECK**-toh-mee
☐ bursectomy   ber-**SEK**-toh-mee
☐ bursitis   ber-**SIGH**-tis
☐ bursotomy   ber-**SOT**-oh-mee
☐ chiropractor   **KIGH**-roh-prak-tor
☐ chondromalacia   kon-droh-mah-**LAY**-she-ah
☐ Colles' fracture   **KALL**-eez fracture
☐ comminuted fracture   **KOM**-ih-noo-ted
☐ condyle   **KON**-dill
☐ cranial   **KRAY**-nee-al
☐ craniotomy   kray-nee-**OT**-oh-mee
☐ crepitation   crep-ih-**TAY**-shun
☐ diskectomy   disk-**EK**-toh-mee
☐ dislocation   **diss**-loh-**KAY**-shun
☐ dual-energy x-ray absorptiometry   dual-energy x-ray ab-**sorp**-she-**AH**-meh-tree

☐ femoral   **FEM**-or-al
☐ fissure   **FIH**-sher
☐ foramen   foh-**RAY**-men
☐ fossa   **FOSS**-ah
☐ gout   GOWT
☐ herniated disk   **HER**-nee-ay-ted disk
☐ humeral   **HYOO**-mor-al
☐ intercostal   **in**-ter-**KOSS**-tal
☐ intervertebral   **in**-ter-**VER**-teh-bral
☐ ischiopubic   **ih**-shee-oh-**PYOO**-bik
☐ kyphosis   kigh-**FOH**-sis
☐ laminectomy   lam-in-**EK**-toh-mee
☐ lordosis   lor-**DOH**-sis
☐ lumbar   **LUM**-bar
☐ lumbosacral   **lum**-boh-**SAY**-kral
☐ myeloma   **my**-eh-**LOH**-mah
☐ orthopedics   **or**-thoh-**PEE**-diks
☐ orthopedist   **or**-thoh-**PEE**-dist
☐ osteitis   **oss**-tee-**EYE**-tis
☐ osteoblast   **OSS**-tee-oh-blast
☐ osteochondritis   **oss**-tee-oh-kon-**DRIGH**-tis
☐ osteoclasis   **oss**-tee-oh-**KLAY**-sis
☐ osteocyte   **OSS**-tee-oh-sight
☐ osteofibroma   **oss**-tee-oh-fih-**BROH**-mah
☐ osteomalacia   **oss**-tee-oh-mah-**LAY**-she-ah
☐ osteomyelitis   **oss**-tee-oh-my-eh-**LIGH**-tis
☐ osteoplasty   **OSS**-tee-oh-plass-tee
☐ osteoporosis   **oss**-tee-oh-poh-**ROH**-sis
☐ osteosarcoma   **oss**-tee-oh-sar-**KOH**-mah
☐ osteotomy   **oss**-tee-**OT**-oh-mee
☐ rheumatoid arthritis   **ROO**-may-toyd ar-**THRIGH**-tis
☐ scoliosis   skoh-lee-**OH**-sis
☐ spondylitis   spon-dih-**LIGH**-tiss

Muscular System Medical Terminology

Muscular system medical terms are organized into three main categories: (1) general medical terms; (2) diseases and conditions; and (3) diagnostic procedure, surgery, and laboratory test terms. The prefixes and suffixes associated with this system are listed in Table 5-3. Review these word parts and complete the related exercises.

TABLE 5-3 COMBINING FORMS, PREFIXES, AND SUFFIXES FOR MUSCULAR SYSTEM TERMS

Prefix	Meaning	Suffix	Meaning
brady-	slow	-algia	pain
dys-	abnormal; difficult	-asthenia	without feeling or sensation
intra-	within	-dynia	pain
poly-	many	-kinesia	movement
		-lysis	destruction, breakdown
		-oma	tumor
		-tonia	muscle tone
		-trophy	growth; development

EXERCISE 7

Write the prefixes, suffixes, and their meanings. Based on the meanings, write a definition for each term.

1. bradykinesia

   PREFIX: _____ MEANING: _____

   SUFFIX: _____ MEANING: _____

   DEFINITION: _____

2. dystrophy

   PREFIX: _____ MEANING: _____

   SUFFIX: _____ MEANING: _____

   DEFINITION: _____

3. dystonia

   PREFIX: _____ MEANING: _____

   SUFFIX: _____ MEANING: _____

   DEFINITION: _____

4. hyperkinesia

   PREFIX: _____ MEANING: _____

   SUFFIX: _____ MEANING: _____

   DEFINITION: _____

5. intramuscular

   PREFIX: _____ MEANING: _____

   SUFFIX: _____ MEANING: _____

   DEFINITION: _____

6. myasthenia

   PREFIX: _____   MEANING: _____

   SUFFIX: _____   MEANING: _____

   DEFINITION: _____

7. myoma

   PREFIX: _____   MEANING: _____

   SUFFIX: _____   MEANING: _____

   DEFINITION: _____

8. polymyositis

   PREFIX: _____   MEANING: _____

   SUFFIX: _____   MEANING: _____

   DEFINITION: _____

9. polymyalgia

   PREFIX: _____   MEANING: _____

   SUFFIX: _____   MEANING: _____

   DEFINITION: _____

Muscular System General Medical Terms

Review the pronunciation and meaning of each term in Table 5-4. Note that most of the terms describe body movement. When one muscle, or set of muscles, flexes, the opposing muscle or set extends and movement occurs. Many of the movement terms can be paired. For example, abduction is movement away from the midline and body, and adduction is movement toward the midline and body. Review the terms in Table 5-4 and complete the exercises.

TABLE 5-4   MUSCULAR SYSTEM GENERAL MEDICAL TERMS

Pronunciation	Meaning
abduction (ab-**DUCK**-shun)	movement away from the midline of the body
adduction (ad-**DUCK**-shun)	movement toward the midline of the body
circumduction (**sir**-kum-**DUCK**-shun)	movement in a circular motion
dorsiflexion (**dor**-see-**FLEX**-shun)	moving the foot upward toward the leg (Figure 5-7)

TABLE 5-4   MUSCULAR SYSTEM GENERAL MEDICAL TERMS (continued)

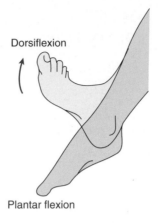

Figure 5-7   Dorsiflexiion

Pronunciation	Meaning
extension (ecks-**TEN**-shun)	straightening motion; movement to increase the angle between bones
flexion (**FLEK**-shun)	bending motion; movement to decrease the angle between bones
intramuscular (**in**-trah-**MUSS**-kyoo-lar) intra- = within muscul/o = muscle -ar = pertaining to	pertaining to within the muscle or muscle tissue
plantar flexion (**PLAN**-tar **FLEK**-shun)	moving the foot in a downward position away from the leg; pointing the toes downward (Figure 5-8)

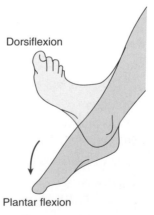

Figure 5-8   Plantar flexion

pronation (proh-**NAY**-shun)	moving the palm face down or toward the back; palms down
rotation (roh-**TAY**-shun)	moving or turning on an axis or pivot point, usually in a left-to-right motion
supination (**soo**-pih-**NAY**-shun)	moving the palms face up or toward the front; palms up

EXERCISE 8

Write the term that describes the "paired" or opposite movement of the listed term.

1. adduction _____

2. dorsiflexion _____

3. extension _____

4. pronation _____

EXERCISE 9

Replace the italicized word or phrase with the correct muscular term.

1. Jorge received a *within the muscle tissue* injection of a potent antibiotic.

   _____

2. *Pointing the toes downward* shortens the Achilles tendon.

   _____

3. *Palms up* allow(s) us to take change from the cashier.

   _____

4. Because of a reaction to her prescription, Neesha was unable to accomplish *moving her head from left to right.*

   _____

5. *Movement in a circular motion* is often used as a warm-up exercise before a tennis match.

   _____

6. *Moving the foot upward toward the leg* stretches the Achilles tendon.

   _____

Muscular System Disease and Disorder Terms

Muscular system diseases include common aches and pains due to overexertion and obscure diagnoses such as Werdnig-Hoffman disease, also known as floppy infant syndrome. Review the pronunciation and definition for each term in Table 5-5 and complete the exercises.

TABLE 5-5 MUSCULAR SYSTEM DISEASE AND DISORDER TERMS

Term with Pronunciation	Definition
atrophy (**AT**-troh-fee) a- = without -trophy = growth; development	wasting or decrease in size of an organ or tissue

2. myoplasty

root	combining vowel	suffix

3. myorrhaphy

root	combining vowel	suffix

4. tenomyoplasty

root	combining vowel	suffix

5. tenorrhaphy

root	combining vowel	suffix

6. tenosynovectomy

root	combining vowel	suffix

7. electromyogram

root	combining vowel	suffix

8. fasciotomy

root	combining vowel	suffix

9. ganglionectomy

root	combining vowel	suffix

Abbreviations

Review the muscular system abbreviations in Table 5-8. Practice writing the meaning of each abbreviation.

TABLE 5-8   ABBREVIATIONS

Abbreviation	Meaning
DTR	deep tendon reflexes
EMG	electromyography
FM	fibromyalgia
IM	intramuscular
MD	muscular dystrophy

CHAPTER REVIEW

The Chapter Review can be used as a self-test. Go through each exercise and answer as many questions as you can without referring to previous exercises or earlier discussions within this chapter. Check your answers and fill in any blanks. Practice writing any terms you might have misspelled.

EXERCISE 17

Analyze each term. Separate the root, combining vowel, and suffix with vertical slashes. Write a definition for each term.

1. bradykinesia

   _____
   root   *combining vowel*   *suffix*
   DEFINITION: _____

2. dyskinesia

   _____
   root   *combining vowel*   *suffix*
   DEFINITION: _____

3. dystonia

   _____
   root   *combining vowel*   *suffix*
   DEFINITION: _____

4. electromyogram

   _____
   root   *combining vowel*   *suffix*
   DEFINITION: _____

5. electromyography

   _____
   root   *combining vowel*   *suffix*
   DEFINITION: _____

6. hyperkinesia

   _____
   root   *combining vowel*   *suffix*
   DEFINITION: _____

7. leiomyofibroma

   _____
   root   *combining vowel*   *suffix*
   DEFINITION: _____

8. myasthenia

   _____
   root   *combining vowel*   *suffix*
   DEFINITION: _____

9. polymyositis

   _____
   root   *combining vowel*   *suffix*
   DEFINITION: _____

10. rhabdomyosarcoma

_____
root   *combining vowel*   *suffix*

DEFINITION: _____

11. tenodynia

_____
root   *combining vowel*   *suffix*

DEFINITION: _____

12. tenosynovitis

_____
root   *combining vowel*   *suffix*

DEFINITION: _____

13. rhabdomyolysis

_____
root   *combining vowel*   *suffix*

DEFINITION: _____

14. fibromyalgia

_____
root   *combining vowel*   *suffix*

DEFINITION: _____

15. dermatomyositis

_____
root   *combining vowel*   *suffix*

DEFINITION: _____

EXERCISE 18

Write the medical term for each definition.

1. extremely slow movement   _____

2. abnormal development   _____

3. tumor of connective tissue   _____

4. surgical repair of muscle tissue   _____

5. tendon pain   _____

6. increased muscle movement and physical activity   _____

7. genetic disorder characterized by progressive atrophy of skeletal muscles   _____

8. hereditary or acquired condition characterized by destruction of skeletal muscle fibers   _____

9. hereditary condition characterized by degeneration of lower leg muscles   _____

10. genetic disorder characterized by progressive weakness and degeneration of muscles   _____

11. process of recording muscle contractions _____

12. muscle weakness and abnormal fatigue _____

13. malignant tumor of skeletal muscle _____

14. benign tumor of smooth muscle _____

15. destruction of muscle tissue and puritic
    inflammation of the skin _____

EXERCISE 19

Read the following progress note and spell out each boldface abbreviation.

> **PATIENT NAME:** GERVAIS, SARA M. **DOB:** 08/05/1978
> Ms. Gervais is a 28-year-old female who presents today with flaccid
> (1) **DTR**s. She states that she stepped on a rusty nail yesterday and received
> an (2) **IM** tetanus injection. After a complete history and physical exami-
> nation, an (3) **EMG** was scheduled. Differential diagnoses at this time
> include (4) **MD** and (5) **FM**. Treatment and prognosis will be decided by
> test results.
> SIGNED: Marilyn Shaski, MD

1. _____

2. _____

3. _____

4. _____

5. _____

EXERCISE 20

Select the best answer for each statement or question.

1. Select the term that means muscle pain.
   a. dyskinesia
   b. myositis
   c. myasthenia
   d. myalgia

2. Choose the term for tissue that connects muscle to bones.
   a. fascia
   b. ligament
   c. tendon
   d. suture

3. Which tissue connects bone to bone?
   a. tendon
   b. fascia
   c. ligament
   d. suture

4. Which tissue holds muscle fibers together?
   a. tendon
   b. ligament
   c. suture
   d. fascia

5. Select the term for suturing a muscle.
   a. myoplasty
   b. myopexy
   c. myorrhaphy
   d. myorrhexis

6. Choose the medical term for recording the electrical activity of muscles.
   a. electromyogram
   b. electromyograph
   c. electrocardiography
   d. electromyography

7. Select the genetic/hereditary disease known as floppy infant syndrome.
   a. muscular dystrophy
   b. Werdnig-Hoffman disease
   c. Charcot-Marie-Tooth disease
   d. rhabdomyolitis

8. Which disease is categorized as a chronic pain illness with widespread muscle aches?
   a. Charcot-Marie-Tooth disease
   b. myasthenia gravis
   c. myodynia
   d. fibromyalgia

9. A malignant tumor of skeletal muscle is called
   a. rhabdomyolitis
   b. leiomyofibroma
   c. rhabdosarcoma
   d. myoma

10. Select the medical term for repetitive stress syndrome.
    a. carpal tunnel syndrome
    b. contracture
    c. hypertrophy
    d. dystonia

11. Which medical term has the opposite meaning of abduction?
    a. circumduction
    b. adduction
    c. pronation
    d. suppination

12. The muscle movement that opposes extension is called
    a. dorsiflexion
    b. plantar flexion
    c. rotation
    d. flexion

13. Moving the foot and toes upward toward the leg is called
    a. dorsiflexion
    b. plantar flexion
    c. rotation
    d. flexion

14. Left-to-right movement on an axis or pivot point is called
    a. circumduction
    b. rotation
    c. supination
    d. pronation

15. Moving the palms forward or upward is called
    a. rotation
    b. pronation
    c. supination
    d. flexion

Pronunciation Review

Review the terms in the chapter. Pronounce each term using the following phonetic pronunciations. Check off each term when you are comfortable saying it.

TERM	PRONUNCIATION
☐ abduction	ab-**DUCK**-shun
☐ adduction	ad-**DUCK**-shun
☐ atrophy	**AT**-troh-fee
☐ bradykinesia	**brad**-ee-kih-**NEE**-see-ah
☐ circumduction	**sir**-kum-**DUCK**-shun
☐ contraction	con-**TRACK**-shun
☐ contracture	con-**TRACK**-cher
☐ disuse atrophy	**DISS**-yoos **AT**-troh-fee
☐ dorsiflexion	**dor**-see-**FLEX**-shun
☐ dyskinesia	**diss**-kih-**NEE**-see-ah
☐ dystonia	dis-**TOH**-nee-ah
☐ dystrophy	**DIS**-troh-fee
☐ electromyogram	ee-**lek**-troh-**MY**-oh-gram
☐ electromyography	ee-**lek**-troh-my-**OG**-rah-fee
☐ extension	ecks-**TEN**-shun
☐ fascia	**FASH**-ee-ah
☐ fasciotomy	fash-ee-**OTT**-oh-mee
☐ fibroma	fih-**BROH**-mah
☐ fibromyalgia	**figh**-broh-my-**AL**-jee-ah
☐ flexion	**FLEK**-shun
☐ ganglion	**GANG**-lee-on

☐ ganglionectomy	**gang**-lee-oh-**NEK**-toh-mee
☐ hyperkinesia	**high**-per-kih-**NEE**-see-ah
☐ hypertrophy	high-**PER**-troh-fee
☐ intramuscular	**in**-trah-**MUSS**-kyoo-lar
☐ leiomyofibroma	**ligh**-oh-**my**-oh-fih-**BROH**-mah
☐ ligament	**LIG**-ah-ment
☐ muscular dystrophy	**MUSS**-kyoo-lar **DIS**-troh-fee
☐ myalgia	my-**AL**-jee-ah
☐ myasthenia	**my**-ass-**THEE**-nee-ah
☐ myasthenia gravis	**my**-ass-**THEE**-nee-ah **GRAV**-is
☐ myoplasty	**MY**-oh-plass-tee
☐ myorrhaphy	my-**OR**-ah-fee
☐ myositis	**my**-oh-**SIGH**-tis
☐ plantar flexion	**PLAN**-tar **FLEK**-shun
☐ polymyositis	**pall**-ee-**my**-oh-**SIGH**-tis
☐ pronation	proh-**NAY**-shun
☐ rhabdomyosarcoma	**rab**-doh-**my**-oh-sar-**KOH**-mah
☐ rotation	roh-**TAY**-shun
☐ striated muscle	**STRIGH**-ay-ted muscle
☐ supination	**soo**-pin-**AY**-shun
☐ tendinitis, tenditis	**ten**-din-**EYE**-tis, ten-**DIGH**-tis
☐ tendon	**TEN**-don
☐ tenodynia	ten-oh-**DIN**-ee-ah
☐ tenomyoplasty	**ten**-oh-**MY**-oh-plass-tee
☐ tenorrhaphy	ten-**OR**-ah-fee
☐ tenosynovectomy	**ten**-oh-**sin**-oh-**VEK**-toh-mee
☐ tenosynovitis	**ten**-oh-**sin**-oh-**VIGH**-tis
☐ torticollis	tor-tih-**KALL**-lis

Chapter 6
Cardiovascular System

OBJECTIVES

At the completion of this chapter, the student should be able to:

1. Identify, define, and spell word roots associated with the cardiovascular system.
2. Label the basic structures of the cardiovascular system.
3. Discuss the functions of the cardiovascular system.
4. Provide the correct spelling of cardiovascular terms, given the definition of the terms.
5. Analyze cardiovascular terms by defining the roots, prefixes, and suffixes of these terms.
6. Identify, define, and spell disease, disorder, and procedure terms related to the cardiovascular system.

OVERVIEW

The cardiovascular system is made up of the heart and blood vessels. The blood vessels include arteries, arterioles, veins, venules, and capillaries. The structures of the cardiovascular system function together for the following purposes: (1) to pump blood to the tissue and cells of the body; (2) to distribute oxygen and nutrients to the tissue and cells; and (3) to remove carbon dioxide and other waste products from the tissues and cells.

Cardiovascular System Word Roots

To understand and use the cardiovascular system medical terms, it is necessary to acquire a thorough knowledge of the associated word roots. Word roots associated with the cardiovascular system are listed with the combining vowel in Table 6-1. Review the word roots and complete the exercises that follow.

TABLE 6-1   CARDIOVASCULAR SYSTEM ROOT WORDS

Word Root/Combining Form	Meaning
aneurysm/o	aneurysm
angi/o	vessel
arter/o; arteri/o	artery
arteriol/o	arteriole
ather/o	fatty, yellowish plaque
cardi/o	heart

(continues)

TABLE 6-1 CARDIOVASCULAR SYSTEM ROOT WORDS (continued)

Word Root/Combining Form	Meaning
coron/o	heart; heart vessel; coronary artery
ech/o	sound
electr/o	electrical
my/o	muscle
phleb/o	vein
ven/o	vein
ventricul/o	ventricle of the heart

EXERCISE 1

Write the definitions of the following word roots.

1. cardi/o   _____

2. my/o   _____

3. angi/o   _____

4. arter/o   _____

5. coron/o   _____

6. ventricul/o   _____

7. arteriol/o   _____

8. ech/o   _____

9. ather/o   _____

10. phleb/o   _____

EXERCISE 2

Write and define the word root in each medical term.

1. cardiologist

    ROOT: _____   MEANING: _____

2. myocardium

    ROOT: _____   MEANING: _____

3. angiography

    ROOT: _____   MEANING: _____

4. endocarditis

    ROOT: _____   MEANING: _____

5. electrocardiography

    ROOT: _____   MEANING: _____

6. coronary

    ROOT: _____   MEANING: _____

7. arteriole

ROOT: _____   MEANING: _____

8. cardiomegaly

ROOT: _____   MEANING: _____

9. tachycardia

ROOT: _____   MEANING: _____

10. phlebitis

ROOT: _____   MEANING: _____

EXERCISE 3

Write the correct word root(s) for the following definitions.

1. electrical   _____

2. artery   _____

3. fatty, yellowish plaque   _____

4. muscle   _____

5. heart   _____

6. sound   _____

7. vessel   _____

8. aneurysm   _____

9. vein   _____

Structures of the Cardiovascular System

The major structures of the cardiovascular system are the heart and blood vessels, which include arteries, capillaries, and veins. The unique characteristics of cardiovascular system structures are presented individually.

Heart

The heart is about the size of a fist and is located in the **mediastinum** (**mee**-dee-ah-**STIGH**-num), the space between the lungs. Figure 6-1 illustrates the atria, ventricles, and septum. Figure 6-2 illustrates the chambers of the heart and the coronary arteries. Refer to these figures as you read about the structures of the heart.

The heart is divided into four chambers. The right and left upper chambers are the (1) **atria** (**atrium**, singular), and the right and left lower chambers are the (2) **ventricles**. A wall called the (3) **septum** separates the chambers. (4) **Coronary arteries** bring oxygen and nutrients to the heart tissue, and (5) **coronary veins** take waste-filled blood away from heart tissue.

The heart wall has three layers of tissue as shown in Figure 6-3. Refer to this figure as you read about the layers of the heart wall.

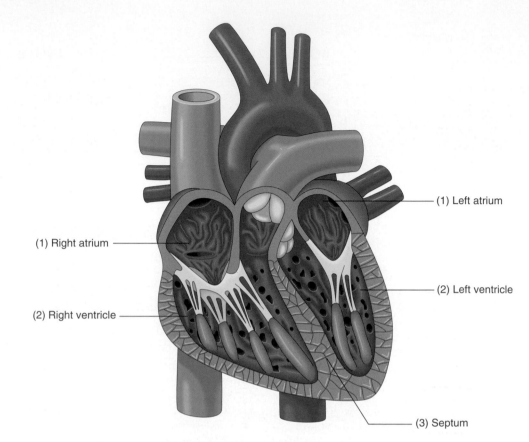

(1) Right atrium

(1) Left atrium

(2) Right ventricle

(2) Left ventricle

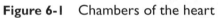

(3) Septum

Figure 6-1 Chambers of the heart

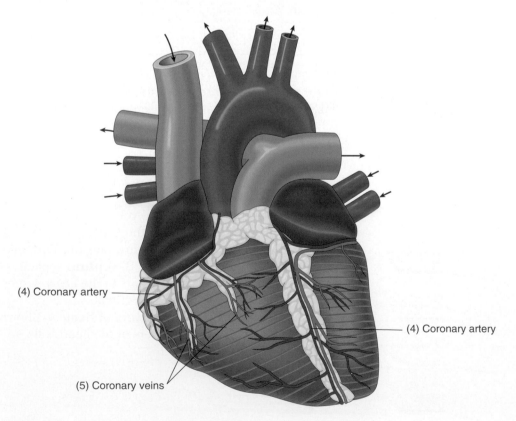

(4) Coronary artery

(4) Coronary artery

(5) Coronary veins

Figure 6-2 Coronary arteries and veins

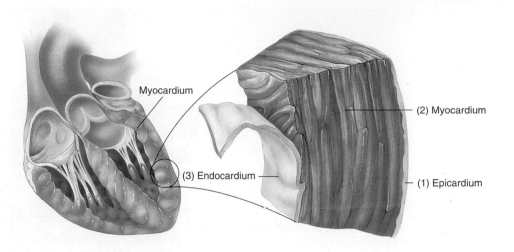

Figure 6-3 Layers of the heart wall

The (1) **epicardium** (ep-ih-**KAR**-dee-um) is the outer layer of the heart wall. The (2) **myocardium** (my-oh-**KAR**-dee-um) is the thick, muscular, middle layer of the heart wall. The (3) **endocardium** (en-doh-**KAR**-dee-um) is the inner layer of the heart wall. A membrane sac, the **pericardium** (pair-ih-**KAR**-dee-um), surrounds and encloses the heart. The pericardium is double-folded membrane that covers the heart and lines the mediastinum. The space between the two folds is called the **pericardial cavity**, and this space is filled with **pericardial fluid**.

Electrical System of the Heart

The pumping action of the heart is controlled by a complex electrical system. The heart's electrical system consists of specialized cardiac muscle tissue that generates the electric impulses, which cause the heart to contract and relax. Figure 6-4 illustrates the key structures of the heart's electrical system. Refer to this figure as you read about the heart's electrical system.

The (1) **sinoatrial** (**sigh**-noh-**AY** tree-al) **node (SA node)** is located in the right atrium. The sinoatrial node is often called the pacemaker because it starts the electrical impulse. The (2) **atrioventricular** (ay-tree-oh-ven-**TRIK**-yoo-lar) **node (AV node)** is located between the right atrium and right ventricle. The AV node carries the impulse to the (3) **atrioventricular bundle**. The atrioventricular bundle, also called the **bundle of His**, is located in the septum between the atria and ventricles.

The atrioventricular bundle divides into the right and left (4) **bundle branches**, which are located in the septum between the ventricles. The bundle branches carry the electrical impulse to the right and left ventricles. The bundle branches cause the ventricles to contract, which pushes blood out of the heart to all parts of the body.

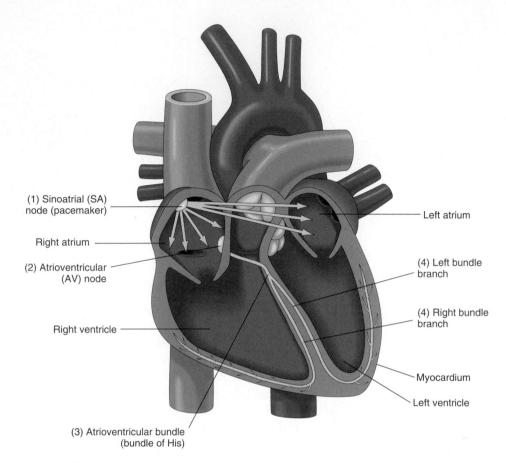

(1) Sinoatrial (SA) node (pacemaker)

Right atrium

(2) Atrioventricular (AV) node

Right ventricle

(3) Atrioventricular bundle (bundle of His)

Left atrium

(4) Left bundle branch

(4) Right bundle branch

Myocardium

Left ventricle

Figure 6-4 Electrical system of the heart

Blood Vessels

Blood vessels carry blood to and from the heart as the blood circulates through the body. The blood vessels include arteries, arterioles, capillaries, and veins. Figure 6-5 illustrates the relationship between arteries, capillaries, and veins. Refer to this figure as you read about the blood vessels.

(1) **Arteries** are large, thick-walled vessels that carry the blood away from the heart. (2) **Veins** have thinner walls and carry blood to the heart. Arteries branch into smaller vessels called (3) **arterioles**. Arterioles branch into minute vessels called (4) **capillaries**. Capillaries deliver oxygen and nutrients to the cells and allow carbon dioxide and waste products from cells to enter (5) **venules**. Venules are the smallest veins.

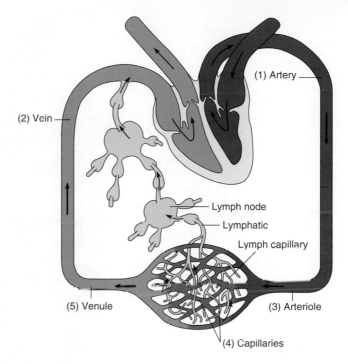

Figure 6-5 Blood vessels

Circulation

Circulation is the movement of blood to and from the heart. Oxygen-rich blood must be delivered to all parts of the body. Waste-filled blood must be removed from all parts of the body. Refer to Figure 6-6 as you read the description of the circulation process.

- Waste-filled blood is carried to the right atrium by way of the (1) **superior vena cava** and the (2) **inferior vena cava**, the largest veins in the body.
- When the right atrium contracts, the waste-filled blood is pushed through the (3) **tricuspid valve** into the right ventricle.
- The right ventricle contracts and pushes the waste-filled blood through the (4) **pulmonary valve** into the right and left (5) **pulmonary arteries** that lead to the lungs.
- In the lungs, waste products are removed from the blood and the blood picks up oxygen and becomes **oxygenated**.
- The oxygenated blood is sent to the left atrium by way of the right and left (6) **pulmonary veins**.
- When the left atrium contracts, the blood is pushed through the (7) **bicuspid** or **mitral valve** into the left ventricle.
- The left ventricle contracts and sends the blood through the (8) **aortic valve** into the (9) **aorta**, the largest artery in the body.
- The aorta branches into arteries that distribute blood to all parts of the body.

The circulation of blood from the heart to the lungs and back to the heart is called **pulmonary circulation**. The circulation of blood from the heart to the rest of the body and back to the heart is called **systemic circulation**.

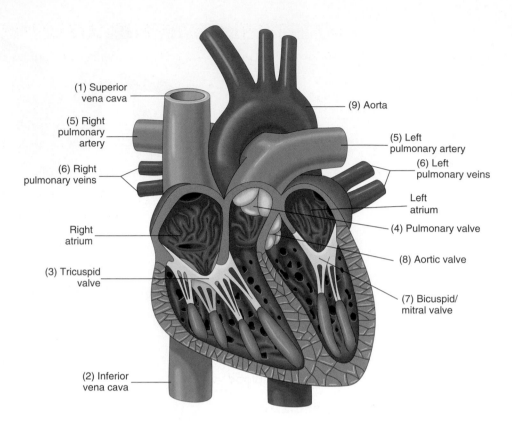

(1) Superior vena cava

(5) Right pulmonary artery

(6) Right pulmonary veins

Right atrium

(3) Tricuspid valve

(2) Inferior vena cava

(9) Aorta

(5) Left pulmonary artery

(6) Left pulmonary veins

Left atrium

(4) Pulmonary valve

(8) Aortic valve

(7) Bicuspid/ mitral valve

Figure 6-6 Circulation through the heart

Blood Pressure

Blood pressure is defined as the pressure that circulating blood exerts on the walls of arteries, the veins, and the chambers of the heart. A routine blood pressure check identifies the pressure exerted on arterial walls. The instrument used to measure this pressure is called a **sphygmomanometer** (**sfig**-moh-man-**AH**-meh-ter), commonly known as a blood pressure cuff. This instrument measures two pressures: (1) **systolic** (sis-**TALL**-ik) pressure; and (2) **diastolic** (**digh**-ah-**STALL**-ik) pressure. Systolic pressure is defined as arterial wall pressure during heart muscle contraction. Diastolic pressure is defined as arterial wall pressure during heart muscle relaxation, or rest period.

Blood pressure measurements are recorded as millimeters (mm) of mercury (Hg). The systolic pressure is given first and the diastolic pressure is given second, as in 120/80mmHg. In this example, the systolic pressure is 120 and the diastolic pressure is 80. Many factors, such as age, gender, weight, physical health, and emotional state might affect your blood pressure. In general, a normal systolic pressure ranges from 90 to less than 140mmHg, and a normal diastolic pressure ranges from 50 to less than 90mmHg.

EXERCISE 4

Match the cardiovascular system structures in Column 1 with the correct definition in Column 2.

COLUMN 1

_____ 1. aorta

_____ 2. arteries

_____ 3. atria

_____ 4. capillaries

_____ 5. endocardium

_____ 6. epicardium

_____ 7. myocardium

_____ 8. pulmonary arteries

_____ 9. pulmonary veins

_____ 10. septum

_____ 11. veins

_____ 12. vena cava

_____ 13. ventricles

COLUMN 2

a. carry blood away from the heart

b. carry blood from the lungs to the left atrium

c. inner layer of the heart

d. largest artery in the body

e. carry blood from the right ventricle to the lungs

f. carry blood to the heart

g. largest vein in the body

h. lower chambers of the heart

i. muscle layer of the heart wall

j. outer layer of the heart wall

k. smallest, minute blood vessels

l. upper chambers of the heart

m. wall between the heart chambers

EXERCISE 5

Circle the term that best fits the definition.

DEFINITION	**CIRCLE ONE TERM**
1. cause ventricular contraction	*bundle branches* OR *sinoatrial node*
2. between the right atrium and right ventricle	*sinoatrial node* OR *atrioventricular node*
3. located in the septum between the atria and ventricles	*atrioventricular bundle* OR *sinoatrial node*
4. pacemaker of the heart	*sinoatrial node* OR *bundle branches*
5. between the left atrium and left ventricle	*aortic valve* OR *bicuspid valve*
6. between the left ventricle and the aorta	*aortic valve* OR *bicuspid valve*
7. between the right atrium and right ventricle	*pulmonary valve* OR *tricuspid valve*
8. between the right ventricle and pulmonary arteries	*pulmonary valve* OR *tricuspid valve*

EXERCISE 6

Label the structures of the heart in Figure 6-7. Write your answers on the spaces provided.

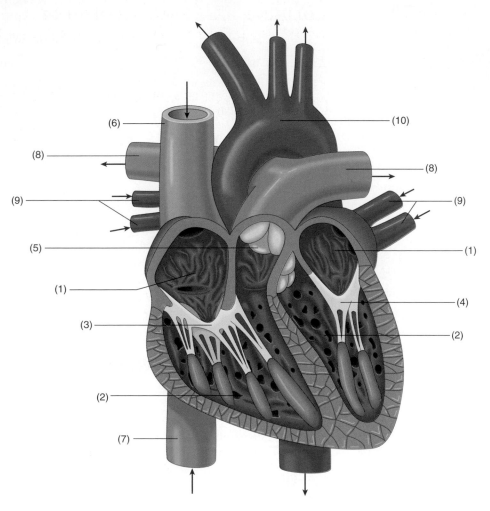

Figure 6-7 Structures of the heart

1. _____

2. _____

3. _____

4. _____

5. _____

6. _____

7. _____

8. _____

9. _____

10. _____

Cardiovascular System Medical Terminology

Cardiovascular medical terms are organized into three main categories: (1) general medical terms; (2) disease and condition terms; and (3) diagnostic procedure, surgery, and laboratory test terms. There are several roots, prefixes, and suffixes commonly used in many cardiovascular terms. The roots, with the combining vowel, prefixes, and suffixes, are listed in Table 6-2. Review these word parts and complete the related exercises.

TABLE 6-2 ROOTS, PREFIXES, AND SUFFIXES FOR CARDIOVASCULAR SYSTEM TERMS

Word Root	Meaning	Prefix	Meaning	Suffix	Meaning
ischi/o	deficiency, blockage	brady-	slow	-graph	instrument to record
sphygm/o	pulse	poly-	many	-graphy	process of recording
steth/o	chest	tachy-	fast	-gram	record, picture
thromb/o	clot			-megaly	enlarged
				-pathy	disease
				-sclerosis	hardening
				-stenosis	narrowing

EXERCISE 7

Write the word root, prefix, suffix, and their meanings on the space provided.

EXAMPLE: thrombosclerosis
ROOT: thromb/o   MEANING: clot
PREFIX: no prefix   MEANING: none
SUFFIX: -sclerosis   MEANING: hardening

1. sphygmomanometer

   ROOT: _____ MEANING: _____

   PREFIX: _____ MEANING: _____

   SUFFIX: _____ MEANING: _____

2. angiopathy

   ROOT: _____ MEANING: _____

   PREFIX: _____ MEANING: _____

   SUFFIX: _____ MEANING: _____

3. thrombosis

   ROOT: _____ MEANING: _____

   PREFIX: _____ MEANING: _____

   SUFFIX: _____ MEANING: _____

4. stethoscope

ROOT: _____ MEANING: _____

PREFIX: _____ MEANING: _____

SUFFIX: _____ MEANING: _____

5. bradycardia

ROOT: _____ MEANING: _____

PREFIX: _____ MEANING: _____

SUFFIX: _____ MEANING: _____

6. tachycardia

ROOT: _____ MEANING: _____

PREFIX: _____ MEANING: _____

SUFFIX: _____ MEANING: _____

7. arteriosclerosis

ROOT: _____ MEANING: _____

PREFIX: _____ MEANING: _____

SUFFIX: _____ MEANING: _____

8. angiostenosis

ROOT: _____ MEANING: _____

PREFIX: _____ MEANING: _____

SUFFIX: _____ MEANING: _____

9. angiography

ROOT: _____ MEANING: _____

PREFIX: _____ MEANING: _____

SUFFIX: _____ MEANING: _____

10. cardiogram

ROOT: _____ MEANING: _____

PREFIX: _____ MEANING: _____

SUFFIX: _____ MEANING: _____

EXERCISE 8

Analyze each term by writing the prefix, root, combining vowel, and suffix separated by vertical slashes. Based on the meaning of the word parts, write a definition for each term.

EXAMPLE: thrombosclerosis

	thromb	*/ o*	*/ sclerosis*
prefix	*root*	*combining vowel*	*suffix*

DEFINITION: hardening of clots

1. angiopathy

prefix	*root*	*combining vowel*	*suffix*

DEFINITION: _____

2. thrombosis

prefix	*root*	*combining vowel*	*suffix*

DEFINITION: _____

3. stethoscope

prefix	*root*	*combining vowel*	*suffix*

DEFINITION: _____

4. bradycardia

prefix	*root*	*combining vowel*	*suffix*

DEFINITION: _____

5. tachycardia

prefix	*root*	*combining vowel*	*suffix*

DEFINITION: _____

6. arteriosclerosis

prefix	*root*	*combining vowel*	*suffix*

DEFINITION: _____

7. angiostenosis

prefix	*root*	*combining vowel*	*suffix*

DEFINITION: _____

8. angiography

prefix	*root*	*combining vowel*	*suffix*

DEFINITION: _____

9. cardiogram

prefix	root	combining vowel	suffix

DEFINITION: _____

Cardiovascular System General Medical Terms

Review the cardiovascular system general medical terms listed in Table 6-3. Complete the exercises for these terms.

TABLE 6-3 CARDIOVASCULAR SYSTEM GENERAL MEDICAL TERMS

Term with Pronunciation	Definition
blood pressure (BP)	the pressure exerted by circulating blood on the walls of the arteries, the veins, and the chambers of the heart
bruits (broo-**EEZ**)	abnormal blowing sounds or murmurs heard while listening to the blood flow through the arteries
cardiologist (**kar**-dee-**ALL**-oh-jist) cardi/o = heart -(o)logist = specialist	physician who specializes in diseases, disorders, and treatments related to the cardiovascular system
cardiology (**kar**-dee-**ALL**-oh-jee) cardi/o = heart -(o)logy = study of	study of the functions, structures, and disorders of the heart
diastole (digh-**ASS**-toh-lee)	period of time when the ventricles relax between contractions
occlusion (oh-**KLOO**-shun)	a blockage in a vessel, cavity, or passage of the body
sphygmomanometer (**sfig**-moh-man-**AH**-meh-ter) sphygm/o = pulse -meter = instrument to measure	instrument used to measure blood pressure
stethoscope (**STETH**-oh-skohp)	instrument used to listen to the sounds of the heart, chest, and lungs
systole (**SISS**-toh-lee)	period of time during ventricular contraction

EXERCISE 9

Write the medical term for each definition.

1. abnormal blowing sounds _____

2. blockage in a vessel or cavity _____

3. instrument used to listen to chest/heart sounds _____

4. instrument used to measure blood pressure _____

5. period of time during ventricular contraction   _____

6. period of time of ventricular relaxation   _____

7. physician heart specialist   _____

8. pressure blood exerts on arterial walls   _____

9. study of the heart   _____

Cardiovascular System Disease and Disorder Terms

Cardiovascular system diseases and disorders include familiar problems such as hypertension and high blood pressure as well as more complex and less familiar diagnoses such as patent ductus arteriosis (i.e., an abnormal opening between the pulmonary artery and aorta). The medical terms are presented in alphabetical order. Review the pronunciation and definition for each term in Table 6-4 and complete the exercises.

TABLE 6-4 CARDIOVASCULAR SYSTEM DISEASE AND DISORDER TERMS

Term with Pronunciation	Definition
aneurysm (**AN**-yoo-rizm)	localized dilatation or ballooning of an artery at a weak point in the vessel wall
angina pectoris (**AN**-jin-ah, *or* an-**JIGH**-nah, **PECK**-tor-is)	severe pain and constriction around the heart; feeling of extreme pressure in the anterior chest
angiocarditis (an-jee-oh-kar-**DIGH**-tis) angi/o = vessels cardi/o = heart -itis = inflammation	Inflammation of the blood vessels of the heart
angiospasm (**AN**-jee-oh-spazm) angi/o = vessel -spasm = involuntary contraction	abnormal contraction of the blood vessels, primarily the arteries
aortic stenosis (ay-**OR**-tik sten-**OH**-sis)	abnormal narrowing of the aorta
arrhythmia (ah-**RITH**-mee-ah)	any irregular heartbeat
arteriosclerosis (ar-**tee**-ree-oh-skleh-**ROH**-sis) arteri/o = artery -sclerosis = hardening	hardening of the arteries
arteriosclerotic heart disease (ASHD) (ar-**tee**-ree-oh-skleh-**RAH**-tic) arteri/o = artery -sclerosis = hardening -ic = pertaining to	heart disease caused by hardening of the arteries

(*continues*)

TABLE 6-4   CARDIOVASCULAR SYSTEM DISEASE AND DISORDER TERMS
(continued)

Term with Pronunciation	Definition
atherosclerosis (**ath**-eh-roh-skleh-**ROH**-sis) ather/o = fat -sclerosis = hardening	hardening and narrowing of the arteries due to deposits of fat and other debris along arterial walls (Figure 6-8)

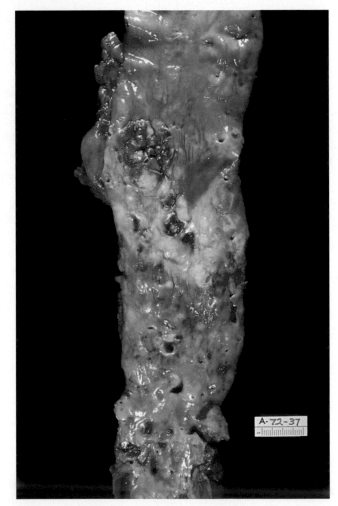

Figure 6-8   Atherosclerosis in the aorta (Centers for Disease Control/Dr. Edwin P. Ewing, Jr.)

atrioventricular defect (**ay**-tree-oh-ven-**TRIK**-yoo-lar)	an abnormal opening between the atria and ventricles
bradycardia (**brad**-ih-**KAR**-dee-ah) brady = slow cardi/o = heart -ia = condition	slow heart rate

(continues)

TABLE 6-4   CARDIOVASCULAR SYSTEM DISEASE AND DISORDER TERMS
(continued)

Term with Pronunciation	Definition
bundle branch block (BBB)	interruption of the electrical impulse of the heart to the right or left bundle branch
cardiac arrest	a sudden and immediate cessation of the heart's pumping action
cardiac tamponade (**KAR**-dee-ak tam-poh-**NAYD**)	compression of the heart due to the accumulation of blood in the pericardial sac
cardiomegaly (**kar**-dee-oh-**MEG**-ah-lee) cardi/o = heart -megaly = enlargement	enlargement of the heart; enlarged heart
cardiomyopathy (**kar**-dee-oh-my-**OP**-ah-thee) cardi/o = heart my/o = muscle -pathy = disease	any disease that affects the structure and function of the heart, and the heart muscle in particular

EXERCISE 10

Analyze each term. Write and define the root, prefix, and suffix, and their meanings. Using the word part definitions, write a definition for the term. Use a medical dictionary to check your definition.

EXAMPLE: cardiologist
ROOT: cardi/o   MEANING: heart
PREFIX: none   MEANING: none
SUFFIX: -logist   MEANING: specialist in the study of
DEFINITION: specialist in the study of the heart

1. angiocarditis

ROOT: _____ MEANING: _____

PREFIX: _____ MEANING: _____

SUFFIX: _____ MEANING: _____

DEFINITION: _____

2. arteriosclerosis

ROOT: _____ MEANING: _____

PREFIX: _____ MEANING: _____

SUFFIX: _____ MEANING: _____

DEFINITION: _____

4. Li was taking a common steroid medication for *inflammation of several medium and small arteries.*

   _____

5. *Inflammation of the pericardium* treatment includes complete bedrest and a light diet.

   _____

6. *Enlarged and twisted veins* might be painful to the touch.

   _____

7. Anticoagulants are often used to treat *inflammation of a vein with a blood clot.*

   _____

8. An *abnormally rapid heartbeat* might involve the atria or ventricles.

   _____

EXERCISE 18

Write out the following abbreviations.

1. PAT   _____

2. PAC   _____

3. PVC   _____

4. RHD   _____

Cardiovascular System Diagnostic, Surgical, and Treatment Terms

Review the pronunciation and definition of the diagnostic, surgical, and treatment terms in Table 6-7. Complete the exercises.

TABLE 6-7 CARDIOVASCULAR SYSTEM DIAGNOSTIC, SURGICAL, AND TREATMENT TERMS

Term with Pronunciation	Definition
anastomosis (ah-**nas**-toh-**MOH**-sis) ana- = without stom/o = mouth, opening -osis = condition	surgical connection of two vessels or other tubular structures
aneurysmectomy (**an**-yoo-rizm-**EK**-toh-mee)	surgical removal of an aneurysm
angiography (an-jee-**OG**-rah-fee) angi/o = vessel -graphy = process of recording	process of recording an x-ray picture of blood vessels

TABLE 6-7 CARDIOVASCULAR SYSTEM DIAGNOSTIC, SURGICAL, AND TREATMENT TERMS (continued)

Term with Pronunciation	Definition
arteriogram (ar-**TEER**-ee-oh-gram) arteri/o = artery -gram = record; picture	x-ray record or picture of an artery
arteriography (ar-**teer**-ee-**OG**-rah-fee) arteri/o = artery -graphy = process of recording	process of recording an x-ray picture of arteries
cardiac catheterization (**KAR**-dee-ak **kath**-eh-ter-ih-**ZAY**-shun)	an x-ray procedure during which a catheter is guided into the heart through a blood vessel for the purpose of injecting a contrast medium to view and image the heart chambers and coronary arteries; also called left heart catheterization or coronary arteriography
cardiopulmonary resuscitation (CPR) (**kar**-dee-oh-**PULL**-mon-air-ee ree-**suss**-ih-**TAY**-shun)	procedure for life support consisting of artificial respiration and manual external cardiac compression
coronary artery bypass graft (CABG) (**KOR**-oh-nair-ee **AR**-ter-ee)	surgical procedure that requires implanting a piece of vein onto the heart to bypass a blockage in a coronary artery and to improve blood flow to the heart; commonly called bypass surgery (Figure 6-9)

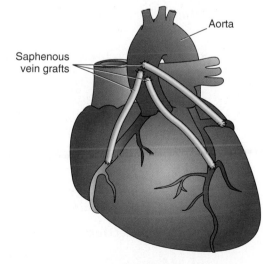

Aorta

Saphenous vein grafts

Figure 6-9 Coronary artery bypass graft (CABG)

(continues)

TABLE 6-7 CARDIOVASCULAR SYSTEM DIAGNOSTIC, SURGICAL, AND TREATMENT TERMS (continued)

Term with Pronunciation	Definition
cardioversion (**kar**-dee-oh-**VER**-zhun)	restoration of a normal heart rhythm by delivering synchronized electric shocks through paddles placed on the chest
defibrillation (dee-**fib**-rih-**LAY**-shun)	technique used to interrupt ventricular fibrillation and restore a normal heart rhythm by delivering electric shocks to specific areas around the heart
echocardiogram (**ek**-oh-**KAR**-dee-oh-gram) echo- = sound cardi/o = heart -gram = record	graphic record of an ultrasound visualization of the heart
echocardiography (**ek**-oh-**kar**-dee-**OG**-rah-fee) echo- = sound cardi/o = heart -graphy = process of recording	ultrasound diagnostic procedure for the purpose of evaluating and recording the structures and motion of the heart
electrocardiogram (EKG, ECG) (ee-**lek**-troh-**KAR**-dee-oh-gram) electr/o = electricity cardi/o = heart -gram = record	graphic record of the electrical activity of the heart (Figure 6-10)

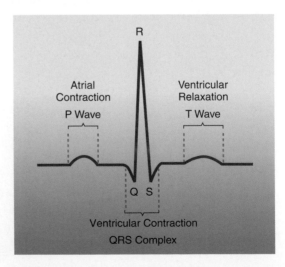

Figure 6-10 Electrocardiogram showing the contraction and relaxation of the heart

(continues)

TABLE 6-7 CARDIOVASCULAR SYSTEM DIAGNOSTIC, SURGICAL, AND TREATMENT TERMS (continued)

Term with Pronunciation	Definition
electrocardiography (ee-**lek**-troh-**kar**-dee-**OG**-rah-fee) electr/o = electricity cardi/o = heart -graphy = process of recording	process of recording the electrical activity of the heart
endarterectomy (**end**-ar-ter-**EK**-toh-mee) end/o = within arter/i = artery -ectomy = surgical removal	surgical removal of the lining of an artery that is occluded due to fatty deposits
Holter monitoring	process of recording and monitoring heart rate and rhythms over a specific period, usually 24 hours
percutaneous transluminal coronary angioplasty (PTCA) (per-kyoo-**TAY**-nee-us trans-**LOO**-min-al **KOR**-oh-nair-ee **AN**-jee-oh-**plass**-tee)	surgical repair of a coronary artery by inserting a balloon on the end of a catheter into the artery, inflating the balloon, flattening the fatty deposits on the arterial wall, and stretching or increasing the diameter of the artery (Figure 6-11)
thallium stress test (**THAL**-ee-um)	assessment of cardiovascular health and function during and after the application of stress
transesophageal echocardiography (TEE) (**trans**-eh-soff-ah-**JEE**-al **ek**-oh-**kar**-dee-**OG**-rah-fee) trans- = through esophag/o = esophagus -al = pertaining to	process of viewing and recording the structures of the heart using ultrasound and placing the recording device into the esophagus
valvoplasty (**VAL**-voh-**plass**-tee)	surgical repair of a heart valve

(continues)

TABLE 6-7 CARDIOVASCULAR SYSTEM DIAGNOSTIC, SURGICAL, AND TREATMENT TERMS (continued)

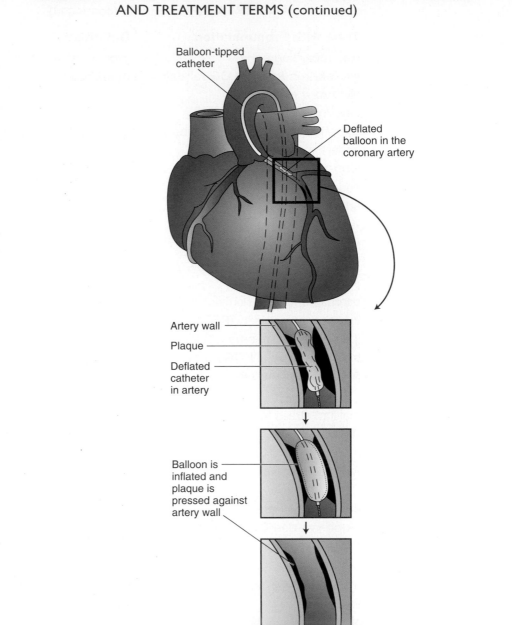

Figure 6-11 Percutaneous transluminal coronary angioplasty (PTCA)

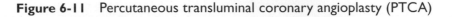

EXERCISE 19

Change the suffix -graphy *to* -gram. *Rewrite the medical term. Based on the meaning of the new root, write a definition for the new term. Check the definition in a medical dictionary.*

EXAMPLE: cardiography   cardiogram   x-ray film of the heart

1. angiography   NEW TERM: _____

    DEFINITION: _____

2. echocardiography NEW TERM: _____

DEFINITION: _____

3. electrocardiography NEW TERM: _____

DEFINITION: _____

4. arteriography NEW TERM: _____

DEFINITION: _____

EXERCISE 20

Analyze each term by writing the prefix, root, combining vowel, and suffix separated by vertical slashes. Based on the meaning of the word parts, write a definition for each term. Check your definition in a medical dictionary.

1. angiography

prefix	*root*	*combining vowel*	*suffix*

DEFINITION: _____

2. arteriogram

prefix	*root*	*combining vowel*	*suffix*

DEFINITION: _____

3. echocardiography

prefix	*root*	*combining vowel*	*suffix*

DEFINITION: _____

4. echocardiogram

prefix	*root*	*combining vowel*	*suffix*

DEFINITION: _____

5. electrocardiogram

prefix	*root*	*combining vowel*	*suffix*

DEFINITION: _____

6. electrocardiography

prefix	*root*	*combining vowel*	*suffix*

DEFINITION: _____

7. endarterectomy

prefix	*root*	*combining vowel*	*suffix*

DEFINITION: _____

8. valvoplasty

_____
prefix   _root_   _combining vowel_   _suffix_

DEFINITION: _____

EXERCISE 21

Write out the following abbreviations.

1. CPR   _____

2. CABG   _____

3. EKG, ECG   _____

4. PTCA   _____

5. TEE   _____

Abbreviations

Review the cardiovascular system abbreviations in Table 6-8. Practice writing out the meaning of each abbreviation.

TABLE 6-8   ABBREVIATIONS

Abbreviation	Meaning
ASHD	arteriosclerotic heart disease
BBB	bundle branch block
BP	blood pressure
CABG	coronary artery bypass graft
CAD	coronary artery disease
CHF	congestive heart failure
CPR	cardiopulmonary resuscitation
DVT	deep vein thrombosis
HHD	hypertensive heart disease
PAC	premature atrial contraction
PAT	paroxysmal atrial tachycardia
PTCA	percutaneous transluminal coronary angioplasty
PVC	premature ventricular contraction
RHD	rheumatic heart disease
TEE	transesophageal echocardiography

CHAPTER REVIEW

The Chapter Review can be used as a self-test. Go through each exercise and answer as many questions as you can without referring to previous exercises or earlier discussions within this chapter. Check your answers and fill in any blanks. Practice writing any terms you might have misspelled.

EXERCISE 22

Analyze each term. Write and define the root, prefix, and suffix. Using the word part definitions, write a definition for the term. Use a medical dictionary to check your definition.

1. cardiology

   ROOT: _____ MEANING: _____

   PREFIX: _____ MEANING: _____

   SUFFIX: _____ MEANING: _____

   DEFINITION: _____

2. cardiologist

   ROOT: _____ MEANING: _____

   PREFIX: _____ MEANING: _____

   SUFFIX: _____ MEANING: _____

   DEFINITION: _____

3. angiocarditis

   ROOT: _____ MEANING: _____

   PREFIX: _____ MEANING: _____

   SUFFIX: _____ MEANING: _____

   DEFINITION: _____

4. bradycardia

   ROOT: _____ MEANING: _____

   PREFIX: _____ MEANING: _____

   SUFFIX: _____ MEANING: _____

   DEFINITION: _____

5. cardiomegaly

   ROOT: _____ MEANING: _____

   PREFIX: _____ MEANING: _____

   SUFFIX: _____ MEANING: _____

   DEFINITION: _____

6. cardiomyopathy

   ROOT: _____ MEANING: _____

   PREFIX: _____ MEANING: _____

   SUFFIX: _____ MEANING: _____

   DEFINITION: _____

7. endocarditis

ROOT: _____ MEANING: _____

PREFIX: _____ MEANING: _____

SUFFIX: _____ MEANING: _____

DEFINITION: _____

8. polyarteritis

ROOT: _____ MEANING: _____

PREFIX: _____ MEANING: _____

SUFFIX: _____ MEANING: _____

DEFINITION: _____

9. tachycardia

ROOT: _____ MEANING: _____

PREFIX: _____ MEANING: _____

SUFFIX: _____ MEANING: _____

DEFINITION: _____

10. thrombophlebitis

ROOT: _____ MEANING: _____

PREFIX: _____ MEANING: _____

SUFFIX: _____ MEANING: _____

DEFINITION: _____

EXERCISE 23

Replace the italicized phrase with the correct medical term.

1. During Jackie's physical examination, the physician heard *an abnormal blowing sound.*

   _____

2. Bill was diagnosed with *hardening of the arteries.*

   _____

3. *A sudden and immediate stoppage of heart function* often results in death.

   _____

4. *Rapid and incomplete contractions of the heart* can be corrected with proper medication.

   _____

5. Bette's *abnormally low blood pressure* was due to loss of blood volume.

   _____

6. Jefferson's vascular problem was corrected by *the surgical removal of an aneurysm.*

_____

7. Brad's echocardiogram revealed *an abnormal narrowing of the aorta.*

_____

8. *Any irregular heartbeat* should be brought to the physician's attention.

_____

9. *High blood pressure* can be a symptom of atherosclerosis.

_____

10. A *heart attack* can occur at any age.

_____

EXERCISE 24

Match the medical terms in Column 1 with the definitions in Column 2.

COLUMN 1

_____ 1. anastomosis
_____ 2. angina pectoris
_____ 3. angiospasm
_____ 4. arteriogram
_____ 5. blood pressure
_____ 6. cardiac tamponade
_____ 7. diastole
_____ 8. endarterectomy
_____ 9. ischemia
_____ 10. palpitation
_____ 11. sphygmomanometer
_____ 12. systole
_____ 13. valvoplasty
_____ 14. varicose veins

COLUMN 2

a. pressure exerted on arterial and venous walls

b. period of time when ventricles are relaxed

c. period of time when ventricles contract

d. instrument used to measure blood pressure

e. deficient blood supply to a body part

f. abnormal contraction of blood vessels

g. compression of the heart resulting from blood in the pericardial sac

h. severe chest pain

i. abnormal, rapid throbbing or fluttering of the heart

j. enlarged, twisted, and dilated veins

k. surgical connection of two vessels

l. x-ray record or picture of an artery

m. surgical removal of the lining of an artery

n. surgical repair of a heart valve

EXERCISE 25

Read the following discharge summary. Write the meaning of the italicized terms and phrases on the spaces provided.

DISCHARGE SUMMARY

BRIEF HISTORY: This 61-year-old woman was brought into the emergency room unconscious. (1) *Cardiopulmonary resuscitation* was begun immediately. During the ambulance transport, the portable (2) *electrocardiogram* demonstrated (3) *ventricular fibrillation*. The advanced (4) *cardiac* life support procedure was followed.

HOSPITAL COURSE: The patient was placed on the Coronary Care Unit. Family members confirmed a previous history of (5) *myocardial infarction* and a subsequent (6) *coronary artery bypass graft*. There was also a history of (7) *hypertension*. The patient's condition deteriorated, and she was in a coma during her entire hospitalization. The family was in close attendance and realized the severity of the situation. Consultation with the (8) *cardiologist* confirmed that there was extensive (9) *myocardial* tissue death due to (10) *ischemia*.

LABORATORY DATA: The chest x-ray showed (11) *cardiomegaly* and right upper lobe infiltrate. All laboratory tests were abnormal during the hospitalization. (12) *Arterial* blood gases indicated that mechanical ventilation was marginal at best.

DISPOSITION: The patient expired on November 12 with the family present.

1. _____
2. _____
3. _____
4. _____
5. _____
6. _____
7. _____
8. _____
9. _____
10. _____
11. _____
12. _____

EXERCISE 26

Circle the correct answer for each statement.

1. Which heart valve is also known as the bicuspid valve?
   a. aortic valve
   b. mitral valve
   c. pulmonary valve
   d. tricuspid valve

2. Which heart chamber pumps blood to the lungs?
   a. right atrium
   b. left atrium
   c. right ventricle
   d. left ventricle

3. Which heart chamber pumps blood to the aorta?
   a. right atrium
   b. left atrium
   c. right ventricle
   d. left ventricle

4. Select the term for hardening of the arteries.
   a. arteriosclerosis
   b. atherosclerosis
   c. angioconstriction
   d. angioplasty

5. Select the term that represents the largest artery in the body.
   a. pulmonary artery
   b. coronary artery
   c. vena cava
   d. aorta

6. Which heart valve is located between the right atrium and right ventricle?
   a. mitral valve
   b. tricuspid valve
   c. bicuspid valve
   d. pulmonary valve

7. Select the term for the smallest blood vessel.
   a. venule
   b. arteriole
   c. capillary
   d. vein

8. Select the term for the largest vein in the body.
   a. vena cava
   b. pulmonary vein
   c. aorta
   d. coronary vein

9. Select the phrase that means circulation of blood from the heart to the lungs.
   a. systemic circulation
   b. cardiac circulation
   c. oxygenation circulation
   d. pulmonary circulation

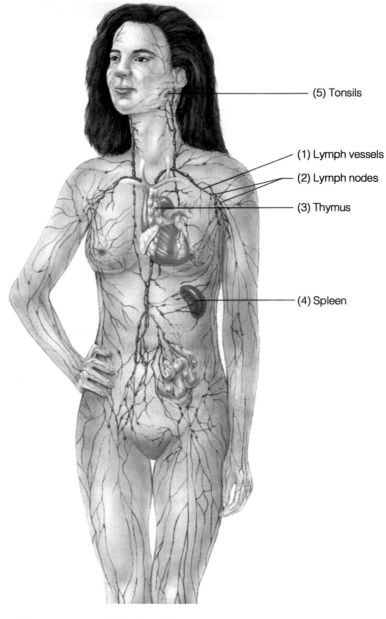

(5) Tonsils

(1) Lymph vessels

(2) Lymph nodes

(3) Thymus

(4) Spleen

Figure 7-5 Components of the lymph system

Lymph Vessels

The smallest lymph vessels are called lymphatic capillaries. Lymph capillaries collect the fluid that filters out of the blood capillaries and into the interstitial (in-ter-**STIH**-shill) spaces. Interstitial spaces are located between the cells of body tissue. Figure 7-6 illustrates the relationship between lymph capillaries and blood capillaries. Once the fluid enters the lymph capillaries, it is called lymph fluid.

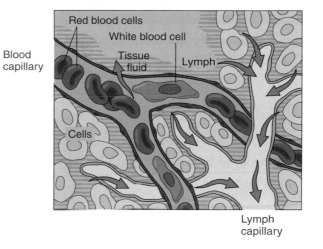

Figure 7-6   Blood and lymph capillaries

The lymph capillaries transport the lymph fluid to the larger lymphatic vessels. The lymphatic vessels allow water and dissolved substances to be returned to the blood. Lymph vessels continue to merge and eventually lead to the two **lymphatic ducts**: the right lymphatic duct and the thoracic duct.

Lymph Nodes

Lymph nodes are collections of lymphatic tissue located at intervals along the course of the lymph vessels. Lymph nodes function as filters for old, dead cells and bacteria that are present in the lymph fluid. **Macrophages** (**MACK**-roh-fay-jezs), phagocytes located in the lymph nodes, engulf and destroy the bacteria. Lymph nodes also produce antibodies and lymphocytes.

Thymus

The **thymus** is a lymph and endocrine gland. It is located in the mediastinum near the middle of the chest. The thymus secretes a hormone called **thymosin** (thigh-**MOH**-sin), which stimulates the production of **T lymphocytes**, also called **T cells**. T cells are an important part of our immune system because they circulate throughout the body and attack foreign and/or abnormal cells.

Spleen

The **spleen** is the largest lymph organ in the body. It is situated in the upper-left quadrant of the abdomen just below the diaphragm and behind the stomach. The spleen filters blood in much the same way the lymph nodes filter lymph fluid. Macrophages in the spleen remove **pathogens** (**PATH**-oh-jens), which are disease-causing substances, from the blood.

Tonsils

The **tonsils**, masses of lymphatic tissue, are located in the mouth at the back of the throat and are divided into three groups. The **pharyngeal tonsils** (**fair**-in-**JEE**-al **TON**-sills), also called the **adenoids** (**ADD**-eh-noydz), are near the opening of the nasal cavity into the pharynx. The **palatine** (**PAL**-ah-tine) **tonsils** are located on each side of the throat at the back of the oral cavity. The **lingual** (**LING**-gwal) **tonsils** are near the base of the tongue. The tonsils are the first lines of defense against bacteria and other harmful substances that might enter the body through the nose and mouth.

☐	pharyngeal tonsils	**fair**-in-**JEE**-al **TON**-sills
☐	plasma	**PLAZ**-mah
☐	platelet	**PLAYT**-let
☐	platelet count	**PLAYT**-let count
☐	polycythemia	**pol**-ee-sigh-**THEE**-mee-ah
☐	polycythemia vera	**pol**-ee-sigh-**THEE**-mee-ah **VAIR**-ah
☐	prothrombin	proh-**THROM**-bin
☐	prothrombin time	proh-**THROM**-bin time
☐	purpura	**PURR**-pyoo-rah
☐	rouleaux	roo-**LOH**
☐	septicemia	**sep**-tih-**SEE**-mee-ah
☐	sickle cell anemia	**SIK**-ul sell ah-**NEE**-mee-ah
☐	spherocytosis	**sfee**-roh-sigh-**TOH**-sis
☐	splenomegaly	splee-neh-**MEG**-ah-lee
☐	thalassemia	thal-ah-**SEE**-mee-ah
☐	thrombocyte	**THROM**-boh-sight
☐	thrombocytopenia	**throm**-boh-**sigh**-toh-**PEE**-nee-ah
☐	thrombosis	throm-**BOH**-sis
☐	thrombus	**THROM**-bus
☐	thymosin	thigh-**MOH**-sin
☐	thymus	**THIGH**-mus
☐	tonsillitis	**ton**-sih-**LIGH**-tis
☐	tonsils	**TON**-sills
☐	white blood cell differential	white blood cell diff-er-**EN**-shal

Chapter 8
Respiratory System

OBJECTIVES

At the completion of this chapter, the student should be able to:

1. Identify, define, and spell word roots associated with the respiratory system.
2. Label the basic structures of the respiratory system.
3. Discuss the functions of the respiratory system.
4. Provide the correct spelling of respiratory terms, given the definition of the terms.
5. Analyze respiratory terms by defining the roots, prefixes, and suffixes of these terms.
6. Identify, define, and spell disease, disorder, and procedure terms related to the respiratory system.

OVERVIEW

The respiratory system is made up of the nose, pharynx, larynx, trachea, bronchi, and lungs. The structures of the respiratory system function together for the following purposes: to provide oxygen to all body cells, to remove the waste product carbon dioxide from all body cells, to assist the body's defense mechanisms against foreign material, and to produce sound necessary for speech. The respiratory system moves oxygen and carbon dioxide by external respiration and internal respiration.

External respiration is the exchange of air between the lungs and the external environment. When a person inhales, the oxygen in the air is drawn into the lungs and distributed, by way of the blood, to all body cells. During exhalation, carbon dioxide is released into the environment.

Internal respiration is the exchange of oxygen and carbon dioxide between the cells and the blood. The blood delivers oxygen to every cell and picks up carbon dioxide. The carbon dioxide is then returned to the lungs and, as previously noted, expelled from the body when you exhale.

Respiratory System Word Roots

To understand and use respiratory system medical terms, it is necessary to acquire a thorough knowledge of the associated word roots. Word roots associated with the respiratory system are listed with the combining vowel. Review the word roots in Table 8-1 and complete the exercises that follow.

TABLE 8-1 RESPIRATORY SYSTEM ROOT WORDS

Word Root/Combining Form	Meaning
alveol/o	alveolus
bronch/o; bronch/i	bronchus
bronchiol/o	bronchus
epiglott/o	epiglottis
laryng/o	larynx
nas/o	nose
orth/o	straight
pector/o	chest
pharyng/o	pharynx
phren/o	diaphragm
pleur/o	pleura
pneum/o	lung; air
pulmon/o	lungs
rhin/o	nose
sinus/o	sinus
spir/o	breathe; breath
tonsill/o	tonsils
thorac/o	chest
trache/o	trachea

EXERCISE 1

Write the definitions of the following word roots.

1. alveol/o _____

2. bronch/o _____

3. bronchiol/o _____

4. epiglott/o _____

5. laryng/o _____

6. nas/o _____

7. orth/o _____

8. pector/o _____

9. pharyng/o _____

10. phren/o _____

11. pleur/o _____

12. pneum/o _____

13. pneumon/o _____

14. pulmon/o _____

15. rhin/o _____

16. sinus/o _____

17. thorac/o   _____

18. trache/o   _____

EXERCISE 2

Write the word root and its meaning on the space provided.

1. alveolar

   ROOT: _____   MEANING: _____

2. sinusitis

   ROOT: _____   MEANING: _____

3. pleurisy

   ROOT: _____   MEANING: _____

4. rhinitis

   ROOT: _____   MEANING: _____

5. pneumothorax

   ROOT: _____   MEANING: _____

6. nasopharynx

   ROOT: _____   MEANING: _____

7. bronchopneumonia

   ROOT: _____   MEANING: _____

8. laryngitis

   ROOT: _____   MEANING: _____

9. thoracocentesis

   ROOT: _____   MEANING: _____

10. epiglottis

    ROOT: _____   MEANING: _____

11. tonsillitis

    ROOT: _____   MEANING: _____

12. phrenic

    ROOT: _____   MEANING: _____

EXERCISE 3

Write the correct word root(s) for the following definitions.

1. lungs   _____

2. nose   _____

3. diaphragm   _____

4. chest   _____

5. straight   _____

6. pleura   _____

7. alveolus   _____

8. trachea   _____

9. breathe; breath   _____

10. tonsils   _____

Structures of the Respiratory System

The structures of the respiratory system include the (1) **nose**, (2) **nasal cavity**, (3) **paranasal sinuses**, (4) **pharynx** (**FAIR**-inks), (5) **larynx** (**LAIR**-inks), (6) **trachea** (**TRAY**-kee-ah), (7) **lungs**, (8) **bronchi** (**BRONG**-kigh), (9) **alveoli** (al-**VEE**-oh-ligh), and (10) **diaphragm** (**DIGH**-ah-fram). Figure 8-1 illustrates these structures. Refer to this figure as you read about each structure.

Nose

The (1) nose and mouth direct air into the body. The entrances to the nose are the **nares** (**NAIRZ**), also called *nostrils*. Air enters the nose through the right and left chambers of the (2) nasal cavity. A cartilage wall called the **septum** divides the chambers. Air also passes through the (3) paranasal sinuses, which are cavities in the skull that open into the nasal cavity. The nose and sinuses are lined with mucous membranes and hair-like projections called **cilia**. The mucous membranes warm the air on its way into the lungs. The cilia sweep dirt and foreign particles toward the throat away from the lungs.

Pharynx and Larynx

The (4) pharynx, or throat, connects the nose and mouth to the (5) larynx, or voice box. The pharynx has three sections: the (11) **nasopharynx** (**nay**-zoh-**FAIR**-inks), the upper section; the (12) **oropharynx** (**or**-oh-**FAIR**-inks), the middle section; and the (13) **laryngopharynx** (lah-**ring**-oh-**FAIR**-inks), the lower portion. These sections are illustrated in Figure 8-1. The pharynx serves as the passageway for both air and food. As food passes through the pharynx, it must be prevented from entering the lungs. A small flap of cartilage, called the (14) **epiglottis** (ep-ih-**GLOT**-iss), closes over the trachea and prevents food from entering the larynx. The adenoids and tonsils are located in the pharynx.

The larynx, also called the voice box, contains vocal cords that make vocal sounds. As air passes through the spaces between the vocal cords, sound is produced. The spaces between the vocal cords are called the **glottis** (**GLOT**-iss). The larynx is made up of cartilage. The most prominent cartilage, usually seen on men, is actually the thyroid cartilage, often called the "Adam's apple." The larynx is connected to the trachea.

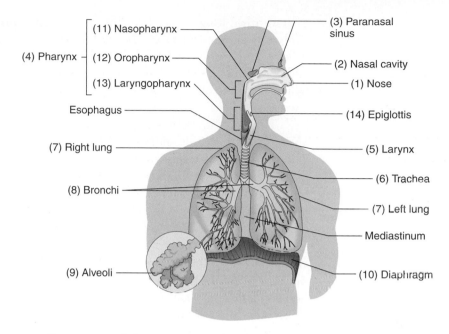

Figure 8-1   Structures of the respiratory system

Trachea, Bronchi, and Lungs

The trachea, bronchi, lungs, and related structures are illustrated in Figure 8-2. Refer to this figure as you read about these structures.

The (1) **trachea** is commonly called the windpipe. It is the passageway for air and consists of muscular tissue that is kept open by a series of C-shaped cartilage rings. Before entering the lungs, the trachea branches into two tubes, called (2) **bronchi** (**BRONG**-kigh). One **bronchus** (**BRONG**-kus) enters the right lung, and the other enters the left lung. Bronchi, as well as nerves and blood vessels, enter the lungs at a specific location called the **hilum** (**HIGH**-lum).

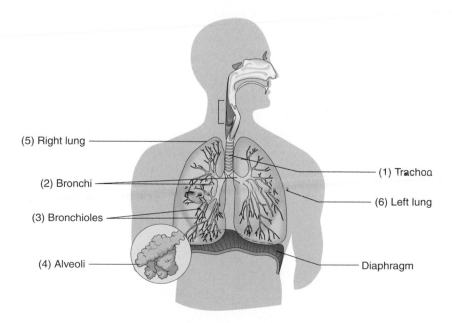

Figure 8-2   Trachea, bronchi, and lungs

In the lungs, the bronchi divide into progressively smaller tubes called (3) **bronchioles** (**BRONG**-kee-ohlz). The bronchioles end in clusters of air sacs called (4) **alveoli** (al-**VEE**-oh-ligh). The alveoli are surrounded by capillaries. Oxygen and carbon dioxide pass between the alveoli and capillaries. The oxygen is delivered, by the blood, to all parts of the body. The carbon dioxide is removed from the body as a waste product.

The lungs are cone-shaped, spongy organs that house the bronchi, bronchioles, alveoli, blood vessels, nerves, and elastic tissue. The lungs are divided into lobes: The (5) **right lung** has three lobes, and the (6) **left lung** has two lobes. The upper part of the lung is called the apex, and the lower part of the lung is called the base. A membrane, the **pleura** (**PLOO**-rah), surrounds the lungs. The pleura consists of two layers. The small space between the layers is the pleural space, which is filled with a fluid that prevents friction between the lungs and ribs during respiration.

The diaphragm is a muscular partition that separates the thoracic and abdominal cavities. During inhalation, the diaphragm drops to enlarge the thoracic cavity and draw air into the lungs. During exhalation, the diaphragm returns to its normal position and helps push air out of the lungs. Drawing air into the lungs is called **inhalation** or **inspiration**. Pushing air out of the lungs is called **exhalation** or **expiration**.

EXERCISE 4

Match the respiratory system structures in Column 1 with the correct definition in Column 2.

COLUMN 1

_____ 1. alveoli

_____ 2. bronchi

_____ 3. bronchioles

_____ 4. capillaries

_____ 5. diaphragm

_____ 6. hilum

_____ 7. larynx

_____ 8. lungs

_____ 9. nares

_____ 10. pharynx

_____ 11. pleura

_____ 12. trachea

COLUMN 2

a. muscular partition between the thoracic and abdominal cavities

b. entrances to the nose

c. entrance into the lungs for bronchi, nerves, and blood vessels

d. very small blood vessel in the lungs

e. membranes surrounding the lungs

f. voice box

g. throat

h. tubes leading to the lungs

i. airway; windpipe

j. air sacs

k. cone-shaped, spongy organs

l. "little" bronchi

EXERCISE 5

Label the structures of the respiratory system identified in Figure 8-3. Write your answer on the spaces provided.

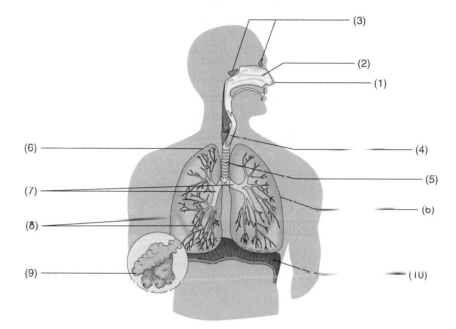

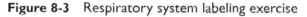

Figure 8-3   Respiratory system labeling exercise

1. _____
2. _____
3. _____
4. _____
5. _____
6. _____
7. _____
8. _____
9. _____
10. _____

Respiratory System Medical Terminology

Respiratory system medical terms are organized into three main categories: (1) general medical terms; (2) disease and condition terms; and (3) diagnostic procedure, surgery, and laboratory test terms. Word roots, prefixes, and suffixes that are often a part of respiratory medical terms are listed in Table 8-2. Review these word parts and complete the related exercises.

9. oximetry

ROOT: _____ MEANING: _____

PREFIX: _____ MEANING: _____

SUFFIX: _____ MEANING: _____

DEFINITION: _____

Respiratory System General Medical Terms

Review the pronunciation and meaning of each term in Table 8-3. Note that some terms are built from word parts and some are not. Complete the exercises for these terms.

TABLE 8-3 RESPIRATORY SYSTEM GENERAL MEDICAL TERMS

Term with Pronunciation	Definition
aspirate (**ASS**-pih-rayt)	to withdraw or suction fluid; to draw foreign material into the lungs
nebulizer (**NEB**-yoo-ligh-zer)	mechanic device for delivering a fine spray or mist into the respiratory tract
oximeter (ock-**SIM**-eh-ter) ox/o = oxygen -meter = instrument to measure	instrument for measuring oxygen saturation in the blood
patent (**PAY**-tent)	open
pulmonologist (**pull**-mon-**ALL**-oh-jist) pulmon/o = lungs -(o)logist = specialist	physician who specializes in respiratory diseases
respiratory therapist (RT)	allied health professional who administers respiratory therapy treatments
spirometer (spigh-**ROM**-eh-ter) spir/o = breathing -meter = instrument to measure	instrument used to measure breathing
ventilator (**VENT**-ih-lay-tor)	mechanical device used to assist with or substitute for patient's breathing

EXERCISE 8

Replace the italicized phrase with the correct respiratory term.

1. The respiratory therapist instructed Beth on the use of the *piece of equipment that creates a fine spray or mist.*

   _____

2. Brian set a goal to become a *physician who specializes in respiratory diseases.*

   _____

3. The *instrument that measures oxygen saturation* was placed on the patient's finger.

_____

4. The hospital board of directors decided it was time to purchase a new *instrument that measures breathing*.

_____

5. As part of Juan's treatment, the physician decided to *withdraw or suction* the fluid from his bronchi.

_____

6. An *open* trachea is necessary for a successful surgical intervention.

_____

7. The *machine to assist breathing* is a piece of medical equipment that sustains life.

_____

Respiratory System Disease and Disorder Terms

Respiratory system diseases and disorders include familiar problems such as influenza as well as more complex and less familiar diagnoses such as *Pneumocystis carinii* pneumonia. The medical terms are presented in alphabetical order in Table 8-4. Review the pronunciation and definition for each term and complete the exercises.

TABLE 8-4   RESPIRATORY SYSTEM DISEASE AND DISORDER TERMS

Term with Pronunciation	Definition
acapnia (ay-**KAP**-nee-ah) a- = without -capnia = carbon dioxide	absence of carbon dioxide in the blood; less than normal blood levels of carbon dioxide
adenoiditis (**ad**-eh-noyd-**EYE**-tis) adenoid/o = adenoids -itis = inflammation	inflammation of the adenoids
adult respiratory distress syndrome (ARDS)	respiratory failure associated with a variety of acute conditions that directly or indirectly injure the lung, for example, primary bacterial or viral pneumonias, aspiration of gastric contents, and trauma
anoxia (an-**OCKS**-ee-ah) an- = absence; lack of ox/i = oxygen -a = noun ending	absence or lack of the normal level of oxygen in the blood
anthracosis (an-thrah-**KOH**-sis) anthrac/o = coal -osis = condition	accumulation of carbon deposits in the lungs; black lung disease; coal worker's pneumoconiosis

(continues)

TABLE 8-4 RESPIRATORY SYSTEM DISEASE AND DISORDER TERMS
(continued)

Term with Pronunciation	Definition
aphonia (ay-**FOH**-nee-ah) a- = absence; lack of -phonia = sound or voice	inability to produce sound or speech
apnea (ap-**NEE**-ah) a- = absence; lack of -pnea = breathing	absence or lack of breathing; temporary cessation of breathing
asbestosis (as-bess-**TOH**-sis)	accumulation of asbestos particles in the lungs
asphyxia (as-**FICKS**-ee-ah)	oxygen deprivation; suffocation
asthma (**AZ**-mah)	spasm or swelling of the mucous membranes of the bronchial tubes resulting in wheezing and difficultly in breathing
atelectasis (at-eh-**LEK**-tah-sis) atel/o = incomplete -ectasis = expansion; dilatation	incomplete expansion, usually of the lung
bronchiectasis (**brong**-kee-**EK**-tah-sis) bronch/o = bronchus; bronchi -ectasis = expansion; dilatation	abnormal dilatation or expansion of the bronchi
bronchitis (brong-**KIGH**-tis bronch/o = bronchus, bronchi -itis = inflammation	inflammation of the bronchi
bronchogenic carcinoma (**brong**-koh-**JEN**-ic kar-sin-OH-mah) bronch/o = bronchus -genic = pertaining to development carcin- = cancer; malignant -oma = tumor	a malignant lung tumor originating in the bronchi; lung cancer
bronchopneumonia (**brong**-koh-noo-**MOH**-nee-ah) bronch/o = bronchus pneumon/o = lungs; air -ia = noun ending	inflammation of the bronchi and lungs caused primarily by bacteria
bronchospasm (**BRONG**-koh-spasm) bronch/o = bronchus -spasm = involuntary contraction	involuntary spasms of the bronchi

EXERCISE 9

Analyze each term by writing the prefix, root, combining vowel, and suffix separated by vertical slashes. Based on the meaning of the word parts, write a definition for each term.

EXAMPLE: angiography

	/ angi	/ o	/ graphy
prefix	*root*	*combining vowel*	*suffix*

DEFINITION: process of recording an x-ray picture of a vessel

1. apnea

prefix	*root*	*combining vowel*	*suffix*

DEFINITION: _____

2. atelectasis

prefix	*root*	*combining vowel*	*suffix*

DEFINITION: _____

3. bronchiectasis

prefix	*root*	*combining vowel*	*suffix*

DEFINITION: _____

4. bronchitis

prefix	*root*	*combining vowel*	*suffix*

DEFINITION: _____

5. bronchospasm

prefix	*root*	*combining vowel*	*suffix*

DEFINITION: _____

6. anoxia

prefix	*root*	*combining vowel*	*suffix*

DEFINITION: _____

7. acapnia

prefix	*root*	*combining vowel*	*suffix*

DEFINITION: _____

8. anthracosis

prefix	*root*	*combining vowel*	*suffix*

DEFINITION: _____

EXERCISE 10

Write a definition for each medical term.

1. After years of working in construction, Ben developed *asbestosis.*

2. The patient was devastated by the diagnosis of *bronchogenic carcinoma.*

3. A common cause of *bronchopneumonia* is streptococcal bacteria.

4. *Aphonia* was a temporary outcome of the patient's larynx surgery.

5. Because he has *asthma,* Joel brings his inhaler to school.

EXERCISE 11

Write the medical term for the italicized phrases.

1. Arthur had recurrent episodes of *inflamed adenoids.*

   _____

2. *Oxygen deprivation* was listed as the immediate cause of death.

   _____

3. According to the respiratory therapist's progress note, the patient exhibited a *lack of oxygen.*

   _____

4. The 80-year-old woman was hospitalized for *respiratory failure.*

   _____

5. *Absence or lack of breathing* while asleep may cause symptoms of sleep deprivation.

   _____

6. Coal miners are especially susceptible to *black lung disease.*

   _____

7. Because of an *abnormal dilatation of the bronchi,* Tanner had trouble breathing.

   _____

8. Ruby's postoperative complications included an *incomplete expansion* of the right lung.

   _____

Review the pronunciation and definition for each term in Table 8-5 and complete the exercises.

TABLE 8-5   RESPIRATORY SYSTEM DISEASE AND DISORDER TERMS

Term with Pronunciation	Definition
chronic obstructive pulmonary disease (COPD)	a progressive and irreversible condition characterized by diminished lung capacity
coryza; rhinitis (koh-**RIGH**-zuh) (righ-**NIGH**-tis) rhin/o = nose -itis = inflammation	inflammation of the mucous membranes of the nose; a common cold
croup (KROOP)	a childhood disease characterized by a barking cough, dyspnea, and laryngeal spasms
cystic fibrosis (CF) (**SIS**-tik figh-**BROH**-sis)	a hereditary disorder characterized by excess mucus production in the respiratory tract
deviated septum (**DEE**-vee-ay-ted)	misalignment of the nasal septum due to malformation or injury
dysphonia (diss-**FOH**-nee-ah) dys- = difficult -phonia = voice; sound	difficulty producing speech or vocal sounds
dyspnea (disp-**NEE**-ah) dys- = difficult -pnea = breathing	difficulty breathing
emphysema (em-fih-**SEE**-mah)	distention and destruction of alveolar walls causing decreased elasticity of the lungs (Figure 8-4)

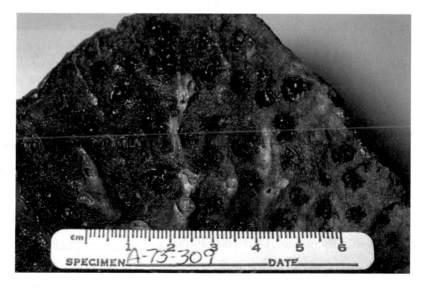

Figure 8-4   Lung tissue with emphysema lesions (Centers for Disease Control/ Edwin P. Ewing, Jr.)

(continues)

3. laryngitis

prefix	root	combining vowel	suffix

DEFINITION: _____

4. laryngospasm

prefix	root	combining vowel	suffix

DEFINITION: _____

5. nasopharyngitis

prefix	root	combining vowel	suffix

DEFINITION: _____

6. mucous

prefix	root	combining vowel	suffix

DEFINITION: _____

7. orthopnea

prefix	root	combining vowel	suffix

DEFINITION: _____

8. pansinusitis

prefix	root	combining vowel	suffix

DEFINITION: _____

9. pleuritis

prefix	root	combining vowel	suffix

DEFINITION: _____

EXERCISE 15

Replace the italicized phrase with the correct medical term.

1. A premature infant might exhibit *a deficiency of oxygen in the blood.*

   _____

2. Cystic fibrosis is often characterized by copious amounts of *a slimy, viscous secretion.*

   _____

3. The symptoms of *whooping cough* are often frightening to the parents.

   _____

4. *The flu* is a highly contagious infection of the respiratory tract.

   _____

5. Albert's sputum sample was *characterized by mucus and pus.*

   _____

6. *Escape of fluid into the pleural space* can be a postoperative complication.

   _____

7. *A temporary absence of breathing during sleep* is more common in men than in women.

   _____

8. Erythromycin is the preferred treatment for *pneumonia caused by the Legionella pneumophila bacteria.*

   _____

   Review the pronunciation and definition for each term in Table 8-7 and complete the exercises.

TABLE 8-7   RESPIRATORY SYSTEM DISEASE AND DISORDER TERMS

Term with Pronunciation	Definition
Pneumocystis carinii pneumonia (**noo**-moh-**SISS**-tis kah-**RIN**-ee-eye noo-**MOH**-nee-ah)	a type of pneumonia caused by a parasite
pneumonia (noo-**MOH**-nee-ah)	an acute inflammation of the lungs
pneumonoconiosis (noo-**mon**-oh-**koh**-nee-**OH**-sis) pneumon/o = lungs con/i = dust -osis = condition	any disease of the lung by chronic inhalation of dust, usually mineral dusts of occupational or environmental origin
pulmonary edema (**PULL**-mon-air-ee eh-**DEE**-mah) pulmon/o = lungs -ary = pertaining to	swelling of the lungs caused by an abnormal accumulation of fluid in the lungs
pulmonary embolism (**PULL**-mon-air-ee **EM**-boh-lizm) pulmon/o = lungs -ary = pertaining to	obstruction of one or more of the pulmonary arteries by a thrombus (clot)
pulmonary heart disease (cor pulmonale) (**PULL**-mon-air-ee) (cor pull-mon-**ALL**-ee)	heart failure caused by pulmonary disease
pyothorax, empyema (pigh-oh-**THOH**-raks, em-pigh-**EE**-mah) py/o = pus -thorax = chest	presence of pus in the chest or pleural space

(continues)

TABLE 8-7 RESPIRATORY SYSTEM DISEASE AND DISORDER TERMS
(continued)

Term with Pronunciaion	Definition
rales (**RALZ**)	abnormal chest sound caused by congested or spasmodic bronchi
respiratory distress syndrome (RDS) of newborns	disorder associated with premature birth and characterized by diffuse atelectasis and immature development of alveolar membranes, also called hyaline membrane disease
rhinorrhea (**righ**-noh-**REE**-ah) rhin/o = nose -(r)rhea = copious discharge; drainage	thin, watery discharge from the nose; runny nose
rhonchi (**RONG**-kigh)	rales or rattling in the throat, resembles snoring
sputum (**SPYOO**-tum)	material coughed up from the lungs
stridor (**STRIGH**-dor)	harsh, high-pitched sound during respiration
tonsillitis (**ton**-sih-**LIGH**-tis) tonsill/o = tonsils -itis = inflammation	inflammation of the palatine tonsils
tracheostenosis (tray-kee-oh-sten-**OH**-sis) trache/o = trachea -stenosis = narrowing	narrowing of the trachea
tuberculosis (TB) (**too**-ber-kyoo-**LOH**-sis)	an infectious disease of the lungs caused by a specific type of bacillus
upper respiratory infection (URI)	infection of the pharynx, larynx, trachea, and bronchi

EXERCISE 16

Write the root, suffix, and their meanings for each term. Using the word part meanings, write a definition for the term. Check the definition in a medical dictionary.

1. pneumonoconiosis

    ROOT: _____ MEANING: _____

    SUFFIX: _____ MEANING: _____

    DEFINITION: _____

2. pulmonary edema

    ROOT: _____ MEANING: _____

    SUFFIX: _____ MEANING: _____

    DEFINITION: _____

3. pyothorax

    ROOT: _____ MEANING: _____

    SUFFIX: _____ MEANING: _____

    DEFINITION: _____

4. rhinorrhea

    ROOT: _____ MEANING: _____

    SUFFIX: _____ MEANING: _____

    DEFINITION: _____

5. tonsillitis

    ROOT: _____ MEANING: _____

    SUFFIX: _____ MEANING: _____

    DEFINITION: _____

6. tracheostenosis

    ROOT: _____ MEANING: _____

    SUFFIX: _____ MEANING: _____

    DEFINITION: _____

EXERCISE 17

Match the medical term in Column 1 with the correct definition in Column 2.

COLUMN 1

_____ 1. pneumonia

_____ 2. pneumonoconiosis

_____ 3. pulmonary heart disease

_____ 4. rales

_____ 5. rhonchi

_____ 6. sputum

_____ 7. stridor

_____ 8. tuberculosis

_____ 9. URI

COLUMN 2

a. abnormal chest sound due to congested bronchi

b. acute inflammation of the lungs

c. harsh, high-pitched sound

d. heart failure caused by lung disease

e. infectious lung disease caused by a type of bacillus

f. infection of the pharynx, larynx, trachea, and bronchi

g. lung disease caused by inhaling dust

h. material coughed up from the lungs

i. rattling in the throat

Respiratory System Diagnostic and Treatment Terms

Review the pronunciation and definition of the surgery and diagnostic procedure terms in Table 8-8. Complete the exercises for each set of terms.

TABLE 8-8 RESPIRATORY SYSTEM DIAGNOSTIC AND TREATMENT TERMS

Term with Pronunciation	Definition
adenoidectomy (**add**-eh-noyd-**EK**-toh-mee) adenoid/o = adenoid gland -ectomy = surgical removal or excision	surgical removal of the adenoid glands
bronchoplasty (**BRONG**-koh-**plass**-tee) bronch/o = bronchi -plasty = surgical repair of	surgical repair of the bronchi
bronchoscope (**BRONG**-koh-skohp) bronch/o = bronchi -scope = instrument for viewing	instrument for viewing the bronchi
bronchoscopy (brong-**KOSS**-koh-pee) bronch/o = bronchi -scopy = process of viewing	visualization of the bronchi with a scope (Figure 8-5)

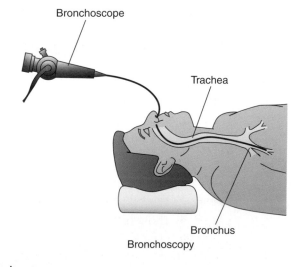

Bronchoscope

Trachea

Bronchus

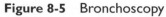
Bronchoscopy

Figure 8-5 Bronchoscopy

chest x-ray	process of recording an x-ray film of the lungs and mediastinum; x-ray film of the lungs and mediastinum

(continues)

TABLE 8-8 RESPIRATORY SYSTEM DIAGNOSTIC AND TREATMENT TERMS (continued)

Term with Pronunciation	Definition
esophagram (eh-**SOFF**-ah-gram) esophag/o = esophagus -gram = record	an x-ray record (picture) of the esophagus obtained by using barium as a contrast medium to visualize and identify abnormalities; also known as a barium swallow
laryngectomy (lair-in-**JEK**-toh-mee) laryng/o = larynx -ectomy = surgical removal or excision	surgical removal of the larynx
laryngocentesis (lah-**ring**-oh-sen-**TEE**-sis) laryng/o = larynx -centesis = surgical puncture to withdraw fluid	surgical puncture into the larynx to withdraw fluid
laryngoplasty (lah-**RING**-oh-**plass**-tee) laryng/o = larynx -plasty = surgical repair	surgical repair of the larynx
laryngoscope (lah-**RING**-oh-skohp) laryng/o = larynx -scope = instrument for viewing	instrument for viewing the larynx
laryngoscopy (lair-in-**GOSS**-koh-pee) laryng/o = larynx -scopy = process of visualization or viewing with a scope	visualization of the larynx with a scope
laryngostomy (lair-in-**GOSS**-toh-mee) laryng/o = larynx -(o)stomy = creation of a new or artificial opening	creation of an artificial opening into the larynx
laryngotracheotomy (lah-**ring**-oh-**tray**-kee-**OT**-oh-mee) laryng/o = larynx trache/o = trachea -(o)tomy = incision into	incision into the larynx and trachea
lobectomy (loh-**BEK**-toh-mee) lob/o = lobe of the lung -ectomy = surgical removal or excision	surgical removal of a lobe of the lung

EXERCISE 18

Analyze each term by writing the root(s), combining vowel, and suffix separated by vertical slashes. Based on the meaning of the word parts, write a definition for each term. Use a medical dictionary to check the definition.

1. adenoidectomy

_____
root   *combining vowel*   *suffix*

DEFINITION: _____

2. bronchoplasty

_____
root   *combining vowel*   *suffix*

DEFINITION: _____

3. bronchoscopy

_____
root   *combining vowel*   *suffix*

DEFINITION: _____

4. laryngectomy

_____
root   *combining vowel*   *suffix*

DEFINITION: _____

5. laryngoscopy

_____
root   *combining vowel*   *suffix*

DEFINITION: _____

6. laryngoplasty

_____
root   *combining vowel*   *suffix*

DEFINITION: _____

7. laryngostomy

_____
root   *combining vowel*   *suffix*

DEFINITION: _____

8. laryngotracheotomy

_____
root   *combining vowel*   *suffix*

DEFINITION: _____

9. lobectomy

_____
root   *combining vowel*   *suffix*

DEFINITION: _____

EXERCISE 19

Write a medical term for each definition.

1. surgical puncture of the larynx to withdraw fluid _____
2. incision into the larynx and trachea _____
3. instrument for viewing the bronchi _____
4. x-ray film of the lungs and mediastinum _____
5. instrument for viewing the larynx _____
6. creation of an artificial opening into the larynx _____
7. surgical removal of a lobe of the lung _____

Review the pronunciation and definition for each term in Table 8-9 and complete the exercises.

TABLE 8-9   RESPIRATORY SYSTEM DIAGNOSTIC AND TREATMENT TERMS

Term with Pronunciation	Definition
pleurocentesis (**ploo**-roh-sen-**TEE**-sis) pleur/o = pleura; pleural space -centesis = surgical puncture to withdraw fluid	surgical puncture into the pleural space to withdraw fluid
pneumonectomy (**noo**-mon-**EK**-toh-mee) pneumon/o = lung; air -ectomy = surgical removal or excision	surgical removal of a lung
rhinoplasty (**RIGH**-noh-**plass**-tee) rhin/o = nose -plasty = surgical repair of	surgical repair of the nose
septoplasty (**SEP**-toh-plass-tee) sept/o = septum; nasal septum -plasty = surgical repair of	surgical repair of the nasal septum
sinusotomy (sigh-nus-**OT**-oh-mee) sinus/o = sinus; nasal sinus -(o)tomy = incision into	incision into the nasal sinuses
thoracentesis (**thor**-ah-sen-**TEE**-sis) thorac/o = thorax; chest -centesis = surgical puncture to withdraw fluid	surgical puncture into the chest or thorax to withdraw fluid

(continues)

TABLE 8-9 RESPIRATORY SYSTEM DIAGNOSTIC AND TREATMENT TERMS (continued)

Term with Pronunciation	Definition
thoracoscopy (**thor**-ah-**KOSS**-koh-pee) thorac/o = thorax; chest -scopy = process of viewing or visualization	visual examination of the thorax
thoracotomy (**thor**-ah-**KOT**-ah-mee) thorac/o = thorax; chest -(o)tomy = incision into	incision into the thorax or chest wall
tonsillectomy (ton-sill-**EK**-toh-mee) tonsil/o = tonsils -ectomy = surgical removal or excision	surgical removal of the tonsils
tracheostomy (**tray**-kee-**OSS**-toh-mee) trache/o = trachea -(o)stomy = creation of a new or artificial opening	creation of a new or artificial opening into the trachea
tracheotomy (tray-kee-**OT**-oh-mee) trache/o = trachea -(o)tomy = incision into	incision into the trachea

EXERCISE 20

Analyze each term by writing the root, combining vowel, and suffix separated by vertical slashes. Based on the meaning of the word parts, write a definition for each term. Use a medical dictionary to check the definition.

1. pleurocentesis

   _____
   root   *combining vowel*   *suffix*

   DEFINITION: _____

2. pneumonectomy

   _____
   root   *combining vowel*   *suffix*

   DEFINITION: _____

3. rhinoplasty

   _____
   root   *combining vowel*   *suffix*

   DEFINITION: _____

4. septoplasty

root	combining vowel	suffix

DEFINITION: _____

5. sinusotomy

root	combining vowel	suffix

DEFINITION: _____

6. thoracentesis

root	combining vowel	suffix

DEFINITION: _____

7. thoracotomy

root	combining vowel	suffix

DEFINITION: _____

8. tonsillectomy

root	combining vowel	suffix

DEFINITION: _____

9. tracheostomy

root	combining vowel	suffix

DEFINITION: _____

10. tracheotomy

root	combining vowel	suffix

DEFINITION: _____

11. thoracoscopy

root	combining vowel	suffix

DEFINITION: _____

EXERCISE 21

Replace the italicized phrase with the correct medical term.

1. *Lung removal* may be the only treatment for lung cancer.

   _____

2. As a result of a sports injury, Jacque was scheduled for *a repair of his nasal septum.*

   _____

3. Katie was hopeful that the *incision into her nasal sinuses* would relieve her pain.

   _____

4. To relieve pressure on the heart, the surgeon performed a *surgical puncture into the pleural space to withdraw fluid*.

   _____

5. After Rosita's motor vehicle accident, she underwent a *surgical repair of the nose*.

   _____

6. *Surgical removal of the tonsils* may be recommended following repeated "strep" infections.

   _____

7. The emergency room physician performed an *incision into the trachea* to restore breathing.

   _____

Review the pronunciation and definition for each pulmonary function test in Table 8-10 and complete the exercises.

TABLE 8-10   RESPIRATORY SYSTEM DIAGNOSTIC AND TREATMENT TERMS

Pulmonary Function Test	Definition
arterial blood gases (ABG) (ar-**TEE**-ree-al)	examination of arterial blood to determine blood levels of oxygen, carbon dioxide, and other gases
lung scan	a nuclear medicine study used to detect abnormalities related to air or blood flow to the lungs
oximeter (ock-**SIM**-eh-ter) ox/i = oxygen -meter = measurement; instrument for measuring	instrument for measuring the oxygen saturation of blood
oximetry (ock-**SIM**-eh-tree) ox/i = oxygen -metry = to measure	measuring the oxygen saturation of blood
perfusion (lung) scan (per-**FYOO**-shun)	a nuclear medicine study used to detect areas of inadequate blood flow to the lungs
pulmonary function tests (PFTs) (**PULL**-mon-air-ee) pulmon/o = lungs -ary = pertaining to	a group of tests designed to measure respiratory function and identify abnormalities
spirometer (spigh-**ROM**-eh-ter) spir/o = breathing -meter = instrument for measuring	instrument used to measure breathing activity or lung volumes

(continues)

TABLE 8-10   RESPIRATORY SYSTEM DIAGNOSTIC AND TREATMENT TERMS (continued)

Pulmonary Function Test	Definition
spirometry (spigh-**ROM**-eh-tree) spir/o = breathing -metry = to measure	the process of measuring breathing or lung volumes
ventilation (lung) scan (vent-ih-**LAY**-shun)	a nuclear medicine study used to detect areas of inadequate air flow to the lungs
ventilation/perfusion (lung) scan (V/Q scan)	a nuclear medicine study used to detect abnormalities of air and blood flow to the lungs

EXERCISE 22

Write the correct term for each definition.

1. an instrument for measuring the oxygen saturation of blood

   _____

2. a group of tests designed to measure respiratory function

   _____

3. a nuclear medicine study of the lungs

   _____

4. the process of measuring breathing or lung volumes

   _____

5. the process of measuring the oxygen saturation of blood

   _____

6. an instrument used to measure breathing or lung volumes

   _____

7. method to determine the levels of oxygen and carbon dioxide in arterial blood

   _____

Abbreviations   Review the respiratory system abbreviations in Table 8-11. Practice writing the meaning of each abbreviation.

TABLE 8-11   ABBREVIATIONS

Abbreviation	Meaning
ABG	arterial blood gases
ARD	acute respiratory distress
ARDS	adult respiratory distress syndrome
ARF	acute respiratory failure
CF	cystic fibrosis

(continues)

☐ pulmonary edema   **PULL**-mon-air-ee eh-**DEE**-mah

☐ pulmonary embolism   **PULL**-mon-air-ee **EM**-boh-lizm

☐ pulmonary heart disease   **PULL**-mon-air-ee heart disease

☐ pulmonologist   **pull**-mon-**ALL**-oh-jist

☐ pyothorax   pigh-oh-**THOH**-raks

☐ rales   **RALZ**

☐ rhinitis   righ-**NIGH**-tis

☐ rhinoplasty   **RIGH**-noh-**plass**-tee

☐ rhinorrhagia   **righ**-noh-**RAY**-jee-ah

☐ rhinorrhea   **righ**-noh-**REE**-ah

☐ rhonchi   **RONG**-kigh

☐ septoplasty   **SEP**-toh-plass-tee

☐ septum   **SEP**-tum

☐ sinusotomy   sigh-nus-**OT**-oh-mee

☐ spirometer   spigh-**ROM**-eh-ter

☐ spirometry   spigh-**ROM**-eh-tree

☐ sputum   **SPYOO**-tum

☐ stridor   **STRIGH**-dor

☐ thoracentesis   **thor**-ah-sen-**TEE**-sis

☐ thoracoscope   thoh-**RAK**-oh-skohp

☐ thoracoscopy   **thor**-ah-**KOSS**-koh-pee

☐ thoracotomy   **thor**-ah-**KOT**-ah-mee

☐ tonsillectomy   ton-sill-**EK**-toh-mee

☐ trachea   **TRAY**-kee-ah

☐ tracheostomy   tray-kee-**OSS**-toh-mee

☐ tracheotomy   tray-kee-**OT**-oh-mee

☐ tuberculosis   **too**-ber-kyoo-**LOH**-sis

☐ ventilation/perfusion scan   vent-ih-**LAY**-shun per-**FYOO**-zhun scan

☐ ventilator   **VENT**-ih-lay-tor

☐ wheeze   **WEEZ**

Chapter 9
Digestive System

OBJECTIVES

At the completion of this chapter, the student should be able to:

1. Identify, define, and spell word roots associated with the digestive system.
2. Label the basic structures of the digestive system.
3. Discuss the functions of the digestive system.
4. Provide the correct spelling of digestive system terms, given the definition of the terms.
5. Analyze digestive system terms by defining the roots, prefixes, and suffixes of these terms.
6. Identify, define, and spell disease, disorder, and procedure terms related to the digestive system.

OVERVIEW

The digestive system, also called the gastrointestinal (GI) tract, alimentary canal, or the digestive tract, is made up of the mouth, pharynx, esophagus, stomach, small intestine, large intestine, and accessory organs, including the salivary glands, liver, gallbladder, and pancreas. The structures of the digestive system function together for the following purposes: (1) to digest food; (2) to absorb nutrients into the bloodstream; and (3) to eliminate solid waste products.

Digestive System Word Roots

To understand and use the digestive system medical terms, it is necessary to acquire a thorough knowledge of the associated word roots. The word roots are listed with the combining vowel in Table 9-1. Review these roots and complete the exercises that follow.

TABLE 9-1   DIGESTIVE SYSTEM ROOT WORDS

Word Root/Combining Form	Meaning
abdomin/o; celi/o	abdomen
an/o	anus
append/o; appendic/o	appendix
bil/I	bile
bucc/o	cheek
cec/o	cecum

(continues)

5. cecum   _____

6. cheek   _____

7. common bile duct   _____

8. fat   _____

9. jejunum   _____

10. lips   _____

11. mouth   _____

12. pharynx   _____

13. rectum   _____

14. salivary gland   _____

15. tongue   _____

Structures of the Digestive System

Structures of the digestive system include the (1) **mouth**, also called the oral cavity, and all that is in it; (2) **salivary glands**; (3) **pharynx** (**FAIR**-inks), commonly called the throat; (4) **esophagus** (eh-**SOFF**-ah-gus), a 10-inch tube that extends from the pharynx to the stomach; (5) **stomach**; (6) **small intestine**; (7) **large intestine**; (8) **anus**; (9) **liver**; (10) **gallbladder**; and (11) **pancreas** (**PAN**-kree-ass). Figure 9-1 illustrates these structures.

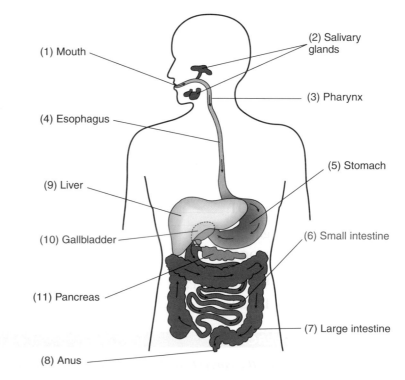

(1) Mouth

(2) Salivary glands

(3) Pharynx

(4) Esophagus

(9) Liver

(5) Stomach

(10) Gallbladder

(6) Small intestine

(11) Pancreas

(7) Large intestine

(8) Anus

Figure 9-1   Digestive system

Mouth/Oral Cavity, Pharynx, Esophagus and Salivary Glands

The mouth, also called the oral cavity, includes the (1) **lips**, (2) **gingiva** (**JIN**-jih-vah), (3) **teeth**, (4) **tongue**, (5) **hard** and (6) **soft palate** (**PAL**-at), and (7) **uvula** (**YOO**-vyoo-lah). Figure 9-2 illustrates the parts of the oral cavity. Refer to this figure as you learn about the mouth.

The lips form the opening to the oral cavity, and the teeth are used to mechanically break down food. The tongue moves the food around the mouth, provides us with our sense of taste, and helps push the food into the throat. The hard palate forms the roof of the mouth, and the soft palate prevents food from entering the nasal cavity. The uvula can trigger our gag reflex and also helps produce sounds and speech.

The salivary glands produce **saliva**, a watery substance that contains digestive enzymes. There are three pairs of salivary glands: **parotid** (pah-**ROT**-id) **glands**, located in front of and slightly below the ear; **sublingual** (sub-**LING**-gwall) **glands**, located underneath the tongue; and **submandibular** (sub-man-**DIB**-yoo-lar) **glands**, located on the posterior floor of the mouth.

The **bolus** (**BOH**-lus), which is foodstuffs mixed with salivary secretions, passes through the pharynx into the esophagus, which is a muscular tube. At this point, the bolus is pushed to the stomach by wave-like muscular contractions called **peristalsis** (pair-ih-**STALL**-sis).

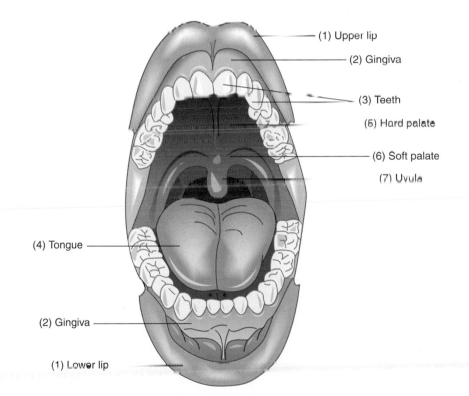

Figure 9-2　Oral cavity

Stomach and Small Intestine

The stomach begins the process of digestion, and the small intestine completes it. In addition, the small intestine is responsible for the absorption of nutrients into the bloodstream. Refer to Figure 9-3 as you learn about these organs.

The bolus of food enters the (1) **stomach** through the (2) **cardiac sphincter** (**KAR**-dee-ak **SFINGK**-ter), a muscular ring at the upper end of the stomach that prevents food from moving back into the esophagus. In the stomach, the bolus mixes with digestive juices and hydrochloric acid. The bulge at the lower end of the stomach is called the (3) **antrum** (**AN**-trum) or **pylorus** (pigh-**LOR**-us). The (4) **pyloric sphincter** (pigh-**LOR**-ik **SFINGK**-ter), a muscular ring at the end of the antrum, allows the partially digested food to move into the small intestine.

The first 10 to 12 inches of the small intestine is the (5) **duodenum** (doo-oh-**DEE**-num, doo-**ODD**-eh-num); it is here that most digestion occurs. The small intestine is approximately 20 feet in length and extends from the pyloric sphincter to the large intestine. The (6) **jejunum** (jeh-**JOO**-num), the second segment of the small intestine, is approximately 8 feet long; and the (7) **ileum** (**ILL**-ee-um), the third segment of the small intestine, is approximately 11 feet long. As the digested food passes through the small intestines, nutrients are passed into the bloodstream. The remaining waste is liquid and is passed into the large intestine.

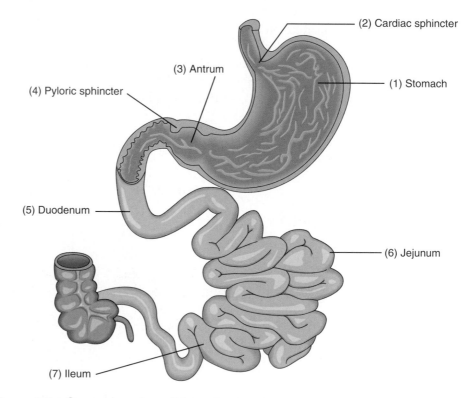

Figure 9-3 Stomach and small intestine

Large Intestine

The large intestine is approximately 5 to 6 feet long and extends from the cecum to the anus. Figure 9-4 illustrates the large intestines. Refer to this figure as you learn about the large intestine.

The large intestine has six distinct segments and two major corners or curves: the (1) **cecum** (**SEE**-kum), (2) **ascending colon**, (3) **hepatic flexure**, (4) **transverse colon**, (5) **splenic flexure**, (6) **descending colon**, (7) **sigmoid colon**, and the (8) **rectum**. The cecum, the pouchlike beginning of the large intestine, is connected to the ileum by the (10) **ileocecal** (ill-ee-oh-**SEE**-kal) **valve**. The valve is a muscular ring that prevents the liquid waste from flowing back into the small intestine. The **vermiform appendix**, commonly called the appendix, is a narrow, wormlike tube connected to the cecum. Inflammation of this tube is called appendicitis.

As the waste product moves through the large intestine, water and minerals are absorbed into the bloodstream. The solid to semisolid waste is stored in the rectum. The (9) **anus**, another sphincter muscle, holds the waste in the rectum until we voluntarily release the waste.

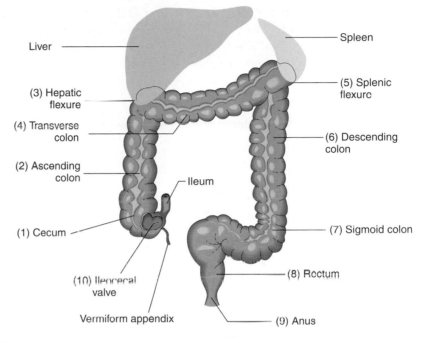

Figure 9-4   Large intestine

Liver, Gallbladder, and Pancreas

The (1) **liver**, (2) **gallbladder**, and (3) **pancreas** are commonly called the accessory organs of the digestive system. Figure 9-5 illustrates these organs. Refer to this figure as you learn about these organs.

The liver produces bile, which is necessary for the digestion of fats. Bile is stored in the gallbladder, a small saclike structure. The pancreas, which functions as a digestive organ and an endocrine gland, produces additional digestive juices that help digest all types of foods.

Bile and pancreatic digestive juices empty into the duodenum by a series of ducts. Note in Figure 9-5 that the (4) **right** and (5) **left hepatic ducts** come together to form the (6) **common hepatic duct**. The common hepatic duct joins with the (7) **cystic duct** to form the (8) **common bile duct**. The common bile duct joins with the (9) **pancreatic ducts** and enters the duodenum.

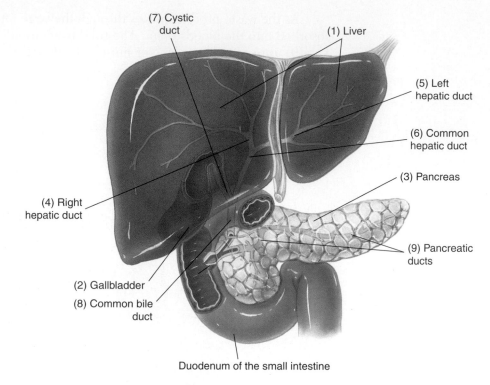

Figure 9-5 Liver, gallbladder, and pancreas

EXERCISE 4

Write the names of the digestive system structures shown in Figure 9-6. Write your answers on the spaces provided.

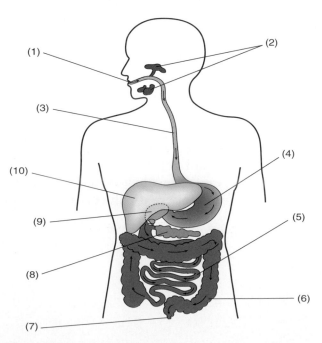

Figure 9-6 Digestive system labeling exercise

1. _____

2. _____

3. _____

4. _____

5. _____

6. _____

7. _____

8. _____

9. _____

10. _____

EXERCISE 5

Write the name of the digestive system organ or structure that fits each description.

1. adds digestive juices to the duodenum _____

2. adds hydrochloric acid to foodstuffs _____

3. nutrients absorbed into the bloodstream _____

4. pouch for storing solid waste _____

5. produces bile _____

6. produce saliva _____

7. stores bile _____

8. water absorbed into the bloodstream _____

EXERCISE 6

Match the sections and structures associated with the small and large intestine in Column 1 with the correct definition in Column 2.

COLUMN 1

_____ 1. anus

_____ 2. ascending colon

_____ 3. cecum

_____ 4. descending colon

_____ 5. duodenum

_____ 6. hepatic flexure

_____ 7. ileocecal valve

_____ 8. ileum

_____ 9. jejunum

_____ 10. rectum

_____ 11. sigmoid colon

_____ 12. splenic flexure

_____ 13. transverse colon

COLUMN 2

a. first segment, small intestine

b. beginning section, large intestine

c. second segment, small intestine

d. stores solid waste

e. last segment, large intestine

f. third segment, small intestine

g. connects small and large intestine

h. located above the cecum

i. located across the abdomen

j. sphincter muscle, holds waste

k. located on the left side

l. curve between the ascending and transverse colon

m. curve between the transverse and descending colon

Digestive System Medical Terminology

Digestive system medical terms are organized into three main categories: (1) general medical terms; (2) disease and condition terms; and (3) diagnostic procedure, surgery, and laboratory test terms. The roots, prefixes, and suffixes associated with digestive system terms are listed in Table 9-2. Review these word parts and complete the exercises.

TABLE 9-2   COMBINING FORMS, PREFIXES, AND SUFFIXES FOR DIGESTIVE SYSTEM TERMS

Root	Meaning	Prefix	Meaning	Suffix	Meaning
leuk/o	white	endo-	within	-centesis	surgical puncture
polyp/o	polyp	retro-	backward	-gram	record of
				-graphy	process of recording
				-iasis	abnormal condition
				-(o)stomy	creating a new or artificial opening
				-pepsia	digestion
				-plasty	surgical repair
				-(r)rhaphy	to suture
				-scope	instrument for viewing
				-scopy	process of viewing
				-tripsy	crushing

EXERCISE 7

Write the root, prefix, suffix, and their meanings for each medical term.

1. duodenoplasty

    ROOT: _____ MEANING: _____

    PREFIX: _____ MEANING: _____

    SUFFIX: _____ MEANING: _____

2. endoscope

    ROOT: _____ MEANING: _____

    PREFIX: _____ MEANING: _____

    SUFFIX: _____ MEANING: _____

3. endoscopy

    ROOT: _____ MEANING: _____

    PREFIX: _____ MEANING: _____

    SUFFIX: _____ MEANING: _____

4. gastroplasty

    ROOT: _____ MEANING: _____

    PREFIX: _____ MEANING: _____

    SUFFIX: _____ MEANING: _____

5. glossorrhaphy

ROOT: _____   MEANING: _____

PREFIX: _____   MEANING: _____

SUFFIX: _____   MEANING: _____

6. ileostomy

ROOT: _____   MEANING: _____

PREFIX: _____   MEANING: _____

SUFFIX: _____   MEANING: _____

7. lithotripsy

ROOT: _____   MEANING: _____

PREFIX: _____   MEANING: _____

SUFFIX: _____   MEANING: _____

8. pancreatography

ROOT: _____   MEANING: _____

PREFIX: _____   MEANING: _____

SUFFIX: _____   MEANING: _____

9. polypectomy

ROOT: _____   MEANING: _____

PREFIX: _____   MEANING: _____

SUFFIX: _____   MEANING: _____

10. retrograde

ROOT: _____   MEANING: _____

PREFIX: _____   MEANING: _____

SUFFIX: _____   MEANING: _____

EXERCISE 8

Based on your knowledge of the meanings of roots, prefixes, and suffixes, write a brief definition for each term. Use a medical dictionary to check your definition.

1. gastrocentesis _____

2. colonoscopy _____

3. endoscope _____

4. choledochogram _____

5. colostomy _____

6. gingivoplasty _____

7. glossorrhaphy _____

8. cholecystography _____

9. retroversion _____

10. polypectomy _____

Digestive System General Medical Terms

Review the pronunciation and meaning of each term in Table 9-3. Note that some terms are built from word parts and some are not. Complete the exercises for these terms.

TABLE 9-3 DIGESTIVE SYSTEM GENERAL MEDICAL TERMS

Term with Pronunciation	Definition
abdominal (ab-**DOM**-ih-nal) abdomin/o = abdomen -al = pertaining to	pertaining to the abdomen
anal (**AY**-nal) an/o = anus -al = pertaining to	pertaining to the anus
buccal (**BUCK**-al) bucc/o = cheek -al = pertaining to	pertaining to the cheek or mouth
fecal (**FEE**-kal) fec/o = feces -al = pertaining to	pertaining to feces
feces (**FEE**-seez)	stool; excrement; body waste from the large intestine
gastric (**GASS**-trik) gastr/o = stomach -ic = pertaining to	pertaining to the stomach
gastroenterologist (**gass**-troh-**en**-ter-**ALL**-oh-jist) gastr/o = stomach enter/o = intestines -(o)logist = specialist in the study of	physician who specializes in diseases and treatments of the digestive system
gastroenterology (**gass**-troh-**en**-ter-**ALL**-oh-jee) gastr/o = stomach enter/o = intestines -(o)logy = study of	study of the diseases and treatments related to the digestive system
ileocecal (**ill**-ee-oh-**SEE**-kal) ile/o = ileum cec/o = cecum -al = pertaining to	pertaining to the ileum and the cecum

(continues)

TABLE 9-3   DIGESTIVE SYSTEM GENERAL MEDICAL TERMS (continued)

Term with Pronunciation	Definition
nasogastric (nay-zoh-**GASS**-trik) nas/o = nose gastr/o = stomach -ic = pertaining to	pertaining to the nose and stomach
oral (**OR**-al) or/o = mouth -al = pertaining to	pertaining to the mouth
pancreatic (pan-kree-**AT**-ik) pancreat/o = pancreas -ic = pertaining to	pertaining to the pancreas
peritoneal (**pair**-ih-toh-**NEE**-al) peritone/o = peritoneum -al = pertaining to	pertaining to the peritoneum or the peritoneal membrane
proctologist (prok-**TALL**-oh-jist) proct/o = rectum; anus -(o)logist = specialist in the study of	physician who specializes in diseases and treatments of the anus and rectum
proctology (prok-**TALL**-oh-jee) proct/o = rectum, anus -(o)logy = study of	study of the diseases and treatments of the anus and rectum
sublingual (sub-**LING**-gwall) sub- = beneath; under ling/o = tongue -al = pertaining to	under the tongue; pertaining to under the tongue

EXERCISE 9

Analyze each term by writing the root, suffix, and their meanings. Based on the meaning of the word parts, write a definition of each term. Check the definition in a medical dictionary.

EXAMPLE: abdominal
ROOT: abdomin/o   MEANING: abdomen
SUFFIX: -al   MEANING: pertaining to
DEFINITION: pertaining to the abdomen

1. anal

ROOT: _____   MEANING: _____

SUFFIX: _____   MEANING: _____

DEFINITION: _____

2. buccal

ROOT: _____ MEANING: _____

SUFFIX: _____ MEANING: _____

DEFINITION: _____

3. fecal

ROOT: _____ MEANING: _____

SUFFIX: _____ MEANING: _____

DEFINITION: _____

4. gastric

ROOT: _____ MEANING: _____

SUFFIX: _____ MEANING: _____

DEFINITION: _____

5. ileocecal

ROOT: _____ MEANING: _____

SUFFIX: _____ MEANING: _____

DEFINITION: _____

6. oral

ROOT: _____ MEANING: _____

SUFFIX: _____ MEANING: _____

DEFINITION: _____

7. pancreatic

ROOT: _____ MEANING: _____

SUFFIX: _____ MEANING: _____

DEFINITION: _____

8. sublingual

ROOT: _____ MEANING: _____

SUFFIX: _____ MEANING: _____

DEFINITION: _____

EXERCISE 10

Write the medical term for each definition.

1. stool, excrement _____

2. physician specialist, digestive diseases _____

3. study of diseases, treatments, digestive system _____

4. pertaining to the peritoneum _____

5. pertaining to the nose and stomach _____

6. physician specialist, anus and rectum _____

7. study of diseases, treatments, anus and rectum   _____

8. pertaining to the ileum and cecum   _____

Digestive System Disease and Disorder Terms

Digestive system diseases and disorders include familiar problems such as diarrhea as well as more complex and less familiar diagnoses such as volvulus. The medical terms are presented in alphabetical order in Table 9-4. Review the pronunciation and definition for each term and complete the exercises.

TABLE 9-4   DIGESTIVE SYSTEM DISEASE AND DISORDER TERMS

Term with Pronunciation	Definition
achalasia (ak-ah-**LAY**-zee-ah)	decreased mobility of the lower two-thirds of the esophagus with lower esophageal sphincter constriction
anorexia nervosa (an-oh-**REK**-see-ah ner-**VOH**-sah)	loss of appetite and emaciation accompanied by an extreme and unfounded fear of obesity
aphagia (ah-**FAY**-jee-ah) a- = lack of; without -phagia = to swallow	loss of the ability to swallow
aphthous stomatitis (**AFF**-thuss **stoh**-mah-**TIGH**-tis) stomat/o = mouth itis = inflammation	inflammatory, noninfectious ulcerated lesion of the lips, tongue, and mouth; canker sore
appendicitis (ah-pen-dih-**SIGH**-tis) appendic/o = appendix -itis = inflammation	inflammation of the vermiform appendix
ascites (ah-**SIGH**-teez)	abnormal accumulation of fluid in the peritoneal cavity
bulimia (buh-**LIM**-ee-ah)	condition characterized by alternately overeating and inducing vomiting
cholecystitis (**koh**-lee-sist-**EYE**-tis) cholecyst/o = gallbladder -itis = inflammation	inflammation of the gallbladder
choledocholithiasis (koh-lee-**doh**-koh-lih-**THIGH**-ah-sis) choledoch/o = bile duct lith/o = stones; calculi -iasis = abnormal condition	presence of calculi (stones) in the common bile duct (Figure 9-7)

(continues)

TABLE 9-4 DIGESTIVE SYSTEM DISEASE AND DISORDER TERMS (continued)

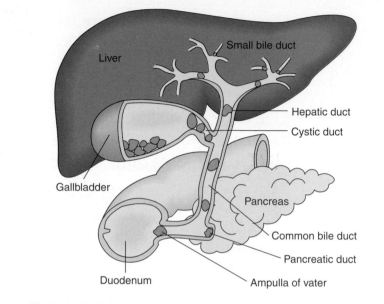

Figure 9-7 Choledocholithiasis and cholelithiasis

Term with Pronunciation	Definition
cholelithiasis (**koh**-lee-lih-**THIGH**-ah-sis) chole/o = bile lith/o = stones -iasis = abnormal condition	formation or presence of bile stones in the gallbladder; gallstones (Figure 9-7)
cirrhosis (sih-**ROH**-sis)	chronic disease of the liver characterized by the destruction of liver cells
colorectal carcinoma (cancer) (koh-loh-**REK**-tal kar-sin-**OH**-mah) col/o = colon rect/o = rectum -al = pertaining to carcin- = cancer; malignant -oma = tumor	malignant neoplasm of the colon and rectum
Crohn's disease (KROHNZ)	chronic inflammation of the ileum characterized by ulcerations along the intestinal wall and the formation of scar tissue; also called regional ileitis or regional enteritis
diarrhea (digh-ah-**REE**-ah)	frequent passage of loose, watery stools
diverticulitis (**digh**-ver-**tik**-yoo-**LIGH**-tis) diverticul/o = diverticulum -itis = inflammation	inflammation of a diverticulum or several diverticula

(continues)

TABLE 9-4 DIGESTIVE SYSTEM DISEASE AND DISORDER TERMS (continued)

Term with Pronunciation	Definition
diverticulosis (**digh**-ver-**tik**-yoo-**LOH**-sis) diverticul/o = diverticulum -osis = condition	presence of diverticula in the colon
diverticulum (**digh**-ver-**TIK**-yoo-lum)	a sac or pouch in the walls of an organ; often exhibited in the large intestine

EXERCISE 11

Write the root, prefix, suffix, and their meanings for each term. Based on the meanings of the word parts, write a definition for the term. Check the definitions using a medical dictionary.

1. aphagia

   ROOT: _____ MEANING: _____

   PREFIX: _____ MEANING: _____

   SUFFIX: _____ MEANING: _____

   DEFINITION: _____

2. appendicitis

   ROOT: _____ MEANING: _____

   PREFIX: _____ MEANING: _____

   SUFFIX: _____ MEANING: _____

   DEFINITION: _____

3. cholecystitis

   ROOT: _____ MEANING: _____

   PREFIX: _____ MEANING: _____

   SUFFIX: _____ MEANING: _____

   DEFINITION: _____

4. choledocholithiasis

   ROOT: _____ MEANING: _____

   PREFIX: _____ MEANING: _____

   SUFFIX: _____ MEANING: _____

   DEFINITION: _____

5. cholelithiasis

   ROOT: _____ MEANING: _____

   PREFIX: _____ MEANING: _____

   SUFFIX: _____ MEANING: _____

   DEFINITION: _____

6. diverticulitis

ROOT: _____ MEANING: _____

PREFIX: _____ MEANING: _____

SUFFIX: _____ MEANING: _____

DEFINITION: _____

7. diverticulosis

ROOT: _____ MEANING: _____

PREFIX: _____ MEANING: _____

SUFFIX: _____ MEANING: _____

DEFINITION: _____

EXERCISE 12

Replace the italicized phrase with the correct medical term.

1. Carlos' lower GI series identified the presence of *sacs or pouches in his large intestine.*

   _____

2. As a result of Marjorie's *overeating and induced vomiting,* Marjorie's parents requested a mental health consultation.

   _____

3. *Canker sores* may be caused by poor dietary habits.

   _____

4. Because of a family history of *malignancy of the colon and rectum,* Jerald made an appointment with his family physician.

   _____

5. Regina's *regional ileitis* was treated with prednisone.

   _____

6. *Decreased esophageal mobility and sphincter constriction* made it difficult for Luke to swallow.

   _____

7. Chronic alcoholism often leads to *abnormal accumulation of fluid in the peritoneal cavity.*

   _____

8. Repeated episodes of *loose, watery stools* caused baby Rosita's dehydration.

   _____

9. *Inflammation of the appendix* usually requires surgical intervention.

   _____

10. *Loss of appetite, emaciation, and an extreme fear of obesity* are more common in young women than in young men.

    _____

Review the pronunciation and definition for each term in Table 9-5 and complete the exercises.

TABLE 9-5 DIGESTIVE SYSTEM DISEASE AND DISORDER TERMS

Term with Pronunciation	Definition
duodenal ulcer (doo-oh-**DEE**-nal, doo-**OD**-eh-nal **ULL**-sir) duoden/o = duodenum -al = pertaining to	ulceration of the mucous membrane of the duodenum; peptic ulcer
dysentery (**DISS**-en-ter-ee)	infection of the intestinal track by bacteria, virus, or microbes that cause an inflammation of the intestinal mucosa characterized by loose, bloody, mucuslike stools
dyspepsia (diss-**PEP**-see-ah) dys- = abnormal; painful; difficult -pepsia = digestion	painful or abnormal digestion; indigestion
dysphagia (diss-**FAY**-jee-ah) dys- = abnormal; painful; difficult -phagia = swallowing	difficulty in swallowing
emaciation (ee-**may**-she-**AY**-shun)	state of being abnormally and extremely lean
eructation (eh-ruk-**TAY**-shun)	producing gas from the stomach and expelling it through the mouth; belch, burp
flatus (**FLAY**-tus)	gas in the digestive tract; expelling gas from the anus
gastric ulcer (**GASS**-trik **ULL**-sir)	ulcer of the mucosa of the stomach; peptic ulcer
gastrodynia, gastralgia (gass-troh-**DIN**-ee-ah, gass-**TRAL**-jee-ah) gastr/o = stomach -dynia, -algia = pain	pain in the stomach; stomachache
gastroenteritis (**gass**-troh-**en**-ter-**EYE**-tis) gastr/o = stomach enter/o = intestines -itis = inflammation	inflammation of the stomach and intestinal tract

(continues)

TABLE 9-5 DIGESTIVE SYSTEM DISEASE AND DISORDER TERMS (continued)

Term with Pronunciation	Definition
gastroesophageal reflux disease (GERD) (**gass**-troh-eh-**soff**-oh-**JEE**-al **REE**-flux) gastr/o = stomach esophag/o = esophagus -eal = pertaining to	reflux or moving backward of gastric contents into the esophagus
gingivitis (jin-jih-**VIGH**-tis) gingiv/o = gingiva; gums -itis = inflammation	inflammation of the gums or gingiva
hematemesis (hem-at-**EM**-eh-sis) hemat/o = blood -emesis = vomiting	vomiting blood
hepatitis (hep-ah-**TIGH**-tis) hepat/o = liver -itis = liver	inflammation of the liver
hernia (**HER**-nee-ah)	protrusion of an organ or part of an organ through the wall of a cavity; usually refers to some part of the intestinal tract protruding through the abdominal wall
herpetic stomatitis (her-**PEH**-tik **stoh**-mah-**TIGH**-tis) stomat/o = mouth -itis = inflammation	inflammatory infectious lesions of the oral cavity caused by the herpes simplex virus; cold sores, fever blisters
hiatal hernia (high-**AY**-tal **HER**-nee-ah)	herniation of a portion of the stomach through the esophageal opening in the diaphragm (Figure 9-8)

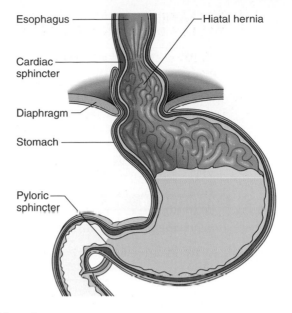

Figure 9-8 Hiatal hernia

EXERCISE 13

Analyze each term by writing the prefix, root, combining vowel, and suffix separated by vertical slashes. Based on the meaning of the word parts, write a definition for each term. Check your definition in a medical dictionary.

EXAMPLE: abdominoplasty

	/ abdomin	/ o	/ plasty
prefix	*root*	*combining vowel*	*suffix*

DEFINITION: surgical repair of the abdomen

1. dyspepsia

prefix	*root*	*combining vowel*	*suffix*

DEFINITION: _____

2. gastrodynia

prefix	*root*	*combining vowel*	*suffix*

DEFINITION: _____

3. gastroenteritis

prefix	*root*	*combining vowel*	*suffix*

DEFINITION: _____

4. gingivitis

prefix	*root*	*combining vowel*	*suffix*

DEFINITION: _____

5. hepatitis

_____
prefix   *root*   *combining vowel*   *suffix*

DEFINITION: _____

6. hematemesis

_____
prefix   *root*   *combining vowel*   *suffix*

DEFINITION: _____

EXERCISE 14

Replace the italicized phrase with the correct medical term.

1. Marilyn developed a *peptic ulcer* for no apparent reason.

   _____

2. Surgery was scheduled to repair the *protrusion of the small intestine through the abdominal wall.*

   _____

3. After visiting a remote tropical village, Ling-Ling had *loose, bloody, mucuslike stools.*

   _____

4. *The state of being abnormally and extremely lean* is often associated with anorexia nervosa.

   _____

5. Gastric hypersecretion was the cause of Rodney's *belching.*

   _____

6. Many hospitals required immunization for *inflammation of the liver* for all employees.

   _____

7. *Fever blisters* often occur around the lips.

   _____

8. "Heartburn" might be caused by a *herniation of the stomach into the esophagus.*

   _____

9. *Vomiting blood* is a good indication of a gastrointestinal problem.

   _____

10. *GERD* causes a burning sensation in the upper gastrointestinal tract.

    _____

EXERCISE 15

Circle the medical term that best fits the definition.

DEFINITION	**CIRCLE ONE TERM**
1. indigestion	*flatus* OR *dyspepsia*
2. extremely, abnormally lean	*emaciation* OR *anorexia nervosa*
3. herniation through the diaphragm	*gastroesophageal reflux disease* OR *hiatal hernia*
4. belch, burp	*flatus* OR *eructation*
5. cold sore	*herpetic stomatitis* OR *gingivitis*
6. stomachache	*gastric ulcer* OR *gastrodynia*
7. expelling gas from the anus	*eructation* OR *flatus*
8. peptic ulcer	*gastroenteritis* OR *gastric ulcer*
9. flow of gastric contents into the esophagus	*GERD* OR *hiatal hernia*
10. inflammation of the liver	*hepatitis* OR *gingivitis*

Review the pronunciation and definition for each term in Table 9-6 and complete the exercises.

TABLE 9-6 DIGESTIVE SYSTEM DISEASE AND DISORDER TERMS

Term with Pronunciation	**Definition**
ileus (**ILL**-ee-us)	obstruction of the intestine
intestinal obstruction (in-**TESS**-tin-al ob-**STRUK**-shun)	complete or partial interruption of the movement of the contents of the small or large intestine
intussusception (in-**tuh**-suh-**SEP**-shun)	telescoping of one portion of the large intestine into another portion of the large intestine (Figure 9-9)

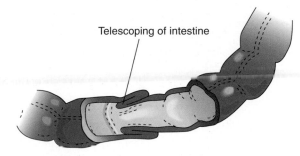

Telescoping of intestine

Figure 9-9 Intussusception

(continues)

TABLE 9-6 DIGESTIVE SYSTEM DISEASE AND DISORDER TERMS (continued)

Term with Pronunciation	Definition
irritable bowel syndrome (IBS)	increased motility of the small or large intestines resulting in abdominal pain, flatulence, nausea, anorexia, and trapped gas throughout the intestines; spastic colon
melena (**MELL**-eh-nah)	abnormal, black, tarry stool containing digested blood
nausea (**NAW**-zee-ah)	unpleasant sensation usually preceding vomiting
oral leukoplakia (**OR**-al **loo**-koh-**PLAY**-kee-ah)	presence of white spots or patches on the mucous membrane of the tongue or cheek; lesions may become malignant
pancreatitis (**pan**-kree-ah-**TIGH**-tis) pancreat/o = pancreas -itis = inflammation	inflammation of the pancreas
peritonitis (**pair**-ih-toh-**NIGH**-tis) peritone/o = peritoneum -itis = inflammation	inflammation of the peritoneum
polyp (**PALL**-ip)	a small growth projecting from the mucous membrane of organs such as the colon, nose, or uterus
polyposis, chronic (pall-ee-**POH**-sis) polyp/o = polyp -osis = condition	presence of a large number of polyps in the large bowel
pruritus ani (proo-**RIGH**-tus **AN**-eye)	severe itching around the anus
sialolithiasis (**sigh**-ah-loh-lih-**THIGH**-ah-sis) sial/o = saliva; salivary glands lith/o = stones; calculi -iasis = abnormal condition	presence of salivary stones or calculi in the salivary gland or duct
thrush	a fungal infection of the mouth and throat that produces creamy white patches on the tongue and other oral surfaces (Figure 9-10)

(continues)

TABLE 9-6   DIGESTIVE SYSTEM DISEASE AND DISORDER TERMS (continued)

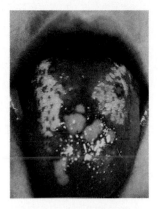

Figure 9-10   Thrush (Centers for Disease Control)

Term with Pronunciation	Definition
ulcerative colitis (**ULL**-ser-ah-tiv koh-**LIGH**-tis) col/o = colon; large intestine -itis = inflammation	a chronic inflammatory condition characterized by the formation of ulcerated lesions in the mucous membrane lining of the colon; inflammatory bowel disease (IBD)
volvulus (**VOL**-vyoo-lus)	twisting of loops of the bowel or colon that results in an intestinal obstruction (Figure 9-11)

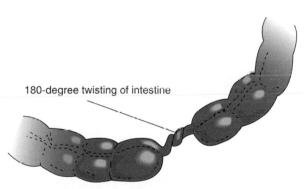

180-degree twisting of intestine

Figure 9-11   Volvulus

EXERCISE 16

Replace the italicized phrase with the correct medical term.

1. Jackson's postoperative course was complicated by an *intestinal obstruction.*

   _____

2. Gita was scheduled for surgery to correct *telescoping of the large intestine.*

   _____

3. Choton eliminated dairy products from his diet to relieve *spastic colon.*

   _____

4. A *twisting of loops of the bowel* might cause an intestinal obstruction.

   _____

5. Marie received high-dose, oral prednisone for her *chronic inflammatory condition of the colon.*

   _____

6. *Black, tarry stools* might be symptomatic of a bleeding ulcer.

   _____

7. Ella received a topical medication for *the creamy, white patches on her tongue.*

   _____

8. The oral surgeon informed Wade that he had *salivary calculi.*

   _____

9. *Severe itching around the anus* might be caused by pinworms.

   _____

10. *Inflammation of the pancreas* complicated Isun's postoperative treatment.

    _____

11. A ruptured appendix might lead to *inflammation of the peritoneum.*

    _____

12. After eating poorly cooked chicken, Bill experienced *a sensation that vomiting might occur.*

    _____

EXERCISE 17

Match the conditions in Column 1 with the correct descriptions in Column 2.

COLUMN 1

_____ 1. IBD
_____ 2. IBS
_____ 3. ileus
_____ 4. intussusception
_____ 5. melena
_____ 6. oral leukoplakia
_____ 7. polyp
_____ 8. sialolithiasis
_____ 9. thrush
_____ 10. volvulus

COLUMN 2

a. black, tarry stools
b. chronic inflammatory condition of the lining of the colon
c. fungal infection of the oral cavity; creamy, white patches
d. growth projecting from the mucous membrane of the colon
e. obstruction of the intestine
f. salivary stones or calculi
g. spastic colon
h. telescoping of the large intestine into itself
i. twisted loops of the bowel or colon
j. white patches of the oral mucous membrane

Digestive System Diagnostic Medical Terms

Review the pronunciation and definition of the diagnostic terms in Table 9-7. Complete the exercises for each set of terms. Diagnostic procedures such as colonoscopy also function as a surgical or treatment approach. For example, during a diagnostic colonoscopy, the gastroenterologist discovers several suspicious looking polyps. With the patient's consent, she removes the polyps. In this example, the diagnostic colonoscopy has become the surgical approach for a polypectomy.

TABLE 9-7   DIGESTIVE SYSTEM DIAGNOSTIC MEDICAL TERMS

Term with Pronunciation	Definition
abdominocentesis (ab-**dom**-ih-noh-sen-**TEE**-sis) abdomin/o = abdomen -centesis = surgical puncture to remove fluid	surgical puncture into the abdominal/ peritoneal cavity to remove excess fluid; also known as paracentesis
cholangiogram (kohl-**AN**-jee-oh-gram) cholangi/o — bile ducts -gram = picture; x-ray	x-ray of the bile ducts
cholangiography (**kohl**-an-jee-**OG**-rah-fee) cholangi/o — bile ducts -graphy = process of recording; x-ray examination	x-ray examination of the bile ducts
cholecystogram (**koh**-lee-**SISS**-toh-gram) cholecyst/o = gallbladder -gram = picture; x-ray	x-ray of the gallbladder
cholecystography (**koh**-lee-sist-**OG**-rah-fee) cholecyst/o = gallbladder -graphy = process of recording; x-ray examination	x-ray examination of the gallbladder
colonoscopy (koh-lon-**OSS**-koh-pee) colon/o = colon; large intestine -scopy = process of visualization with a scope	endoscopic visualization and examination of the large intestine from the anus to the ileocecal junction

(*continues*)

TABLE 9-7 DIGESTIVE SYSTEM DIAGNOSTIC MEDICAL TERMS (continued)

Term with Pronunciation	Definition
endoscopic retrograde cholangiopancreatogram (ERCP) (en-doh-**SKOP**-ic **REH**-troh-grayd kohl-**an**-jee-oh-**PAN**-kree-**ah**-toh-gram) endo- = within -scopic = pertaining to visualization with a scope cholangi/o = bile duct pancreat/o = pancreas -gram = picture; x-ray	x-ray of the pancreatic ducts and bile ducts
endoscopic retrograde cholangiopancreatography (ERCP) (en-doh-**SKOP**-ic **REH**-troh-grayd kohl-**an**-jee-oh-**pan**-kree-ah-**TOG**-rah-fee) cholangi/o = bile duct pancreat/o = pancreas -graphy = process of recording; x-ray examination	x-ray examination of the pancreatic ducts and bile ducts
esophagogastroduodenoscopy (EGD) (eh-**soff**-ah-goh-**gass**-troh-doo-**wah**-den-**OSS**-koh-pee) esophag/o = esophagus gastr/o = stomach duoden/o = duodenum -scopy = process of visualization with a scope	endoscopic visualization and examination of the esophagus, stomach, and duodenum
esophagoscopy (eh-**soff**-ah-**GOSS**-koh-pee) esophag/o = esophagus -scopy = process of visualization with a scope	endoscopic visualization and examination of the esophagus
gastroscopy (gass-**TROSS**-koh-pee) gastr/o = stomach -scopy = process of visualization with a scope	endoscopic visualization and examination of the stomach

(continues)

TABLE 9-7   DIGESTIVE SYSTEM DIAGNOSTIC MEDICAL TERMS (continued)

Term with Pronunciation	Definition
Helicobacter pylori (H. pylori) (hee-lih-koh-**BAK**-ter pigh-**LOR**-eye)	a blood test to determine the presence of *H. pylori* antibodies, which indicate infection with the bacteria; *H. pylori* is also found in the lining of the stomach and causes duodenal ulcers
laparoscopy (lap-ah-**ROSS**-koh-pee) lapar/o = abdominal wall -scopy = process of visualization with a scope	endoscopic visualization and examination of the abdominal and pelvic cavities
lower gastrointestinal series; barium (**gass**-troh-in-**TESS**-tin-al) gastr/o = stomach intestin/o = intestines -al = pertaining to	x-ray examination of the rectum and large intestine aided by a contrast medium
occult blood test (uh-**KULT**)	microscopic examination of feces to detect the presence of blood that is not otherwise visible; screen for colorectal cancer
proctoscopy (prok-**TOSS**-koh-pee) proct/o = rectum, anus -scopy = process of visualization with a scope	endoscopic visualization and examination of the anus and rectum
sigmoidoscopy (sig-moyd-**OSS**-koh-pee) sigmoid/o = sigmoid colon -scopy = process of visualization with a scope	endoscopic visualization and examination of the sigmoid colon
small bowel follow-through (SBF)	x-ray examination of the small intestine aided by a contrast medium; often done with an upper gastrointestinal series (Figure 9-12)
upper gastrointestinal series (**gass**-troh-in-**TESS**-tin-al) gastr/o = stomach intestin/o = intestines -al = pertaining to	x-ray examination of the esophagus, stomach, and small intestine aided by a contrast medium (Figure 9-12)

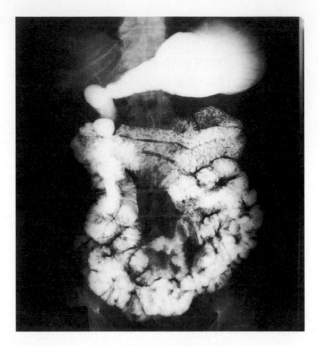

Figure 9-12 Upper gastrointestinal series and small bowel follow-through

EXERCISE 18

Analyze each term by writing the root, combining vowel, and suffix separated by vertical slashes. Based on the meaning of the word parts, write a definition for each term. Check your definition in a medical dictionary.

1. abdominocentesis

   _____
   root   *combining vowel*   *suffix*

   DEFINITION: _____

2. cholecystogram

   _____
   root   *combining vowel*   *suffix*

   DEFINITION: _____

3. cholecystography

   _____
   root   *combining vowel*   *suffix*

   DEFINITION: _____

4. cholangiography

   _____
   root   *combining vowel*   *suffix*

   DEFINITION: _____

5. colonoscopy

   _____
   root   *combining vowel*   *suffix*

   DEFINITION: _____

6. esophagoscopy

_____
root   _combining vowel_   _suffix_

DEFINITION: _____

7. esophagogastroduodenoscopy

_____
root   _combining vowel_   _suffix_

DEFINITION: _____

8. gastroscopy

_____
root   _combining vowel_   _suffix_

DEFINITION: _____

9. laparoscopy

_____
root   _combining vowel_   _suffix_

DEFINITION: _____

10. proctoscopy

_____
root   _combining vowel_   _suffix_

DEFINITION: _____

11. sigmoidoscopy

_____
root   _combining vowel_   _suffix_

DEFINITION: _____

EXERCISE 19

Replace the italicized phrase or abbreviation with the correct medical term.

1. Tom's _barium enema_ revealed an obstruction in the descending colon.

_____

2. The _microscopic screen for colorectal cancer_ is usually ordered for all patients age 50 and older.

_____

3. Elizabeth had a _barium swallow_ that revealed no abnormalities.

_____

4. The _x-ray examination of the small intestine_ identified several hernias.

_____

5. A patient is sedated but conscious during the _endoscopic examination of the entire large intestine._

_____

6. The *x-ray of the bile ducts* showed several large gallstones in the common bile duct.

   _____

7. Kwan was told not to eat or drink the night before his scheduled *ERCP*.

   _____

8. An upper GI series often includes an *SBF*.

   _____

Digestive System Surgery and Treatment Terms

Digestive system surgery and treatment terms cover a range of procedures, from an appendectomy to proctocolectomy (i.e., the surgical removal of the entire large intestine, including the rectum). Review the pronunciation and definition of the terms in Table 9-8 and complete the exercises.

TABLE 9-8   DIGESTIVE SYSTEM SURGERY AND TREATMENT TERMS

Term with Pronunciation	Definition
abdominoplasty (ab-**dom**-in-oh-**PLASS**-tee) abdomin/o = abdomen -plasty = surgical repair	plastic surgery of the abdomen
anoplasty (**AY**-noh-**plass**-tee) an/o = anus -plasty = surgical repair	surgical repair of the anus
appendectomy (ap-en-**DEK**-toh-mee) append/o = appendix -ectomy = surgical removal	surgical removal of the appendix
bariatric surgery (bair-ee-**AT**-rik)	weight-loss surgical procedure accomplished by gastric bypass or adjustable gastric banding
celiotomy (see-lee-**OT**-oh-mee) celi/o = abdomen -(o)tomy = incision into	surgical incision into the abdominal cavity
cheiloplasty (**KIGH**-loh-**plass**-tee) cheil/o = lip -plastic = surgical, plastic repair	surgical or plastic repair of the lip
cheilorrhaphy (kigh-**LOR**-ah-fee) cheil/o = lip -(r)rhaphy = to suture	suturing the lip

(continues)

TABLE 9-8 DIGESTIVE SYSTEM SURGERY AND TREATMENT TERMS
(continued)

Term with Pronunciation	Definition
cholecystectomy (**koh**-lee-sist-**EK**-toh-mee) cholecyst/o = gallbladder -ectomy = surgical removal	surgical removal of the gallbladder
choledocholithotomy (koh-leh-**doh**-koh-lith-**OT**-oh-mee) choledoch/o = bile duct lith/o = stones; calculi -(o)tomy = incision into	removal of gallstones through an incision into the common bile duct
choledocholithotripsy (koh-leh-**doh**-koh-**LITH**-oh-trip-see) choledoch/o = bile duct lith/o = stones; calculi -tripsy = crushing	crushing of gallstones in the common bile duct
colectomy (koh-**LEK**-toh-mee) col/o = colon; large intestine -ectomy = surgical removal	surgical removal of all or part of the colon or large intestine
colostomy (koh-**LOSS**-toh-mee) col/o = colon; large intestine -(o)stomy = creating a new or artificial opening	creation of a new or artificial opening for the colon through the abdominal wall to its outside surface
diverticulectomy (**digh**-ver-**tik**-yoo-**LEK**-toh-mee) diverticul/o = diverticulum -ectomy = surgical removal	surgical removal of diverticulum or diverticula
esophagogastroplasty (eh-**soff**-ah-goh-**GASS**-troh-plass-tee) esophag/o = esophagus gastr/o = stomach -plasty = surgical repair	surgical repair of the esophagus and stomach
extracorporeal shock wave lithotripsy (ESWL) (**eks**-trah-kor-**POR**-ee-al shock wave **LITH**-oh-trip-see) lith/o = stones; calculi -tripsy = crushing	crushing of gallstones using ultrasound and shock waves; nonsurgical treatment for gallstones

(continues)

TABLE 9-8 DIGESTIVE SYSTEM SURGERY AND TREATMENT TERMS
(continued)

Term with Pronunciation	Definition
gastrectomy (gass-**TREK**-toh-mee) gastr/o = stomach -ectomy = surgical removal	surgical removal of all or a portion of the stomach; also known as gastric resection
gastric lavage (**GASS**-trik lah-**VAHZ**) gastr/o = stomach -ic = pertaining to	washing out the contents of the stomach; commonly called "pumping the stomach"

EXERCISE 20

Analyze each term by writing the root, combining vowel, and suffix separated by vertical slashes. Based on the meaning of the word parts, write a definition for each term. Check your definition in a medical dictionary.

1. abdominoplasty

root	combining vowel	suffix

DEFINITION: _____

2. anoplasty

root	combining vowel	suffix

DEFINITION: _____

3. appendectomy

root	combining vowel	suffix

DEFINITION: _____

4. cheilorrhaphy

root	combining vowel	suffix

DEFINITION: _____

5. cholecystectomy

root	combining vowel	suffix

DEFINITION: _____

6. choledocholithotomy

root	combining vowel	suffix

DEFINITION: _____

7. choledocholithotripsy

_____
root   _combining vowel_   _suffix_

DEFINITION: _____

8. colectomy

_____
root   _combining vowel_   _suffix_

DEFINITION: _____

9. colostomy

_____
root   _combining vowel_   _suffix_

DEFINITION: _____

10. esophagogastroplasty

_____
root   _combining vowel_   _suffix_

DEFINITION: _____

EXERCISE 21

Match the procedures in Column 1 with the descriptions in Column 2.

COLUMN 1

_____ 1. celiotomy

_____ 2. cheiloplasty

_____ 3. choledocholithotomy

_____ 4. choledocholithotripsy

_____ 5. colectomy

_____ 6. colostomy

_____ 7. diverticulectomy

_____ 8. ESWL

_____ 9. gastrectomy

_____ 10. gastric lavage

COLUMN 2

a. creation of a new or artificial opening for the colon

b. crushing of gallstones

c. excision of diverticula

d. incision into the abdomen or abdominal cavity

e. incision into the common bile duct to remove stones

f. pumping the stomach

g. removal of all or part of the large intestine

h. removal of all or part of the stomach

i. surgical repair of the lip

j. ultrasound crushing of gallstones

Review the pronunciation and definition of the terms in Table 9-9 and complete the exercises.

TABLE 9-9 DIGESTIVE SYSTEM SURGERY AND TREATMENT TERMS

Term with Pronunciation	Definition
gastric banding, bariatric	restrictive bariatric surgical procedure during which a silicone band is placed around a portion of the stomach to limit the volume of the contents of the stomach
gastric bypass, bariatric	weight-loss surgical procedure characterized by reducing the size of the stomach and connecting it to a portion of the small intestine; part of the stomach and the first segment of the small intestine are bypassed
gastroduodenostomy (**gass**-troh-doo-**wah**-den-**OSS**-toh-mee) gastr/o = stomach duoden/o = duodenum -(o)stomy = creation of a new or artificial opening	creation of a new or artificial opening between the stomach and the duodenum, usually after a portion of the stomach is removed
gavage (gah-**VAHZ**)	feeding through a stomach tube
gingivectomy (jin-jih-**VEK**-toh-mee gingiv/o = gingiva -ectomy = surgical removal	surgical removal of the gingiva (gums)
glossorrhaphy (gloss-**OR**-ah-fee) gloss/o = tongue -(r)rhaphy = to suture	suture of a wound of the tongue
herniorrhaphy (her-nee-**OR**-ah-fee)	suture repair of a hernia
ileostomy (ill-ee-**OSS**-toh-mee) ile/o = ileum -(o)stomy = creation of a new or artificial opening	surgical creation of a new or artificial opening for the ileum through the abdominal wall to its outside surface
laparoscopic adjustable gastric banding (LAGB) (**lap**-ah-roh-**SKAH**-pic) lapar/o = abdominal wall -scopy = process of viewing -ic = pertaining to gastr/o = stomach	bariatric surgical procedure in which a silicone band is placed around a portion of the stomach; the band, which is inserted via laparoscope, can be tightened or loosened

(continues)

TABLE 9-9 DIGESTIVE SYSTEM SURGERY AND TREATMENT TERMS
(continued)

Term with Pronunciation	Definition
laparotomy (lap-ah-**ROT**-oh-mee) lapar/o = abdomen; abdominal wall -(o)tomy = incision into	surgical incision into the abdominal wall
nasogastric intubation (nay-zoh-**GASS**-trik in-too-**BAY**-shun) nas/o = nose gastr/o = stomach -ic = pertaining to	insertion of a tube through the nose into the stomach
palatoplasty (**PAL**-at-oh-plass-tee) palat/o = palate -plasty = surgical repair	surgical repair of the palate, usually to repair a cleft palate
polypectomy (pall-ih-**PEK**-toh-mee) polyp/o = polyp -ectomy = surgical removal	surgical removal of a polyp
proctocolectomy (**prock**-toh-koh-**LEK**-toh-mee) proct/o = rectum; anus col/o = colon; large intestine -ectomy = surgical removal	surgical removal of the large intestine and rectum
pyloroplasty (pigh-**LOR**-oh-plass-tee) pylor/o = pylorus -plasty = surgical repair	surgical procedure for enlarging the opening between the stomach and duodenum
Roux-en-Y gastric bypass (**ROO**-en-wigh) (RYGBP) gastr/o = stomach -ic = pertaining to	bariatric surgical procedure during which the size of the stomach is reduced and subsequently connected to a portion of the small intestine; also called proximal gastric bypass
total parenteral nutrition (TPN) (par-**EN**-ter-al)	provision of nutritional and caloric needs by an intravenous route in order to bypass the digestive tract
uvulopalatopharyngoplasty (UPPP) (**yoo**-vyoo-loh-**pal**-ah-toh-fah-**RING**-oh-plass-tee) uvul/o = uvula palat/o = palate pharyng/o = pharynx -plasty = surgical repair	plastic surgery of the soft palate, uvula, and other structures of the oropharynx to correct sleep apnea

EXERCISE 22

Analyze each term by writing the root, combining vowel, and suffix separated by vertical slashes. Based on the meaning of the word parts, write a definition for each term. Check your definition in a medical dictionary.

1. gastroduodenostomy

_____
root   *combining vowel*   *suffix*

DEFINITION: _____

2. gingivectomy

_____
root   *combining vowel*   *suffix*

DEFINITION: _____

3. herniorrhaphy

_____
root   *combining vowel*   *suffix*

DEFINITION: _____

4. ileostomy

_____
root   *combining vowel*   *suffix*

DEFINITION: _____

5. palatoplasty

_____
root   *combining vowel*   *suffix*

DEFINITION: _____

6. polypectomy

_____
root   *combining vowel*   *suffix*

DEFINITION: _____

7. proctocolectomy

_____
root   *combining vowel*   *suffix*

DEFINITION: _____

8. uvulopalatopharyngoplasty

_____
root   *combining vowel*   *suffix*

DEFINITION: _____

EXERCISE 23

Replace the italicized phrase or abbreviation with the correct medical term or phrase.

1. Mrs. Wicket's nurse initiated *feeding through a stomach tube* as the physician ordered.

   _____

2. After the anesthesia took effect, the surgical nurse proceeded with *the insertion of a tube through the nose into the stomach*.

   _____

3. *Surgical incision into the abdominal wall* might serve as a diagnostic or treatment procedure.

   _____

4. As a result of the accident, Jennifer underwent *surgical repair of the palate*.

   _____

5. Caleb's physician recommended *the surgical removal of polyps* to correct rectal bleeding.

   _____

6. Removal of the small intestine might result in the need for *TPN*.

   _____

7. As a result of ulcerative colitis, Milton underwent a *removal of the colon, rectum, and anus*.

   _____

8. Jeramiah's obstructive sleep apnea was corrected by *UPPP*.

   _____

Abbreviations

Review the digestive system abbreviations in Table 9-10. Practice writing out the meaning of each abbreviation.

TABLE 9-10 ABBREVIATIONS

Abbreviation	Meaning
BE	barium enema
EGD	esophagogastroduodenoscopy
ERCP	endoscopic retrograde cholangiopancreatography
GERD	gastroesophageal reflux disease
GI	gastrointestinal
LAGBP	laparoscopic adjustable gastric bypass
NG	nasogastric
RYGBP	Roux-en-Y gastric bypass

(continues)

TABLE 9-10 ABBREVIATIONS (continued)

Abbreviation	Meaning
SBF	small bowel follow-through
TPN	total parenteral nutrition
UGI	upper gastrointestinal
UPPP	uvulopalatopharyngoplasty

CHAPTER REVIEW

The Chapter Review can be used as a self-test. Go through each exercise and answer as many questions as you can without referring to previous exercises or earlier discussions within this chapter. Check your answers and fill in any blanks. Practice writing any terms you might have misspelled.

EXERCISE 24

Using your knowledge of roots, prefixes, and suffixes, write the medical term for each definition.

1. specialist in diseases and treatments of the stomach and intestines _____

2. study of the diseases and treatments of the stomach and intestines _____

3. pertaining to the ileum and cecum _____

4. pertaining to the nose and stomach _____

5. specialist in the diseases and treatments of the rectum and anus _____

6. study of the diseases and treatments of the rectum and anus _____

7. loss of the ability to swallow _____

8. inflammation of the gallbladder _____

9. abnormal condition of gallstones _____

10. inflammation of the diverticula _____

11. abnormal or difficult digestion _____

12. inflammation of the stomach and intestines _____

13. vomiting blood _____

14. x-ray examination of the bile ducts _____

15. visualization of the colon with a scope _____

16. surgical removal of the appendix _____

17. surgical removal of the gallbladder _____

18. creation of a new or artificial opening for the colon _____

19. creation of a new or artificial opening for the ileum _____

20. surgical removal of all or part of the stomach _____

21. surgical removal of the gingiva _____

22. surgical removal of the anus, colon, and rectum _____

23. presence of diverticula in the colon _____

24. surgical incision into the abdominal wall
or abdomen _____

25. abnormal condition of gallstones in the common
bile duct _____

EXERCISE 25

Write a brief definition for each term.

1. aphthous stomatitis _____

2. ascites _____

3. bulimia _____

4. cirrhosis _____

5. dysentery _____

6. emaciation _____

7. eructation _____

8. gastric lavage _____

9. hernia _____

10. herpetic stomatitis _____

11. ileus _____

12. melena _____

13. occult blood test _____

14. thrush _____

15. volvulus _____

EXERCISE 26

*Read the following operative report excerpt. Write a brief definition for each
italicized term or phrase.*

PREOPERATIVE DIAGNOSIS: Chronic (1) *cholecystitis* and
(2) *cholelithiasis*.

POSTOPERATIVE DIAGNOSIS: Cholecystitis, cholelithiasis, and common duct stone.

OPERATION PERFORMED: (3) *Cholecystectomy* and common bile duct exploration.

INDICATIONS: The patient is a 48-year-old female who was admitted to the hospital with a chronic history of right upper quadrant pain and with associated (4) *dyspepsia*.

FINDINGS: Surgical intervention revealed numerous cholesterol stones. The initial (5) *cystic duct* (6) *cholangiogram* failed to reveal clear passage of dye into the (7) *duodenum*. There was a concentric defect in the terminal (8) *common bile duct*. After 1 mg of glucagon was given, cholangiograms were repeated and the common duct was open.

1. _____
2. _____
3. _____
4. _____
5. _____
6. _____
7. _____
8. _____

EXERCISE 27

Explain the difference between the following conditions.

1. choledocholithiasis and cholelithiasis

_____

_____

2. diarrhea and dysentery

_____

_____

3. diverticulitis and diverticulosis

_____

_____

4. dyspepsia and dysphagia

_____

_____

5. aphthous stomatitis and herpetic stomatitis

_____

_____

6. irritable bowel syndrome and inflammatory bowel disease

_____

_____

7. intussusception and volvulus

_____

_____

EXERCISE 28

Select the best answer for each question or statement.

1. Which term describes the wavelike movement of the gastrointestinal tract?
   a. bolus
   b. volvulus
   c. involuntary ileus
   d. peristalsis

2. Select the term for foodstuffs mixed with saliva.
   a. volvulus
   b. bolus
   c. chyme
   d. digestion

3. Which accessory organ produces bile?
   a. gallbladder
   b. pancreas
   c. liver
   d. spleen

4. Select the medical term for the "gums" of the oral cavity.
   a. gingiva
   b. buccal ridges
   c. glossorus
   d. hard palate

5. Which structure triggers the gag reflex and assists in the production of sound?
   a. hard palate
   b. soft palate
   c. tongue
   d. uvula

6. Select the area of the gastrointestinal tract where most digestion occurs.
   a. stomach
   b. oral cavity
   c. duodenum
   d. ileum

7. Which accessory organ stores the bile?
   a. liver
   b. common bile duct
   c. pancreatic duct
   d. gallbladder

8. Choose the name of the digestive system structure that secretes hydrochloric acid.
   a. liver
   b. stomach
   c. oral cavity
   d. duodenum

☐ gastroesophageal reflux disease (GERD)	**gass**-troh-eh-**soff**-oh-**JEE**-al reflux disease
☐ gastroscopy	gass-**TROSS**-koh-pee
☐ gavage	gah-**VAHZ**
☐ gingivectomy	jin-jih-**VEK**-toh-mee
☐ gingivitis	jin-jih-**VIGH**-tis
☐ glossorrhaphy	gloss-**OR**-ah-fee
☐ hard palate; soft palate	hard **PAL**-at; soft **PAL**-at
☐ *Helicobacter pylori* antibodies test	hee-lih-koh-**BAK**-ter pigh-**LOR**-eye antibodies test
☐ hematemesis	hem-at-**EM**-eh-sis
☐ hepatitis	hep-ah-**TIGH**-tis
☐ hernia	**HER**-nee-ah
☐ herniorrhaphy	her-nee-**OR**-ah-fee
☐ herpetic stomatitis	her-**PEH**-tik **stoh**-mah-**TIGH**-tis
☐ hiatal hernia	high-**AY**-tal **HER**-nee-ah
☐ ileocecal	**ill**-ee-oh-**SEE**-kal
☐ ileocecal valve	**ill**-ee-oh-**SEE**-kal valve
☐ ileostomy	ill-ee-**OSS**-toh-mee
☐ ileum	**ILL**-ee-um
☐ ileus	**ILL**-ee-us
☐ intussusception	in-**tuh**-suh-**SEP**-shun
☐ jejunum	jeh-**JOO**-num
☐ laparoscopy	lap-ah-**ROSS**-koh-pee
☐ laparotomy	lap-ah-**ROT**-oh-mee
☐ lower gastrointestinal series	**gass**-troh-in-**TESS**-tin-al series
☐ melena	**MELL**-eh-nah
☐ nasogastric	nay-zoh-**GASS**-trik
☐ nasogastric intubation	nay-zoh-**GASS**-trik in-too-**BAY**-shun
☐ nausea	**NAW**-zee-ah
☐ occult blood test	uh-**KULT** blood test
☐ oral	**OR**-al
☐ oral leukoplakia	**OR**-al loo-koh-**PLAY**-kee-ah
☐ palatoplasty	**PAL**-at-oh-**plass**-tee
☐ pancreas	**PAN**-kree-ass
☐ pancreatic	pan-kree-**AT**-ik
☐ pancreatitis	**pan**-kree-ah-**TIGH**-tis
☐ parotid glands	pah-**ROT**-id glands
☐ peristalsis	pair-ih-**STALL**-sis
☐ peritoneal	**pair**-ih-toh-**NEE**-al
☐ pharynx	**FAIR**-inks
☐ polyp	**PALL**-ip
☐ polypectomy	pall-ih-**PEK**-toh-mee
☐ polyposis, chronic	pall-ee-**POH**-sis, chronic
☐ proctocolectomy	**prock**-toh-koh-**LEK**-toh-mee
☐ proctologist	prok-**TALL**-oh-jist
☐ proctology	prok-**TALL**-oh-jee
☐ proctoscopy	prok-**TOSS**-koh-pee
☐ pruritus ani	proo-**RIGH**-tus **AN**-eye
☐ pyloric sphincter	pigh-**LOR**-ik **SFINGK**-ter
☐ pyloroplasty	pigh-**LOR**-oh-**plass**-tee

☐ saliva   sah-**LIGH**-vah
☐ salivary glands   **SAL**-ih-vair-ee glands
☐ sialolithiasis   **sigh**-ah-loh-lih-**THIGH**-ah-sis
☐ sigmoid colon   **SIG**-moyd colon
☐ sigmoidoscopy   sig-moyd-**OSS**-koh-pee
☐ sublingual glands   sub-**LING**-gwall glands
☐ submandibular glands   sub-man-**DIB**-yoo-lar glands
☐ total parenteral nutrition (TPN)   total par-**EN**-ter-al nutrition
☐ ulcerative colitis   **ULL**-ser-ah-tiv koh-**LIGH**-tis
☐ uvula   **YOO**-vyoo-lah
☐ uvulopalatopharyngoplasty   **yoo**-vyoo-loh-**pal**-ah-toh-fah-**RING**-oh-**plass**-tee

☐ volvulus   **VOL**-vyoo-lus

Chapter 10
Urinary System

OBJECTIVES

At the completion of this chapter, the student should be able to:

1. Identify, define, and spell word roots associated with the urinary system.
2. Label the basic structures of the urinary system.
3. Discuss the functions of the urinary system.
4. Provide the correct spelling of urinary terms, given the definition of the terms.
5. Analyze urinary terms by defining the roots, prefixes, and suffixes of these terms.
6. Identify, define, and spell disease, disorder, and procedure terms related to the urinary system.

OVERVIEW

The urinary system is made up of the kidneys, ureters, urinary bladder, and urethra. The structures of the urinary system function together for the following purposes: (1) to filter the blood; (2) to maintain the proper balance of water, salts, and other substances found in our body fluids; and (3) to remove waste and excess fluids from the body. Each urinary system structure and its unique characteristics are presented individually.

Urinary System Word Roots

To understand and use urinary system medical terms, it is necessary to acquire a thorough knowledge of the associated word roots. Word roots associated with the urinary system structures are listed with the combining vowel. The suffix *-uria*, which means "urine," is included on the list. Review the word roots in Table 10-1 and complete the exercises that follow.

TABLE 10-1   URINARY SYSTEM WORD ROOTS

Word Root/Combining Form	Meaning
cyst/o	bladder; sac; urinary bladder
glomerul/o	glomerulus
meat/o	meatus (opening)
nephr/o	kidney
pyel/o	renal pelvis
ren/o	kidney
ur/o	urine; urinary system
ureter/o	ureter

(continues)

TABLE 10-1 URINARY SYSTEM WORD ROOTS (continued)

Word Root/Combining Form	Meaning
urethr/o	urethra
vesic/o	urinary bladder
Suffix	
-uria	urine; urination

EXERCISE 1

Write the meanings of the following word roots.

1. cyst/o _____

2. glomerul/o _____

3. meat/o _____

4. nephr/o _____

5. pyel/o _____

6. ren/o _____

7. ureter/o _____

8. urethr/o _____

9. vesic/o _____

EXERCISE 2

Write the word root and meaning.

1. cystectomy

   ROOT: _____ MEANING: _____

2. ureterocele

   ROOT: _____ MEANING: _____

3. nephritis

   ROOT: _____ MEANING: _____

4. renogram

   ROOT: _____ MEANING: _____

5. pyelogram

   ROOT: _____ MEANING: _____

6. meatotomy

   ROOT: _____ MEANING: _____

7. vesicocele

   ROOT: _____ MEANING: _____

8. glomerulonephritis

ROOT: _____ MEANING: _____

ROOT: _____ MEANING: _____

9. urethritis

ROOT: _____ MEANING: _____

Write the correct word root(s) for the following definitions.

1. bladder; sac; urinary bladder _____

2. glomerulus _____

3. kidney _____

4. meatus (opening) _____

5. renal pelvis _____

6. ureter _____

7. urethra _____

Structures of the Urinary System

The major structures of the urinary system include the kidneys, ureters, urinary bladder, and urethra. The (1) **kidneys** are responsible for filtering the blood and producing urine. The (2) **ureters** transport the urine from the kidney to the (3) **urinary bladder**, which is the storage sac for the urine. Urine leaves the body through the (4) **urethra** (yoo-**REE**-thrah). Figure 10-1 illustrates the major structures of the urinary system.

Kidneys

The kidneys are bean-shaped organs located on the posterior wall of the abdominal cavity. There is one kidney on each side of the spinal column. The kidneys are super-filters for the blood. They remove waste products from the bloodstream and help maintain the proper balance of water, salts, and other necessary substances found in body fluids.

The outer layer of the kidney is called the (1) **cortex** (**KOR**-tecks) and contains the **nephrons** (**NEFF**-ronz), or kidney cells. The inner layer of the kidney is called the (2) **medulla** (meh-**DULL**-ah). The (3) **renal pelvis** is the upper, expanded section of the ureters. Urine collects in the renal pelvis and then travels to the urinary bladder by way of the ureters. Figure 10-2 illustrates the areas of the kidney. Remember, the nephrons are microscopic and are not visible in Figure 10-2.

Nephrons are the filtering unit of the kidney and are responsible for filtering blood and forming urine. There are two important parts of each nephron: the (1) **glomerulus** (glom-**AIR**-yoo-lus) and (2) **renal tubules** (**TOOB**-yoolz). The glomerulus is a cluster or ball of capillaries. The renal tubule has many loops and coils. Figure 10-3 illustrates these structures. Refer to this figure as you read about the nephron.

Blood enters the kidney and passes through the **glomeruli** (glom-**AIR**-yoo-ligh) of the nephrons, which filter the blood. The renal tubules capture water and waste products to form urine. The renal tubules deposit the urine into the renal pelvis. The filtered blood continues to flow through the blood vessels that surround the renal tubules and eventually leaves the kidney.

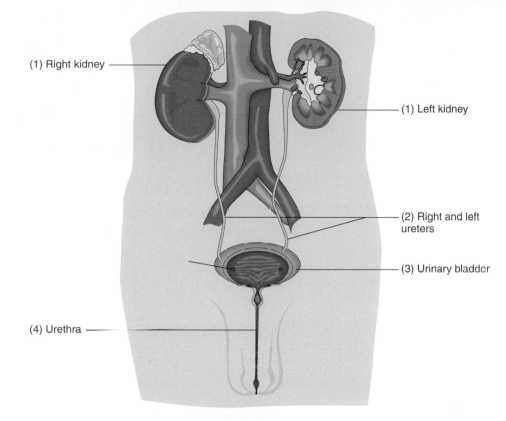

(1) Right kidney

(1) Left kidney

(2) Right and left ureters

(3) Urinary bladder

(4) Urethra

Figure 10-1 Structures of the urinary system

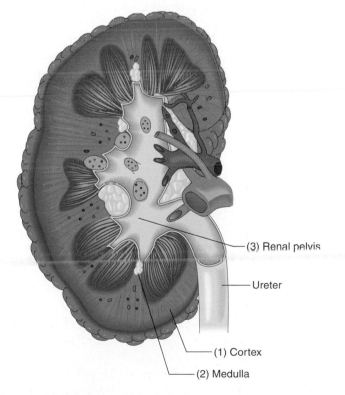

(3) Renal pelvis

Ureter

(1) Cortex

(2) Medulla

Figure 10-2 Areas of the kidney

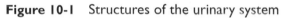

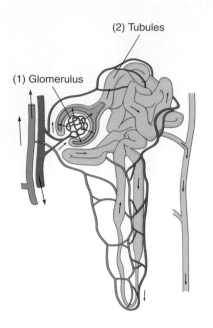

(2) Tubules

(1) Glomerulus

Figure 10-3 Nephron

Urine is the liquid waste of the body. It is made up of 95% water and 5% of other substances. These substances, known as *waste products*, include urea (yoo-**REE**-ah), creatinine (kree-**AT**-in-in), ammonia, and mineral salts.

Ureters, Urinary Bladder, and Urethra

The ureters, urinary bladder, and urethra are responsible for moving urine out of the body. Figure 10-4 illustrates these structures. Refer to this figure as you read about the movement of urine.

The (1) **ureters** are narrow tubes and are about 10 to 12 inches in length. The upper ends of the ureters are located in the kidney. These sections of the ureters are called the (2) **renal pelvis**. From the kidney, the ureters narrow and connect to the (3) **urinary bladder**.

The urinary bladder is a hollow, muscular organ or sac that temporarily stores urine. When the body is ready to release urine, the bladder contracts and expels the urine. *Urination, voiding,* and **micturition** (mick-too-**RIH**-shun) are terms that mean the normal process of expelling urine.

The (4) **urethra** is the tube leading from the urinary bladder to the outside of the body. The male urethra is about 8 inches long, and the female urethra is about 1.5 inches long. The male urethra transports both urine and semen through the penis, but not at the same time. Only urine passes through the female urethra. The **urinary meatus** (mee-**AY**-tus), also called the *urethral meatus,* is the external opening of the urethra. In the male, the urinary meatus is at the tip of the penis; in the female, it is located between the clitoris and the vaginal opening.

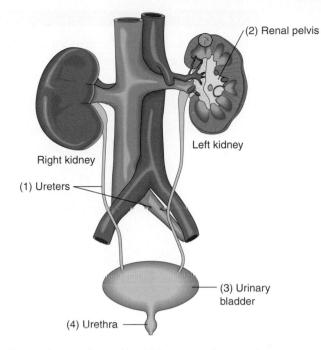

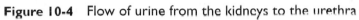

Figure 10-4 Flow of urine from the kidneys to the urethra

Match the urinary system structures in Column 1 with the correct definition in Column 2.

COLUMN 1

_____ 1. glomerulus

_____ 2. nephron

_____ 3. renal pelvis

_____ 4. renal tubule

_____ 5. ureter

_____ 6. urethra

_____ 7. urinary bladder

_____ 8. urinary meatus

COLUMN 2

a. tube that leads to the urinary bladder

b. tube that leads to the outside of the body

c. filtering unit of the kidney

d. storage sac for urine

e. cluster of capillaries

f. external opening of the urethra

g. captures water and waste from blood

h. upper expanded end of the ureters

EXERCISE 5

Label the structures of the urinary system identified in Figure 10-5. Write your answers on the spaces provided.

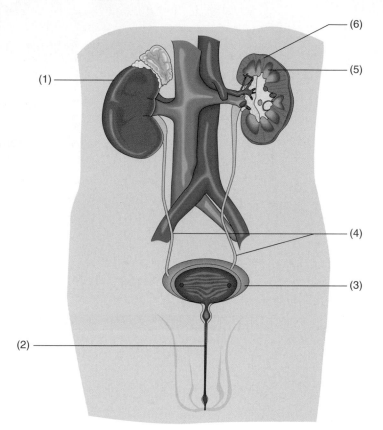

(6)

(5)

(1)

(4)

(3)

(2)

Figure 10-5 Labeling exercise

1. _____
2. _____
3. _____
4. _____
5. _____
6. _____

EXERCISE 6

Write the name of the defined urinary system structure.

1. tube that leads to the outside of the body   _____
2. tubes that bring urine to the bladder   _____
3. outer area of the kidney   _____
4. inner area of the kidney   _____
5. microscopic filtration unit of the kidney   _____
6. cluster or ball of capillaries   _____
7. captures water and waste products   _____

Urinary System Medical Terminology

Urinary medical terms are organized into three main categories: (1) general medical terms; (2) disease and disorder terms; and (3) diagnostic procedure, surgery, and laboratory test terms. The roots, prefixes, and suffixes used in urinary system terms are listed in Table 10-2. Review these word parts and complete the exercises.

TABLE 10-2 COMBINING FORMS, PREFIXES, AND SUFFIXES FOR URINARY SYSTEM TERMS

Root	Meaning	Prefix	Meaning	Suffix	Meaning
hemat/o	blood	an-	without	-cele	hernia; protrusion
lith/o	stone	dys-	abnormal; painful; difficult	-gram	record; x-ray film
noct/o	night	poly-	many	-graph	instrument for recording
olig/o	few; diminished			-graphy	process of recording
py/o	pus			-pexy	surgical fixation
				-ptosis	drooping; sagging
				-scope	instrument for viewing
				-scopy	process of viewing
				-(o)stomy	creation of a new or artificial opening
				-(o)tomy	incision into
				-tripsy	crushing

EXERCISE 7

Write the root, prefix, suffix, and their meanings for each medical term. Based on the meanings of the word parts, write a definition for each term. Check your definition using a medical dictionary. Note: *Not all terms have a root, prefix, and suffix.*

1. pyuria

    ROOT: _____ MEANING: _____

    PREFIX: _____ MEANING: _____

    SUFFIX: _____ MEANING: _____

    DEFINITION: _____

2. anuria

    ROOT: _____ MEANING: _____

    PREFIX: _____ MEANING: _____

    SUFFIX: _____ MEANING: _____

    DEFINITION: _____

3. oliguria

ROOT: _____ MEANING: _____

PREFIX: _____ MEANING: _____

SUFFIX: _____ MEANING: _____

DEFINITION: _____

4. polyuria

ROOT: _____ MEANING: _____

PREFIX: _____ MEANING: _____

SUFFIX: _____ MEANING: _____

DEFINITION: _____

5. hematuria

ROOT: _____ MEANING: _____

PREFIX: _____ MEANING: _____

SUFFIX: _____ MEANING: _____

DEFINITION: _____

6. nocturia

ROOT: _____ MEANING: _____

PREFIX: _____ MEANING: _____

SUFFIX: _____ MEANING: _____

DEFINITION: _____

EXERCISE 8

Write the suffix associated with the following definitions.

1. cut into; incision _____

2. drooping; sagging _____

3. hernia; protrusion _____

4. instrument for recording _____

5. instrument for viewing _____

6. process of recording _____

7. record; x-ray film _____

8. creation of a new or artificial opening _____

9. surgical fixation _____

Urinary System General Medical Terms

Review the pronunciation and meaning of each term in Table 10-3. Note that some terms are built from word parts and some are not. The exercises for these few terms are included with the exercises for urinary system disease terms.

TABLE 10-3   URINARY SYSTEM GENERAL MEDICAL TERMS

Term with Pronunciation	Definition
meatal (mee-**AY**-tal) meat/o = meatus -al = pertaining to	pertaining to the meatus
urine (**YOOR**-in)	liquid waste product
urologist (yoor-**ALL**-oh-jist) ur/o = urinary system -(o)logist = physician specialist	physician who specializes in the urinary system and male reproductive system
urology (yoor-**ALL**-oh-jee) ur/o = urinary system -(o)logy = study of	study of the urinary tract

Urinary System Disease and Disorder Terms

Urinary system diseases and disorders include familiar problems such as urinary tract infection (UTI) as well as other more complex and less familiar diagnoses such as glomerulonephritis. The disease and disorder terms are presented in alphabetical order in Table 10-4. Review the pronunciation and definition for each term and complete the exercises.

TABLE 10-4   URINARY SYSTEM DISEASE AND DISORDER TERMS

Term with Pronunciation	Definition
anuria (an-**YOO**-ree-ah) an- = lack of; without -uria = urine	absence of urine
azoturia (azz-oh-**TOO**-ree-ah)	an increase of urea in urine
cystitis (siss-**TIGH**-tis) cyst/o = urinary bladder -itis = inflammation	inflammation of the urinary bladder
cystocele (**SISS**-toh-seel) cyst/o = urinary bladder -cele = hernia; protrusion	hernia of the urinary bladder through the vaginal wall
diuresis (**digh**-yoo-**REE**-siss)	secretion of large amounts of urine

(continues)

TABLE 10-4 URINARY SYSTEM DISEASE AND DISORDER TERMS (continued)

Term with Pronunciation	Definition
diuretic (**digh**-yoo-**RET**-ik)	increasing the secretion of urine; a substance that increases the secretion of urine
dysuria (diss-**YOO**-ree-ah) dys- = abnormal; painful; difficult -uria = urine	painful or difficult urination
enuresis (en-yoo-**REE**-siss)	involuntary release of urine; bedwetting
epispadias (ep-ih-**SPAY**-dee-as)	congenital defect in which the urinary meatus is on the upper surface of the penis
glomerulonephritis (glom-**air**-yoo-loh-neh-**FRIGH**-tis) glomerul/o = glomerulus nephr/o = kidney -itis = inflammation	inflammation of the glomerulus of the kidneys
glycosuria (**gligh**-kohs-**YOO**-ree-ah) glycos/o = glucose -uria = urine	presence of glucose in the urine
hematuria (**hee**-mah-**TOO**-ree-ah) hemat/o = blood -uria = urine	presence of blood in the urine

EXERCISE 9

Analyze each term by writing the prefix, root, combining vowel, and suffix separated by vertical slashes. Based on the meaning of the word parts, write a definition for each term. Check the definition in a medical dictionary.

EXAMPLE: urologist:

	/ ur	/ o	/ logist
prefix	*root*	*combining vowel*	*suffix*

DEFINITION: specialist in the urinary and male reproductive systems

1. anuria

prefix	*root*	*combining vowel*	*suffix*

DEFINITION: _____

2. cystitis

prefix	*root*	*combining vowel*	*suffix*

DEFINITION: _____

3. cystocele

prefix	root	combining vowel	suffix

DEFINITION: _____

4. dysuria

prefix	root	combining vowel	suffix

DEFINITION: _____

5. glycosuria

prefix	root	combining vowel	suffix

DEFINITION: _____

6. glomerulonephritis

prefix	root	combining vowel	suffix

DEFINITION: _____

7. hematuria

prefix	root	combining vowel	suffix

DEFINITION: _____

8. urologist

prefix	root	combining vowel	suffix

DEFINITION: _____

9. urology

prefix	root	combining vowel	suffix

DEFINITION: _____

EXERCISE 10

Replace the italicized phrase or word with the correct medical term.

1. Victoria's physician said that her history of _secretion of large amounts of urine_ called for special kidney tests.

   _____

2. Thomas was relieved when he learned that _bedwetting_ can be treated.

   _____

3. To relieve fluid overload, the physician might prescribe a _medication that increases the secretion of urine._

   _____

4. _Increased urea in urine_ is associated with kidney failure.

   _____

5. Surgical intervention might correct *a urinary meatus on the upper surface of the penis.*

_____

6. *The presence of glucose in the urine* is seen in uncontrolled diabetes mellitus.

_____

EXERCISE 11

Match the medical term in Column 1 with the correct definition in Column 2.

COLUMN 1	COLUMN 2
_____ 1. anuria	a. blood in the urine
_____ 2. azoturia	b. glucose in the urine
_____ 3. cystitis	c. herniation of the urinary bladder
_____ 4. cystocele	d. absence of urine
_____ 5. diuresis	e. painful urination
_____ 6. dysuria	f. inflammation of the urinary bladder
_____ 7. enuresis	g. pertaining to the meatus
_____ 8. glycosuria	h. increase of urea in the urine
_____ 9. hematuria	i. bedwetting
_____ 10. meatal	j. secretion of large amounts of urine

Review the pronunciation and definition for each term in Table 10-5 and complete the exercises.

TABLE 10-5   URINARY SYSTEM DISEASE AND DISORDER TERMS

Term with Pronunciation	Definition
hydronephrosis (**high**-droh-neh-**FROH**-sis) hydro- = water nephr/o = kidney -osis = condition	distention of the renal pelvis caused by the inability of the urine to leave the kidney (Figure 10-6)
hypospadias (**high**-poh-**SPAY**-dee-as)	a congenital defect in which the urinary meatus is on the under surface of the penis
incontinence (in-**KON**-tin-ents)	loss of urinary bladder control
nephritis (neh-**FRIGH**-tis) nephr/o = kidney -itis = inflammation	inflammation of the kidney

(continues)

TABLE 10-5 URINARY SYSTEM DISEASE AND DISORDER TERMS (continued)

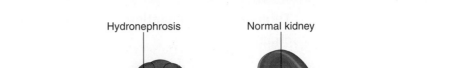

Figure 10-6   Hydroureter and hydronephrosis

Term with Pronunciation	Definition
nephrolithiasis (**neh**-froh-lih-**THIGH**-ah-sis) nephr/o = kidney lith/o = stone -iasis = condition	presence of stones in the kidneys; kidney stones; also called renal calculi
nephroma (neh-**FROH**-mah) nephr/o = kidney -oma = tumor	kidney tumor
nephromegaly (**neh**-froh-**MEG**-ah-lee) nephr/o = kidney -megaly = enlarged; enlargement	enlargement of one or both kidneys
nephroptosis (**neh**-frop-**TOH**-sis) nephr/o = kidney -ptosis = drooping; sagging	downward displacement of the kidney; falling, drooping kidney; also known as a *floating kidney*
nocturia (nok-**TOO**-ree-ah) noct/o = night -uria = urine	excessive urination at night

(continues)

TABLE 10-5 URINARY SYSTEM DISEASE AND DISORDER TERMS (continued)

Term with Pronunciation	Definition
oliguria (all-ig-**YOO**-ree-ah) olig/o = few; diminished -uria = urine	diminished urine secretion
polycystic kidney (pall-ee-**SISS**-tik) poly- = many cyst/o = fluid-filled sac -ic = pertaining to	a hereditary kidney disorder in which fluid-filled cysts or sacs replace normal kidney tissue (Figure 10-7)

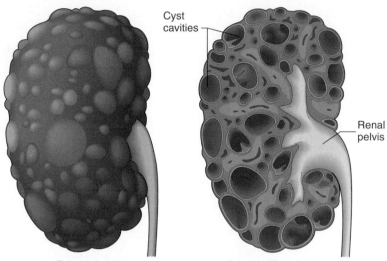

Polycystic kidney   Section through kidney

Figure 10-7 Polycystic kidney disease, external and internal views

polyuria (pall-ee-**YOO**-ree-ah) poly- = many -uria = urine	excessive urination

EXERCISE 12

Analyze each term by writing the prefix, root, combining vowel, and suffix separated by vertical slashes. Based on the meaning of the word parts, write a definition for each term. Check the definition in a medical dictionary.

1. hydronephrosis

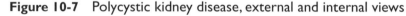

prefix   *root*   *combining vowel*   *suffix*

DEFINITION: _____

2. nephritis

prefix   *root*   *combining vowel*   *suffix*

DEFINITION: _____

3. nephrolithiasis

prefix	root	combining vowel	suffix

DEFINITION: _____

4. nephroptosis

prefix	root	combining vowel	suffix

DEFINITION: _____

5. nocturia

prefix	root	combining vowel	suffix

DEFINITION: _____

6. oliguria

prefix	root	combining vowel	suffix

DEFINITION: _____

7. polyuria

prefix	root	combining vowel	suffix

DEFINITION: _____

8. nephromegaly

prefix	root	combining vowel	suffix

DEFINITION: _____

9. nephroma

prefix	root	combining vowel	suffix

DEFINITION: _____

EXERCISE 13

Write the medical term for each definition.

1. fluid-filled cysts replace normal kidney tissue   _____

2. urinary meatus opens on the under surface
   of the penis   _____

3. loss of urinary bladder control   _____

4. kidney tumor   _____

5. excessive urination   _____

6. enlarged kidney   _____

7. diminished urine secretion   _____

EXERCISE 19

Analyze each term by writing the prefix, root, combining vowel, and suffix separated by vertical slashes. Based on the meaning of the word parts, write a definition for each term. Check the definition in a medical dictionary.

1. cystectomy

prefix	*root*	*combining vowel*	*suffix*

   DEFINITION: _____

2. urethroplasty

prefix	*root*	*combining vowel*	*suffix*

   DEFINITION: _____

3. cystolithotomy

prefix	*root*	*combining vowel*	*suffix*

   DEFINITION: _____

4. urethropexy

prefix	*root*	*combining vowel*	*suffix*

   DEFINITION: _____

5. cystopexy

prefix	*root*	*combining vowel*	*suffix*

   DEFINITION: _____

6. ureterectomy

prefix	*root*	*combining vowel*	*suffix*

   DEFINITION: _____

7. cystoplasty

prefix	*root*	*combining vowel*	*suffix*

   DEFINITION: _____

8. pyelolithotomy

prefix	*root*	*combining vowel*	*suffix*

   DEFINITION: _____

9. cystorrhaphy

prefix	*root*	*combining vowel*	*suffix*

   DEFINITION: _____

10. nephropexy

| prefix | root | combining vowel | suffix |

DEFINITION: _____

11. cystostomy

| prefix | root | combining vowel | suffix |

DEFINITION: _____

12. lithotripsy

| prefix | root | combining vowel | suffix |

DEFINITION: _____

13. nephrolithotomy

| prefix | root | combining vowel | suffix |

DEFINITION: _____

14. meatotomy

| prefix | root | combining vowel | suffix |

DEFINITION: _____

15. nephrectomy

| prefix | root | combining vowel | suffix |

DEFINITION: _____

EXERCISE 20

Circle the medical term that best fits the definition.

DEFINITION	CIRCLE ONE TERM
1. incision into the urinary bladder to remove a stone	*cystotomy* OR *cystolithotomy*
2. surgical repair of the urinary bladder	*cystoplasty* OR *cystorrhaphy*
3. surgical fixation of the kidney	*nephroplasty* OR *nephropexy*
4. surgical creation of a new or artificial opening for the urinary meatus	*meatostomy* OR *meatotomy*
5. surgical excision of the urethra	*urethrectomy* OR *ureterectomy*
6. surgical fixation of the urinary bladder	*cystoplasty* OR *cystopexy*
7. surgical repair of the ureter	*ureteroplasty* OR *ureteropexy*
8. creating a new or artificial opening for the urethra	*urethrotomy* OR *urethrostomy*

☐ cystectomy	siss-**TEK**-toh-mee
☐ cystitis	siss-**TIGH**-tis
☐ cystocele	**SISS**-toh-seel
☐ cystography	siss-**TOG**-roh-fee
☐ cystolithotomy	**siss**-toh-lith-**OT**-oh-mee
☐ cystometrography	**siss**-toh-meh-**TROG**-rah-fee
☐ cystopexy	**SISS**-toh-**pek**-see
☐ cystoplasty	**SISS**-toh-**plass**-tee
☐ cystorrhaphy	sist-**OR**-ah-fee
☐ cystoscopy	sist-**OSS**-koh-pee
☐ cystostomy	sist-**OSS**-toh-mee
☐ diuresis	**digh**-yoo-**REE**-siss
☐ diuretic	**digh**-yoo-**RET**-ik
☐ dysuria	diss-**YOO**-ree-ah
☐ enuresis	en-yoo-**REE**-siss
☐ epispadias	ep-ih-**SPAY**-dee-as
☐ glomeruli	glom-**AIR**-yoo-ligh
☐ glomerulonephritis	glom-**air**-yoo-loh-neh-**FRIGH**-tis
☐ glomerulus	glom-**AIR**-yoo-lus
☐ glycosuria	**gligh**-kohs-**YOO**-ree-ah
☐ hematuria	**hee**-mah-**TOO**-ree-ah
☐ hemodialysis	**hee**-moh-digh-**AL**-ih-sis
☐ hydronephrosis	**high**-droh-neh-**FROH**-sis
☐ hypospadias	**high**-poh-**SPAY**-dee-as
☐ incontinence	in-**KON**-tin-ents
☐ intravenous pyelography	in-trah-**VEE**-nus pigh-eh-**LOG**-rah-fee
☐ lithotripsy	**LITH**-oh-trip-see
☐ meatotomy	mee-ah-**TOT**-oh-mee
☐ medulla	meh-**DULL**-ah
☐ micturition	mick-too-**RIH**-shun
☐ nephrectomy	neh-**FREK**-toh-mee
☐ nephritis	neh-**FRIGH**-tis
☐ nephrolithiasis	**neh**-froh-lih-**THIGH**-ah-sis
☐ nephrolithotomy	**neh**-froh-lith-**OT**-oh-mee
☐ nephroma	neh-**FROH**-mah
☐ nephromegaly	**neh**-froh-**MEG**-ah-lee
☐ nephron	**NEFF**-ron
☐ nephropexy	**NEFF**-roh-pek-see
☐ nephroptosis	**neh**-frop-**TOH**-sis
☐ nocturia	nok-**TOO**-ree-ah
☐ oliguria	oh-lig-**YOO**-ree-ah
☐ peritoneal dialysis	**pair**-ih-toh-**NEE**-al digh-**AL**-ih-sis
☐ polycystic kidney disease	**pall**-ee-**SISS**-tik kidney disease
☐ polyuria	**pall**-ee-**YOO**-ree-ah
☐ pyelitis	**pigh**-eh-**LIGH**-tis
☐ pyelolithotomy	**pigh**-eh-loh-lith-**OT**-oh-mee
☐ pyelonephritis	**pigh**-eh-loh-neh-**FRIGH**-tis
☐ pyuria	pigh-**YOO**-ree-ah
☐ renal hypertension	**REE**-nal hypertension
☐ renal pelvis	**REE**-nal **PELL**-viss
☐ renal tubules	**REE**-nal **TOOB**-yoolz

☐ retrograde pyelography   **REH**-troh-grayd **pigh**-eh-**LOG**-rah-fee

☐ uremia   yoo-**REE**-mee-ah

☐ ureter   **YOO**-reh-ter

☐ ureterectomy   yoo-**ree**-ter-**EK**-toh-mee

☐ ureteritis   yoo-**ree**-ter-**EYE**-tis

☐ ureterocele   yoo-**REE**-ter-oh-seel

☐ ureterolithiasis   yoo-**ree**-ter-oh-lih-**THIGH**-ah-sis

☐ ureterostenosis   yoo-**ree**-ter-oh-sten-**OH**-sis

☐ urethra   yoo-**REE**-thrah

☐ urethrocystitis   yoo-**ree**-throh-siss-**TIGH**-tis

☐ urethropexy   yoo-**REE**-throh-pek-see

☐ urethroplasty   yoo-**REE**-throh-plass-tee

☐ urethrostomy   **yoo**-reh-**THROSS**-toh-mee

☐ urinalysis   yoor-in-**AL**-ih-sis

☐ urinary bladder   **YOOR**-in-air-ee bladder

☐ urinary catheterization   **YOOR**-in-air-ee **kath**-eh-ter-ih-**ZAY**-shun

☐ urinary meatus   **YOOR**-in-air-ee mee-**AY**-tus

☐ urinary retention   **YOOR**-in-air-ee ree-**TEN**-shun

☐ urinary tract infection   **YOOR**-in-air-ee tract in-**FEK**-shun

☐ urine   **YOOR**-in

☐ urologist   yoor-**ALL**-oh-jist

☐ urology   yoor-**ALL**-oh-jee

☐ vesicourethral suspension   **vess**-ih-koh-yoo-**REETH**-ral suspension

☐ voiding cystourethrography   voiding **siss**-toh-yoo-ree-**THROG**-rah-fee

Chapter 11
Endocrine System

OBJECTIVES

At the completion of this chapter, the student should be able to:

1. Identify, define, and spell word roots associated with the endocrine system.
2. Label the basic structures of the endocrine system.
3. Discuss the functions of the endocrine system.
4. Provide the correct spelling of endocrine terms, given the definition of the terms.
5. Analyze endocrine terms by defining the roots, prefixes, and suffixes of these terms.
6. Identify, define, and spell disease, disorder, and procedure terms related to the endocrine system.

OVERVIEW

The endocrine system is made up of the pituitary gland, pineal gland, thyroid gland, parathyroid glands, thymus, adrenal gland, pancreas, ovaries, and testes. Endocrine glands are ductless and release their hormones directly into the bloodstream. Hormones are chemicals that maintain and regulate the growth and activity of specific organs and the body as a whole. For example, hormones from the thyroid gland regulate metabolism, adrenal gland hormones help maintain the body's fluid balance, and the hormones from the testes and ovaries are important to the development of secondary sex characters. In fact, every single aspect of human growth and development is affected by the hormones of the endocrine system.

Endocrine System Word Roots

To understand and use endocrine system medical terms, it is necessary to acquire a thorough knowledge of the associated word roots. The word roots are listed with the combining vowel. Review the word roots in Table 11-1 and complete the exercises that follow.

TABLE 11-1   ENDOCRINE SYSTEM WORD ROOTS

Word Root/Combining Form	Meaning
acr/o	extremities
aden/o	gland
adren/o; adrenal/o	adrenal glands
andr/o	male; man
calc/i	calcium
cortic/o	cortex

(continues)

TABLE 11-1   ENDOCRINE SYSTEM WORD ROOTS (continued)

Word Root/Combining Form	Meaning
endocrin/o	endocrine
gonad/o	sex glands
gluc/o; glyc/o	glucose; sugar; sweet
kal/i	potassium
lact/o	milk
natr/o	sodium
pancreat/o	pancreas
parathyroid/o	parathyroid glands
somat/o	body
toxic/o	poison
thym/o	thymus gland
thyr/o; thyroid/o	thyroid gland

EXERCISE 1

Write the meanings for the following word roots.

1. adrenal/o _____
2. thym/o _____
3. calc/i _____
4. kal/i _____
5. cortic/o _____
6. pancreat/o _____
7. somat/o _____
8. natr/o _____
9. andr/o _____
10. lact/o _____
11. toxic/o _____
12. aden/o _____
13. thyr/o _____

EXERCISE 2

Write the root and meaning on the spaces provided.

1. hypoglycemia

   ROOT: _____ MEANING: _____

2. adrenalectomy

   ROOT: _____ MEANING: _____

3. hypercalcemia

   ROOT: _____ MEANING: _____

4. toxicology

    ROOT: _____   MEANING: _____

5. adrenocortical

    ROOT: _____   MEANING: _____

6. cortisol

    ROOT: _____   MEANING: _____

7. acromegaly

    ROOT: _____   MEANING: _____

8. hyperkalemia

    ROOT: _____   MEANING: _____

9. pancreatitis

    ROOT: _____   MEANING: _____

EXERCISE 3

Write the correct word root(s) for the following definitions.

1. body   _____

2. thymus gland   _____

3. gland   _____

4. sex glands   _____

5. parathyroid glands   _____

6. thyroid gland   _____

7. sweet   _____

8. adrenal glands   _____

9. calcium   _____

10. poisons   _____

11. pancreas   _____

Structures of the Endocrine System

The major structures of the endocrine system include the (1) **pituitary gland**, (2) **pineal gland**, (3) **thyroid gland**, (4) **parathyroid glands**, (5) **thymus**, (6) **adrenal glands**, (7) **pancreas**, (8) **ovaries**, and (9) **testes**. The endocrine system structures are located throughout the body. Figure 11-1 illustrates the location of these structures.

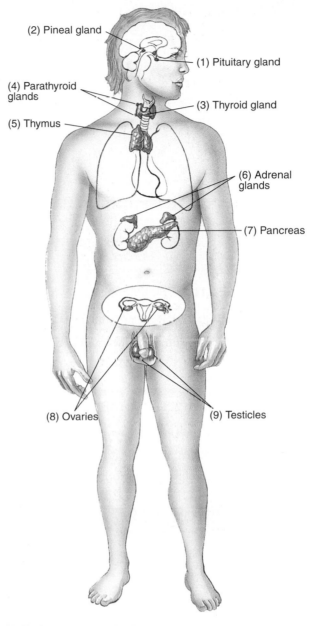

Figure 11-1   Endocrine system glands

Pituitary Gland

The pituitary gland, often called the *master gland,* is a pea-sized structure located at the base of the brain. Figure 11-2 illustrates the pituitary gland and its two lobes.

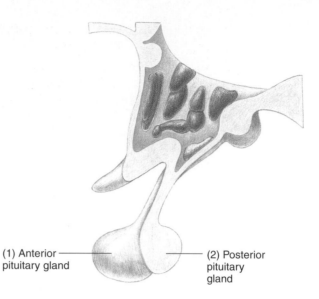

(1) Anterior pituitary gland

(2) Posterior pituitary gland

Figure 11-2 Pituitary gland

The pituitary gland has two lobes, (1) **anterior** and (2) **posterior**, that secrete specific hormones. Table 11-2 describes the hormones of the anterior and posterior lobes of the pituitary gland.

TABLE 11-2   PITUITARY GLAND HORMONES

Anterior Lobe Hormones	Function
adrenocorticotropic hormone (ACTH)	stimulates the adrenal cortex
follicle-stimulating hormone (FSH)	stimulates estrogen secretion, ovum production, and sperm production
growth hormone (GH), or somatotropic hormone (STH)	regulates the growth of body tissues (i.e., muscles and bones)
lactogenic hormone, or prolactin	stimulates breast development and milk production
luteinizing hormone (LH)	stimulates ovulation and testosterone production
melanocyte-stimulating hormone (MSH)	controls the pigmentation of skin cells
thyroid-stimulating hormone (TSH)	stimulates the thyroid gland
Posterior Lobe Hormones	**Function**
antidiuretic hormone (ADH) or vasopressin	regulates urine secretion
oxytocin	stimulates uterine contractions and release of breast milk

Pituitary gland hormones effect nearly all body functions.

Pineal Gland

The pineal gland is a pinecone-shaped gland located in the midbrain. The pineal gland secretes **melatonin** (mell-ah-**TOH**-nin), a hormone that seems to have a role in promoting sleep. Figure 11-1 illustrates the location of the pineal gland. Although the precise function of the pineal gland is not clearly understood, evidence suggests that this gland helps regulate our biological clock.

Thyroid Gland and Parathyroid Glands

The thyroid gland is located in the neck and attached to the trachea. The thyroid gland has two lobes, one on either side of the trachea, that are connected by a strip of tissue called the *isthmus*. The parathyroid glands are four round bodies of tissue on the back of the thyroid gland, two on each thyroid lobe. Figure 11-3 illustrates the (1) **thyroid gland** and the (2) **parathyroid glands**.

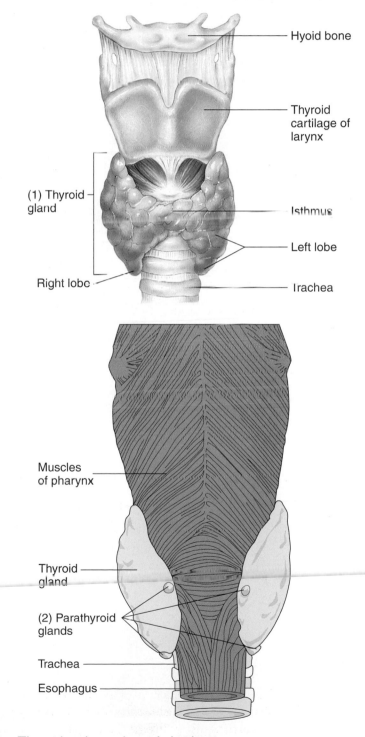

Figure 11-3 Thyroid and parathyroid glands

Thyroid gland hormones include **triiodothyronine** (try-**eye**-oh-doh-**THIGH**-roh-neen) (**T$_3$**), **thyroxine** (thigh-**ROCKS**-in) (**T$_4$**), and **calcitonin** (**kal**-sih-**TOH**-nin). T$_3$ and T$_4$ regulate growth and control body temperature and metabolism. Calcitonin helps regulate the amount of calcium in the blood. The parathyroid glands secrete **parathyroid hormone (PTH)**. This hormone, in partnership with calcitonin, regulates the amount of calcium in the blood.

Thymus Gland

The thymus gland is located in the middle of the pleural cavity. It is large in infants and shrinks as the body ages. The thymus gland is primarily responsible for the development of the immune system. Figure 11-4 illustrates the location of this important gland.

Thymus gland hormones include **thymosin** (thigh-**MOH**-sin) and **thymopoietin** (**thigh**-moh-**POY**-eh-tin), which stimulate the production of T cells. T cells are specialized lymphocytes and are part of the immune system.

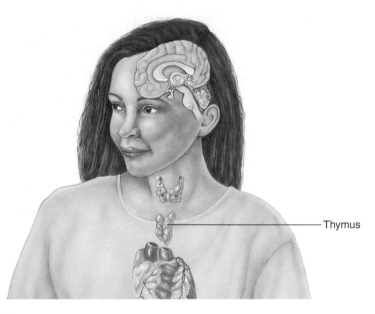

Thymus

Figure 11-4 Thymus

Adrenal Glands

The (1) **adrenal glands** are two small glands that sit on top of each kidney. The adrenal gland consists of two parts: the (2) **adrenal cortex** (outer part) and the (3) **adrenal medulla** (inner part). Figure 11-5 illustrates the location and sections of the adrenal glands.

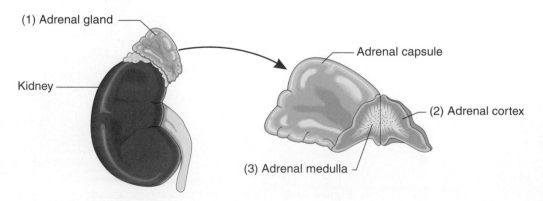

(1) Adrenal gland

Kidney

Adrenal capsule

(2) Adrenal cortex

(3) Adrenal medulla

Figure 11-5 Adrenal glands

Each part of the adrenal gland secretes different hormones. Table 11-3 lists and describes the adrenal gland hormones.

TABLE 11-3 ADRENAL GLAND HORMONES

Steroid Hormones of the Adrenal Cortex

Mineralocorticoids: regulate the fluid and electrolyte balance in the body	**Aldosterone** is the primary mineralocorticoid of the adrenal cortex.
Glucocorticoids: influence the metabolism of carbohydrates, fats, and proteins; maintain normal blood pressure; have an anti-inflammatory effect during times of stress	**Cortisol**, also called **hydrocortisone**, is the primary glucocorticoid of the adrenal cortex and electrolyte balance in the body.
Gonadocorticoids: sex hormones that contribute to the secondary sex characteristics in males and females	**Androgen** is one of the gonadocorticoid hormones secreted by the adrenal cortex.

Nonsteroid Hormones of the Adrenal Medulla

Epinephrine or **adrenaline**: increases heart rate; dilates the bronchioles; raises blood glucose levels	This hormone plays an important role in the body's response to stress by increasing the availability of oxygen and glucose in the blood.
Norepinephrine or **noradrenaline**: causes the blood vessels to constrict and thereby raises the blood pressure	This hormone also plays an important role in the body's response to stress by raising the individual's blood pressure.

The adrenal cortex hormones are classified as steroid hormones, and the adrenal medulla hormones are classified as nonsteroid hormones.

Pancreas

The pancreas is a gland that is located in the upper-left quadrant of the abdomen, under the stomach. Figure 11-6 illustrates the pancreas.

Specialized pancreatic cells called the **islets** (**EYE**-lets) **of Langerhans** (**LONG**-er-honz) produce **insulin** and **glucagon** (**GLOO**-kah-gon), the pancreatic hormones. Insulin is responsible for decreasing the amount of glucose in the blood. Glucagon is responsible for increasing the amount of glucose in the blood.

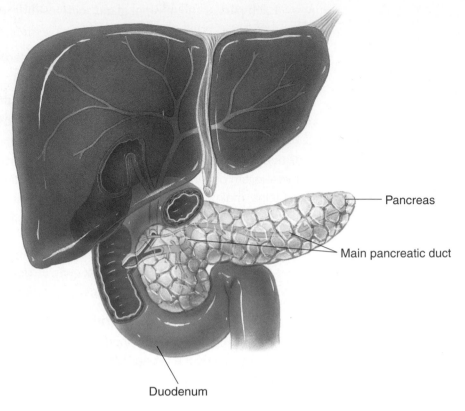

Pancreas

Main pancreatic duct

Duodenum

Figure 11-6 Pancreas

Ovaries and Testes

The ovaries are female sex glands or gonads. There are two ovaries, one on each side of the pelvic cavity. The ovaries produce the hormones **estrogen** (**ESS**-troh-jen) and **progesterone** (proh-**JESS**-ter-ohn). Estrogen promotes the maturation of the ovum (egg) and prepares the uterus for implantation of a fertilized ovum. Estrogen is necessary for the development of female secondary sex characteristics. Progesterone also helps prepare the uterus for implantation and is responsible for the growth and development of the placenta.

Testes are the male sex organs, or gonads, and are contained in the scrotum. The testes produce **testosterone** (tess-**TOSS**-ter-ohn), the hormone responsible for the maturation of sperm and the development of male secondary sex characteristics. A complete discussion of the functions of the ovaries and testes is presented in Chapters 12 and 13.

EXERCISE 4

Match the endocrine gland in Column 1 with the correct definition in Column 2.

COLUMN 1	COLUMN 2
_____ 1. thyroid gland	a. produce male hormones
_____ 2. pancreas	b. primarily functions during childhood
_____ 3. testes	c. produces insulin
_____ 4. parathyroid glands	d. secrete adrenaline
_____ 5. pituitary gland	e. produce female hormones

_____ 6. adrenal glands   f. four round bodies

_____ 7. thymus   g. secretes T_3 and T_4

_____ 8. ovaries   h. the master gland

EXERCISE 5

Label the structures of the endocrine system identified in Figure 11-7. Write your answer on the spaces provided.

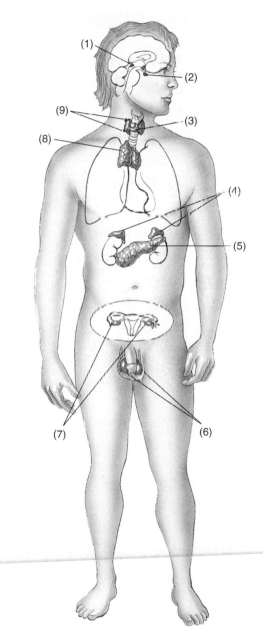

Figure 11-7   Labeling exercise

1. _____

2. _____

3. _____

4. _____

5. _____

6. _____

7. _____

8. _____

9. _____

EXERCISE 6

Match the hormone in Column 1 with the endocrine gland in Column 2. Note that some endocrine glands will be used more than once.

COLUMN 1

_____ 1. adrenocorticotropic hormone

_____ 2. androgen

_____ 3. antidiuretic hormone

_____ 4. calcitonin

_____ 5. cortisol

_____ 6. epinephrine

_____ 7. estrogen

_____ 8. glucagon

_____ 9. growth hormone

_____ 10. insulin

_____ 11. testosterone

_____ 12. PTH

_____ 13. T_3, T_4

_____ 14. thymopoietin

_____ 15. thyroid-stimulating hormone

COLUMN 2

a. adrenal cortex

b. adrenal medulla

c. anterior lobe of the pituitary gland

d. ovaries

e. pancreas

f. parathyroid glands

g. posterior lobe of the pituitary gland

h. testes

i. thymus gland

j. thyroid gland

Endocrine System Medical Terminology

Endocrine system medical terms are organized into three main categories: (1) general medical terms; (2) disease and condition terms; and (3) diagnostic procedure, surgery, and laboratory test terms. The roots, prefixes, and suffixes associated with endocrine system terms are listed in Table 11-4. Review these word parts and complete the related exercises.

TABLE 11-4 ROOTS, PREFIXES, AND SUFFIXES FOR ENDOCRINE SYSTEM TERMS

Root	Meaning	Prefix	Meaning	Suffix	Meaning
acid/o	sour; bitter	eu-	same; normal	-crine	secrete
dips/o	thirst	ex-	out; outward	-ectomy	surgical removal
ket/o	ketone bodies	oxy-	sharp; quick	-emia	blood condition
ophthalm/o	eye	poly-	excessive	-tropin	stimulating effect of a hormone

EXERCISE 7

Write the root, prefix, suffix, and their meanings on the spaces provided.

1. endocrine

    ROOT: _____ MEANING: _____

    PREFIX: _____ MEANING: _____

    SUFFIX: _____ MEANING: _____

2. polydipsia

    ROOT: _____ MEANING: _____

    PREFIX: _____ MEANING: _____

    SUFFIX: _____ MEANING: _____

3. somatotropin

    ROOT: _____ MEANING: _____

    PREFIX: _____ MEANING: _____

    SUFFIX: _____ MEANING: _____

4. acromegaly

    ROOT: _____ MEANING: _____

    PREFIX: _____ MEANING: _____

    SUFFIX: _____ MEANING: _____

5. thyrotoxicosis

    ROOT: _____ MEANING: _____

    PREFIX: _____ MEANING: _____

    SUFFIX: _____ MEANING: _____

6. hypoglycemia

    ROOT: _____ MEANING: _____

    PREFIX: _____ MEANING: _____

    SUFFIX: _____ MEANING: _____

EXERCISE 8

Based on the meaning of the word parts, write a definition for each term.

1. euthyroid _____

2. adrenomegaly _____

3. polydipsia _____

4. hyperglycemia _____

5. somatotropin _____

6. pancreatitis _____

7. thyroidectomy _____

Endocrine System General Medical Terms

Review the pronunciation and meaning of each term in Table 11-5. Note that some terms are built from word parts and some are not. Complete the exercises for these terms.

TABLE 11-5 ENDOCRINE SYSTEM GENERAL MEDICAL TERMS

Term with Pronunciation	Definition
cortical (**KOR**-tih-kal)	pertaining to the cortex
corticoid (**KOR**-tih-koyd)	pertaining to the hormones of the adrenal cortex
endocrinologist (**en**-doh-krin-**ALL**-oh-jist) endocrin/o = endocrine -(o)logist = specialist	physician who specializes in the diseases and disorders of the endocrine system
endocrinology (**en**-doh-krin-**ALL**-oh-jee) endocrin/o = endocrine -(o)logy = study of	study and treatment of endocrine system diseases and disorders
euthyroid (**YOO**-thigh-royd) eu- = normal	normal thyroid function
hormone (**HOR**-mohn)	chemical substance that affects the function of a specific organ
isthmus (**ISS**-mus)	a narrow structure connecting two parts
metabolism (meh-**TAB**-oh-lizm)	the sum of all the chemical changes that take place in the body

EXERCISE 9

Write the medical term for each definition.

1. chemical that affects the function of a specific body structure or organ _____
2. narrow structure that connects two parts _____
3. normal thyroid function _____
4. pertaining to the cortex _____
5. pertaining to the hormones of the adrenal cortex _____
6. physician who specializes in the endocrine system _____
7. study and treatment of endocrine system diseases and disorders _____
8. sum of all chemical changes in the body _____

Endocrine System Disease and Disorder Terms

Endocrine system diseases and disorders include familiar problems such as diabetes as well as more complex and less familiar diagnoses such as virilism. The medical terms are presented in alphabetical order in Table 11-6. Review the pronunciation and definition for each term and complete the exercises.

TABLE 11-6 ENDOCRINE SYSTEM DISEASE AND DISORDER TERMS

Term with Pronunciation	Definition
acidosis (ass-ih-**DOH**-sis) acid/o = sour; bitter -osis = condition	excessive acidity of body fluids
acromegaly (ak-roh-**MEG**-ah-lee) acr/o = extremities -megaly = enlargement	enlargement of the bones of the extremities and face
Addison's disease (**AD**-ih-sons)	deficiency in the secretion of adrenal cortex hormones
adrenalitis (ah-**dree**-nah-**LIGH**-tis) adren/o = adrenal gland -itis = inflammation	inflammation of the adrenal gland
adrenomegaly (ah-**dree**-no-**MEG**-ah-lee) adren/o = adrenal gland -megaly = enlargement	enlargement of the adrenal gland
cretinism (**KREE**-tin-izm)	congenital condition related to the lack of thyroid hormone secretion
Cushing's syndrome (**CUSH**-ings **SIN**-drohm)	hypersecretion of adrenal cortex glucocorticoids

TABLE 11-6 ENDOCRINE SYSTEM DISEASE AND DISORDER TERMS
(continued)

Term with Pronunciation	Definition
diabetes insipidus (**digh**-ah-**BEE**-teez in-**SIP**-ih-dus)	disorder of the pituitary gland due to a deficiency in the secretion of antidiuretic hormone (ADH)
diabetes mellitus (**digh**-ah-**BEE**-teez **MELL**-ih-tus)	disorder of carbohydrate metabolism due to insufficient insulin secretion; diabetes mellitus can be insulin-dependent (IDDM), which means the individual must inject insulin to control blood glucose levels, or non–insulin-dependent (NIDDM)
dwarfism	congenital condition characterized by abnormal underdevelopment due to a deficiency of human growth hormone
exophthalmia (**eks**-off-**THAL**-me-ah) ex- = outward ophthalm/o = eye -ia = condition	abnormal outward protrusion of the eyeball; also called *exophthalmos*
gigantism (**JIGH**-gan-tism)	excessive size and height caused by excessive secretion of growth hormone
goiter (**GOY**-ter)	hyperplasia of the thyroid gland due to a lack of dietary iodine; iodine is necessary for the production of thyroid hormones T_3 and T_4
Graves' disease	hyperthyroidism characterized by excessive secretion of thyroid hormone and exophthalmia
Hashimoto's thyroiditis (**HASH**-ee-moh-toz **thigh**-royd-**EYE**-tis) thyr/o = thyroid gland -itis = inflammation	an autoimmune disease in which the immune system produces antibodies that target thyroid cells; often results in hypothyroidism
hirsutism (**HER**-soot-izm)	excessive body hair, especially on a female in a male distribution pattern

EXERCISE 10

Analyze each term by writing the prefix, root, combining vowel, and suffix separated by vertical slashes. Based on the meaning of the word parts, write a definition for each term. Check the definition in your medical dictionary.

EXAMPLE: endocrinologist:

	/ endocrin	/ o	/ logist
prefix	*root*	*combining vowel*	*suffix*

DEFINITION: physician who specializes in the endocrine system

1. acromegaly

prefix	*root*	*combining vowel*	*suffix*

DEFINITION: _____

2. acidosis

prefix	*root*	*combining vowel*	*suffix*

DEFINITION: _____

3. adrenalitis

prefix	*root*	*combining vowel*	*suffix*

DEFINITION: _____

4. adrenomegaly

prefix	*root*	*combining vowel*	*suffix*

DEFINITION: _____

5. exophthalmia

prefix	*root*	*combining vowel*	*suffix*

DEFINITION: _____

EXERCISE 11

Replace the italicized medical term with its definition.

1. Gina was recently diagnosed with *diabetes mellitus.*

   _____

2. Maintaining iodine in the diet prevents the development of a *goiter.*

   _____

3. Roberta's *hirsutism* was corrected after she began hormone replacement therapy.

   _____

4. *Cretinism* is usually accompanied by arrested physical and mental development.

   _____

5. *Cushing's syndrome* is usually caused by an adrenal tumor.

_____

6. Adrenal gland hemorrhage might result in *Addison's disease*.

_____

EXERCISE 12

Match the medical term in Column 1 with the correct definition in Column 2.

COLUMN 1

____ 1. acidosis

____ 2. acromegaly

____ 3. Addison's disease

____ 4. adrenomegaly

____ 5. diabetes insipidus

____ 6. diabetes mellitus

____ 7. exophthalmos

____ 8. gigantism

____ 9. goiter

____ 10. Graves' disease

COLUMN 2

a. abnormal eyeball protrusion

b. deficient secretion of adrenal cortex hormones

c. disorder of the pituitary gland

d. excessive acidity of body fluids

e. enlarged thyroid gland

f. enlarged adrenal gland

g. excessive size and height

h. enlargement of the extremities

i. hyperthyroidism with exophthalmia

j. insufficient insulin secretion

Review the pronunciation and definition for each term in Table 11-7 and complete the exercises.

TABLE 11-7   ENDOCRINE SYSTEM DISEASE AND DISORDER TERMS

Term with Pronunciation	Definition
hypercalcemia (**high**-per-kal-**SEE**-mee-ah) hyper- = excessive calc/o = calcium -emia = blood condition	excessive amount of calcium in the blood
hyperglycemia (**high**-per-gligh-**SEE**-mee-ah) hyper- = excessive glyc/o = glucose; sugar; sweet -emia = blood condition	excessive amount of glucose in the blood
hyperkalemia (**high**-per-kal-**EE**-mee-ah) hyper- = excessive kal/i = potassium -emia = blood condition	excessive amount of potassium in the blood

TABLE 11-7 ENDOCRINE SYSTEM DISEASE AND DISORDER TERMS
(continued)

Term with Pronunciation	Definition
hyperthyroidism (**high**-per-**THIGH**-royd-izm) hyper- = excessive thyroid/o = thyroid gland -ism = condition	overactivity of the thyroid gland
hypocalcemia (**high**-poh-kal-**SEE**-mee-ah) hypo- = decreased calc/o = calcium -emia = blood condition	decreased amount of calcium in the blood
hypoglycemia (**high**-poh-gligh-**SEE**-mee-ah) hypo- = decreased glyc/o = glucose; sugar; sweet -emia = blood condition	decreased amount of glucose in the blood
hypokalemia (**high**-poh-kal-**EE**-mee-ah) hypo- = decreased kal/i = potassium -emia = blood condition	decreased amount of potassium in the blood
hyponatremia (**high**-poh-nah-**TREE**-mee-ah) hypo- = decreased natr/o = sodium -emia = blood condition	decreased amount of sodium in the blood
hypothyroidism (**high**-poh-**THIGH**-royd-izm) hypo- = decreased thyroid/o = thyroid gland -ism = condition	decreased activity of the thyroid gland
ketoacidosis (**kee**-toh-**ass**-ih-**DOH**-sis) ket/o = ketone bodies acid/o = sour; bitter -osis = condition	accumulation of ketone bodies and an increase in the acidity of the blood
myxedema (miks-eh-**DEE**-mah)	the most severe form of adult hypothyroidism
pancreatitis (**pan**-kree-ah-**TIGH**-tis) pancreat/o = pancreas -itis = inflammation	inflammation of the pancreas

(continues)

TABLE 11-7   ENDOCRINE SYSTEM DISEASE AND DISORDER TERMS
(continued)

Term with Pronunciation	Definition
polydipsia (pall-ee-**DIP**-see-ah) poly- = excessive dips/o = thirst -ia = condition	excessive thirst
thyroiditis (**thigh**-royd-**EYE**-tis) thyr/o = thyroid gland -itis = inflammation	chronic inflammation and enlargement of the thyroid gland
thyrotoxicosis (**thigh**-roh-toks-ih-**KOH**-sis) thyr/o = thyroid toxic/o = poison -osis = condition	toxic condition caused by hyperactivity of the thyroid gland
virilism (**VEER**-il-izm)	development of masculine physical traits in a female

EXERCISE 13

Analyze each term by writing the prefix, root, combining vowel, and suffix separated by vertical slashes. Based on the meaning of the word parts, write a definition for each term. Check the definition in a medical dictionary.

1. hypercalcemia

   _____
   prefix   *root*   *combining vowel*   *suffix*
   DEFINITION: _____

2. hyperglycemia

   _____
   prefix   *root*   *combining vowel*   *suffix*
   DEFINITION: _____

3. hyperkalemia

   _____
   prefix   *root*   *combining vowel*   *suffix*
   DEFINITION: _____

4. hyperthyroidism

   _____
   prefix   *root*   *combining vowel*   *suffix*
   DEFINITION: _____

5. hypocalcemia

   _____
   prefix   *root*   *combining vowel*   *suffix*
   DEFINITION: _____

6. hypoglycemia

prefix	root	combining vowel	suffix

DEFINITION: _____

7. hypokalemia

prefix	root	combining vowel	suffix

DEFINITION: _____

8. hyponatremia

prefix	root	combining vowel	suffix

DEFINITION: _____

9. hypothyroidism

prefix	root	combining vowel	suffix

DEFINITION: _____

10. pancreatitis

prefix	root	combining vowel	suffix

DEFINITION: _____

11. polydipsia

prefix	root	combining vowel	suffix

DEFINITION: _____

12. thyrotoxicosis

prefix	root	combining vowel	suffix

DEFINITION: _____

EXERCISE 14

Replace the italicized phrase with the correct medical term.

1. Uncontrolled diabetes mellitus might result in *an accumulation of ketone bodies and increased acidity in the blood.*

   _____

2. *The most severe form of adult hypothyroidism* is a life-threatening endocrine disease.

   _____

3. Lack of female hormones might contribute to *the development of masculine traits in a female.*

   _____

4. *Excessive thirst* is a symptom of diabetes mellitus.

   _____

5. *A decreased amount of potassium in the blood* has serious implications for heart function.

_____

6. Insufficient insulin secretion leads to *excessive amounts of glucose in the blood.*

_____

7. *Inflammation of the pancreas* might interfere with adequate hormone secretion.

_____

8. Weight control is an issue for individuals who have *decreased activity of the thyroid gland.*

_____

Endocrine System Diagnostic, Laboratory, and Treatment Terms

Review the pronunciation and definition of the diagnostic, laboratory, and treatment terms in Table 11-8 and complete the exercise.

TABLE 11-8 ENDOCRINE SYSTEM DIAGNOSTIC, LABORATORY, AND TREATMENT TERMS

Laboratory/Diagnostic Tests	Definition
fasting blood sugar (FBS)	blood test that measures the amount of glucose in the blood; screening test for diabetes mellitus
glucose tolerance test (GTT)	blood test that measures blood glucose levels over a period of time, usually 2 to 3 hours
hemoglobin A1c (HgA1c)	blood test that evaluates and measures blood glucose levels for the preceeding two or three months; used to monitor blood glucose control in individuals with diabetes
radioactive iodine uptake (RAIU)	thyroid function test that measures thyroid activity by determining the amount of radioactive iodine taken up by the thyroid gland
thyroid function tests	blood tests that measure the blood levels of the thyroid hormones T_3 and T_4
thyroid scan	nuclear medicine imaging scan to determine the size, shape, and function of the thyroid gland
thyroid-stimulating hormone test	blood test that measures the concentration of thyroid-stimulating hormone in the blood

(continues)

TABLE 11-8 ENDOCRINE SYSTEM DIAGNOSTIC, LABORATORY,
AND TREATMENT TERMS (continued)

Treatment Terms with Pronunciation	Definition
adrenalectomy (ah-**dreen**-al-**EK**-toh-mee) adrenal/o = adrenal gland -ectomy = surgical removal	surgical removal of one or both of the adrenal glands
parathyroidectomy (**pair**-ah-**thigh**-royd-**EK**-toh-mee) parathyroid/o = parathyroid gland -ectomy = surgical removal	surgical removal of one or all of the parathyroid glands
thyroidectomy (**thigh**-royd-**EK**-toh-mee) thyroid/o = thyroid gland -ectomy = surgical removal	surgical removal of all or part of the thyroid

EXERCISE 15

Match the diagnostic and treatment terms in Column 1 with the definitions in Column 2.

COLUMN 1

_____ 1. adrenalectomy

_____ 2. fasting blood sugar

_____ 3. glucose tolerance test

_____ 4. parathyroidectomy

_____ 5. radioactive iodine uptake

_____ 6. thyroid function tests

_____ 7. thyroid scan

_____ 8. thyroid-stimulating hormone test

_____ 9. thyroidectomy

COLUMN 2

a. excision of all or part of the thyroid gland

b. measures blood levels of thyroid-stimulating hormone

c. measures the level of T_3 and T_4 in the blood

d. screening test for diabetes mellitus

e. removal of one or both of the adrenal glands

f. nuclear medicine imaging scan of the thyroid

g. measures blood glucose levels over a period of time

h. surgical removal of one or all of the parathyroid glands

i. measures thyroid activity using iodine

Abbreviations

Review the endocrine system abbreviations in Table 11-9. Practice writing out the meaning of each abbreviation.

TABLE 11-9 ABBREVIATIONS

Abbreviation	Meaning
ACTH	adrenocorticotropic hormone
ADH	antidiuretic hormone
FBS	fasting blood sugar
FSH	follicle-stimulating hormone
GH	growth hormone
GTT	glucose tolerance test
IDDM	insulin-dependent diabetes mellitus
LH	luteinizing hormone
MSH	melanocyte-stimulating hormone
NIDDM	non–insulin-dependent diabetes mellitus
PTH	parathyroid hormone
RAIU	radioactive iodine uptake test
STH	somatotropin hormone
T_3	triiodothyronine
T_4	thyroxine
TSH	thyroid-stimulating hormone

CHAPTER REVIEW

The Chapter Review can be used as a self-test. Go through each exercise and answer as many questions as you can without referring to previous exercises or earlier discussions within this chapter. Check your answers and fill in any blanks. Practice writing any terms you might have misspelled.

EXERCISE 16

Write the medical term for each definition.

1. excessive acidity of body fluids _____

2. enlargement of the bones of the extremities and face _____

3. inflammation of the adrenal gland _____

4. enlargement of the adrenal gland _____

5. abnormal outward protrusion of the eyeball _____

6. overactivity of the thyroid gland _____

7. increased glucose in the blood _____

8. most severe form of adult hypothyroidism _____

9. inflammation of the pancreas _____

10. excessive thirst _____

11. toxic condition due to hyperactivity of the
    thyroid gland _____

12. development of masculine physical traits
    in a female _____

13. male-pattern hair distribution in a female _____

14. surgical removal of the thyroid gland _____

15. enlarged thyroid gland due to hypertrophy of
    thyroid cells and tissue _____

EXERCISE 17

Write the names of the following hormones next to the endocrine gland that secretes the hormone.

ACTH	cortisol	insulin	PTH
androgen	epinephrine	noradrenaline	testosterone
aldosterone	FSH	oxytocin	T_3, T_4
antidiuretic hormone	glucagon	prolactin	TSH
calcitonin	growth hormone	progesterone	thymopoietin

1. pituitary gland _____

2. thyroid gland _____

3. parathyroid glands _____

4. thymus _____

5. pancreas _____

6. adrenal glands _____

7. ovaries _____

8. testes _____

EXERCISE 18

Read the following progress notes. For progress notes A and B, define each italicized term in the space provided; for progress note C, write the medical term for the italicized phrase.

PROGRESS NOTE A

Viola was seen today for a (1) *glucose tolerance test*. Her (2) *fasting blood sugar*, which was done two days ago, indicated hyperglycemia, which might indicate diabetes mellitus. The results of the GTT will confirm or rule out that diagnosis.

1. _____

2. _____

PROGRESS NOTE B

Gerald has recent complaints of fatigue, lack of energy, and weight gain. His initial (3) *thyroid function test* showed a decreased level of T_3 and T_4. A follow-up (4) *thyroid-stimulating hormone test* ruled out pituitary malfunction. A (5) *thyroid scan* is scheduled for tomorrow.

3. _____

4. _____

5. _____

PROGRESS NOTE C

Alonzo is seen today for a complete evaluation of endocrine gland function. He is very concerned because his family history is positive for the following: Paternal grandfather underwent (6) *the surgical removal of adrenal glands* at age 54; his mother had a (7) *surgical removal of the thyroid gland* at age 45; and his father, age 62, recently was treated for hyperparathyroidism with (8) *a surgical removal of the parathyroid glands.*

6. _____

7. _____

8. _____

EXERCISE 19

Write out the following endocrine system abbreviations.

1. FBS _____

2. ADH _____

3. GTT _____

4. IDDM _____

5. NIDDM _____

6. FSH _____

7. TSH _____

8. GH _____

9. MSH _____

10. LH _____

EXERCISE 20

Select the best answer for each statement or question.

1. Which endocrine gland has two lobes that secrete different hormones?
   a. parathyroid gland
   b. thyroid gland
   c. pineal gland
   d. pituitary gland

2. Select the hormone that is responsible for stimulating the release of breast milk.
   a. oxytocin
   b. luteinizing hormone
   c. prolactin
   d. follicle-stimulating hormone

3. Choose the hormone that stimulates breast development and milk production.
   a. oxytocin
   b. prolactin
   c. luteinizing hormone
   d. follicle-stimulating hormone

4. Which term means development of masculine physical traits in a female?
   a. hirsutism
   b. testosteronism
   c. virilism
   d. myxedema

5. Select the disease associated with insufficient insulin secretion.
   a. diabetes insipidus
   b. diabetes mellitus
   c. pancreatitis
   d. acromegaly

6. Which term means excessive body hair on a female in a male pattern?
   a. virilism
   b. acromegaly
   c. testosteronism
   d. hirsutism

7. Select the term for an enlarged thyroid gland.
   a. goiter
   b. Graves' disease
   c. exophthalmia
   d. thyroidosis

8. Which disease is caused by an insufficient secretion of ADH?
   a. diabetes mellitus
   b. Graves' disease
   c. acromegaly
   d. diabetes insipidus

9. Select the blood test that is a screening test for diabetes mellitus.
   a. glucose tolerance test
   b. fasting blood sugar
   c. insulin secretion test
   d. pancreatic hormone screening test

10. Which term is defined as the most severe form of adult hypothyroidism?
    a. cretinism
    b. Cushing's syndrome
    c. myxedema
    d. acromegaly

CHALLENGE EXERCISE

Diabetes mellitus is a serious health problem that can affect many organs in the body, especially the eyes and kidneys. Research how this disease affects one of these organ pairs. Information should be available from the local public health department, the local hospital's patient education department, or the American Diabetic Association's Web site. If you search the Internet, keywords are diabetes mellitus or American Diabetic Association.

Pronunciation Review

Review the terms in this chapter. Pronounce each term using the following phonetic pronunciations. Check off the term when you are comfortable saying it.

TERM	PRONUNCIATION
☐ acidosis	ass-ih-**DOH**-sis
☐ acromegaly	ak-roh-**MEG**-ah-lee
☐ Addison's disease	**AD**-ih-sons disease
☐ adrenalectomy	ah-**dree**-nal-**EK**-toh-mee
☐ adrenal gland	ah-**DREE**-nal gland
☐ adrenalitis	ah-**dree**-nah-**LIGH**-tis
☐ adrenomegaly	ah-**dree**-noh-**MEG**-ah-lee
☐ calcitonin	**kal**-sih-**TOH**-nin
☐ cortical	**KOR**-tih-kal
☐ cretinism	**KREE**-tin-izm
☐ Cushing's syndrome	**CUSH**-ings **SIN**-drohm
☐ diabetes insipidus	**digh**-ah-**BEE**-teez in-**SIP**-ih-dus
☐ diabetes mellitus	**digh**-ah-**BEE**-teez **MELL**-ih-tus
☐ dwarfism	**DWARF**-ism
☐ endocrinologist	**en**-doh-krin-**ALL**-oh-jist
☐ endocrinology	**en**-doh-krin-**ALL**-oh-jee
☐ estrogen	**ESS**-troh-jen
☐ euthyroid	**YOO**-thigh-royd
☐ exophthalmia	**eks**-off-**THAL**-mee-ah
☐ exophthalmos	**eks**-off-**THAL**-mohs
☐ gigantism	**JIGH**-gan-tizm
☐ glucagon	**GLOO**-kah-gon
☐ glucose tolerance test (GTT)	**GLOO**-kohs **TALL**-er-ans test
☐ goiter	**GOY**-ter
☐ Hashimoto's thyroiditis	**HASH**-ee-moh-toz **thigh**-royd-**EYE**-tis
☐ hirsutism	**HER**-soot-izm
☐ hormone	**HOR**-mohn
☐ hypercalcemia	**high**-per-kal-**SEE**-mee-ah
☐ hyperglycemia	**high**-per-gligh-**SEE**-mee-ah
☐ hyperkalemia	**high**-per-kal-**EE**-mee-ah
☐ hyperthyroidism	**high**-per-**THIGH**-royd-izm

☐ hypocalcemia	**high**-poh-kal-**SEE**-mee-ah
☐ hypoglycemia	**high**-poh-gligh-**SEE**-mee-ah
☐ hypokalemia	**high**-poh-kal-**EE**-mee-ah
☐ hyponatremia	**high**-poh-nah-**TREE**-mee-ah
☐ hypothyroidism	**high**-poh-**THIGH**-royd-izm
☐ insulin	**IN**-suh-lin
☐ islets of Langerhans	**EYE**-lets of **LONG**-er-honz
☐ isthmus	**ISS**-mus
☐ ketoacidosis	**kee**-toh-**ass**-ih-**DOH**-sis
☐ melatonin	mell-ah-**TOH**-nin
☐ metabolism	meh-**TAB**-oh-lizm
☐ myxedema	miks-eh-**DEE**-mah
☐ ovaries	**OH**-vah-reez
☐ pancreas	**PAN**-kree-as
☐ pancreatitis	**pan**-kree-ah-**TIGH**-tis
☐ parathyroidectomy	**pair**-ah-**thigh**-royd-**EK**-toh-me
☐ parathyroid gland	**pair**-ah-**THIGH**-royd gland
☐ parathyroid hormone	**pair**-ah-**THIGH**-royd **HOR**-mohn
☐ pineal gland	**PIN**-ee-al gland
☐ pituitary gland	pih-**TOO**-ih-tair-ee gland
☐ polydipsia	pall-oo-**DIP**-see-ah
☐ progesterone	proh-**JESS**-ter-ohn
☐ testes	**TESS**-teez
☐ testosterone	tess-**TOSS**-ter-ohn
☐ thymopoietin	**thigh**-moh-**POY**-eh-tin
☐ thymosin	**thigh MOH**-sin
☐ thymus	**THIGH**-mus
☐ thyroidectomy	**thigh**-royd-**EK**-toh-mee
☐ thyroiditis	**thigh**-royd-**EYE**-tis
☐ thyrotoxicosis	**thigh**-roh-toks-ih-**KOH**-sis
☐ thyroxine (T4)	thigh-**ROKS**-in
☐ triiodothyronine	try-**eye**-oh-doh-**THIGH**-roh-neen
☐ virilism	**VEER**-il-izm

Chapter 12
Male Reproductive System

OBJECTIVES

At the completion of this chapter, the student should be able to:

1. Identify, define, and spell word roots associated with the male reproductive system.
2. Label the basic structures of the male reproductive system.
3. Discuss the functions of the male reproductive system.
4. Provide the correct spelling of male reproductive system terms, given the definition of the terms.
5. Analyze the male reproductive system terms by defining the roots, prefixes, and suffixes of these terms.
6. Identify, define, and spell disease, disorder, and procedure terms related to the male reproductive system.
7. Describe the characteristics of sexually transmitted infections.

OVERVIEW

The structures of the male reproductive system include the testes, epididymis, vas deferens, seminal vesicle, ejaculatory duct, prostate gland, Cowper's gland, urethra, and penis. These structures function to produce male hormones and to produce, sustain, and transport **spermatozoa** (sper-**mat**-oh-**ZOH**-ah), usually called *sperm*. The reproductive structures are collectively known as the male **genitalia** (jen-ih-**TAY**-lee-ah).

This chapter also covers sexually transmitted infections. Information includes the characteristics, lesions, and symptoms associated with the infections.

Male Reproductive System Word Roots

To understand and use male reproductive system medical terms, it is necessary to acquire a thorough knowledge of the associated word roots. Word roots associated with the male reproductive system are listed with the combining vowel. Review the word roots in Table 12-1 and complete the exercises that follow.

TABLE 12-1   MALE REPRODUCTIVE SYSTEM WORD ROOTS

Word Root/Combining Form	Meaning
andr/o	male
balan/o	glans penis
hydr/o	water

(continues)

TABLE 12-1   MALE REPRODUCTIVE SYSTEM WORD ROOTS (continued)

Word Root/Combining Form	Meaning
orch/o; orchi/o; orchid/o	testis; testicle
prostat/o	prostate gland
semin/i	semen
sperm/o; spermat/o	sperm; spermatic cord
test/o; testicul/o	testes; testis; testicle
vas/o	vessel

EXERCISE 1

Write the definitions of the following word roots.

1. spermat/o   _____
2. orchid/o   _____
3. prostat/o   _____
4. vas/o   _____
5. test/o   _____
6. crypt/o   _____
7. orch/o   _____
8. epididym/o   _____
9. semin/i   _____
10. andr/o   _____
11. hydr/o   _____

EXERCISE 2

Write the word root and its meaning on the spaces provided.

1. hydrocele

   ROOT:_____   MEANING: _____

2. vasectomy

   ROOT:_____   MEANING: _____

3. android

   ROOT:_____   MEANING: _____

4. prostatectomy

   ROOT:_____   MEANING: _____

5. epididymitis

   ROOT:_____   MEANING: _____

6. balanitis

   ROOT:_____   MEANING: _____

7. cryptorchidism

ROOT: _____   MEANING: _____

8. seminal vesicles

ROOT: _____   MEANING: _____

9. orchidectomy

ROOT: _____   MEANING: _____

EXERCISE 3

Write the correct word root(s) for the following definitions.

1. testicle _____

2. epididymis _____

3. male _____

4. hidden _____

5. prostate gland _____

6. semen _____

7. vessel _____

8. sperm _____

Structures of the Male Reproductive System

The male reproductive system is made up of the (1) **testes** (**TESS**-teez) (pl.), (2) **scrotum** (**SKROH**-tum), (3) **epididymis** (**ep**-ih-**DID**-ih-miss), (4) **vas deferens** (**VAZ DEFF**-er-enz), (5) **seminal vesicle** (**SEM**-ih-nall **VESS**-ih-kal), (6) **ejaculatory** (ee-**JACK**-yoo-lah-**tor**-ee) **duct**, (7) **prostate** (**PROSS**-tayt) **gland**, (8) **Cowper's** (**COW**-perz) **glands**, (9) **urethra**, and (10) **penis**. Figure 12-1 illustrates the structures of the male reproductive system. The structures of this system are discussed individually.

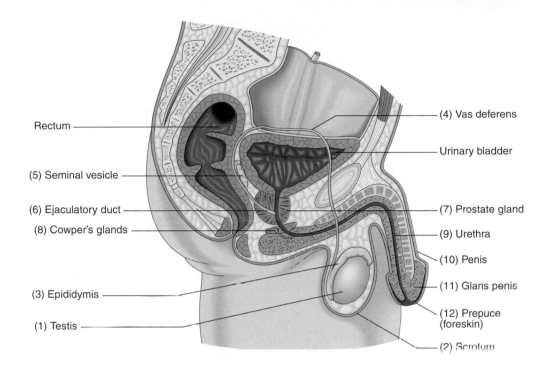

Rectum

(5) Seminal vesicle

(6) Ejaculatory duct

(8) Cowper's glands

(3) Epididymis

(1) Testis

(4) Vas deferens

Urinary bladder

(7) Prostate gland

(9) Urethra

(10) Penis

(11) Glans penis

(12) Prepuce (foreskin)

(2) Scrotum

Figure 12-1   Male reproductive system

Testes, Epididymis, and Vas Deferens

The (1) testes, also called *testicles*, are the male gonads, or sex organs. They develop in the abdominal cavity and eventually descend into the scrotum, the sac that houses the testes. Figure 12-2 illustrates a testis and related structures. Refer to this figure as you learn about the testes.

The (1) testes are composed of tiny, coiled tubules called (2) **seminiferous tubules** (sem-ih-NIFF-er-us TOO-byools), which are responsible for sperm production. The tissue between the tubules secretes the male sex hormone testosterone.

The (3) epididymis, which is a continuation of the seminiferous tubules, is a tightly coiled tube on the testes. Sperm mature and become motile (i.e., able to move) in the epididymis. The (4) vas deferens, which is a continuation of the epididymis, leaves the scrotum, passes around the urinary bladder, and eventually connects with the urethra. Part of the vas deferens is illustrated in Figure 12-2. Refer to Figure 12-1 for an illustration of the entire vas deferens.

Each testicle is suspended by a (5) **spermatic cord** that contains blood and lymph vessels, nerves, and the vas deferens.

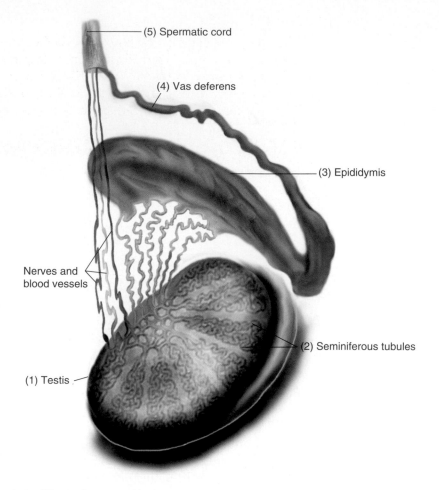

Figure12-2　Testis (testes, pl.)

Seminal Vesicles, Ejaculatory Duct, and Cowper's Gland

Refer to Figure 12-1 for an illustration of the seminal vesicles, ejaculatory duct, and Cowper's glands. The (5) seminal vesicles, two glands located behind the urinary bladder, open into the vas deferens and secrete a thick fluid called seminal fluid. Seminal fluid is part of the **semen**, which is the substance discharged from the penis.

The seminal vesicles narrow into a straight duct that joins with the vas deferens to form the (6) ejaculatory duct. The ejaculatory duct passes through the (7) prostate gland and joins with the urethra.

The (8) Cowper's glands, also called the **bulbourethral** (**bull**-boh-yoo-**REE**-thrall) **glands**, are a pair of glands that lie just below the prostate gland. The Cowper's glands secrete a mucus-like fluid into the urethra. The fluid, which is a component of semen, provides lubrication during intercourse.

Prostate Gland

The (7) prostate gland lies at the base of the bladder and surrounds the urethra. Refer to Figure 12-1 for an illustration of the prostate gland. The prostate gland secretes a milky-colored fluid that enhances sperm motility and helps neutralize vaginal secretions. Prostate fluid is added to the semen via ducts that open into the urethra. During ejaculation, the muscular action of the prostate gland helps propel semen through the urethra into the vagina.

Penis

The (10) penis consists of a base that attaches the penis to the pubic region, a shaft or body that becomes engorged with blood during arousal, and a tip or head called the (11) **glans penis**. Refer to Figure 12-1 for an illustration of the penis. A retractable fold of skin called the (12) **prepuce** (**PREE**-pus), or foreskin, covers the glans penis. The prepuce is often removed by a procedure known as **circumcision**.

EXERCISE 4

Label the structures of the male reproductive system as shown in Figure 12-3. Write your answer in the spaces provided.

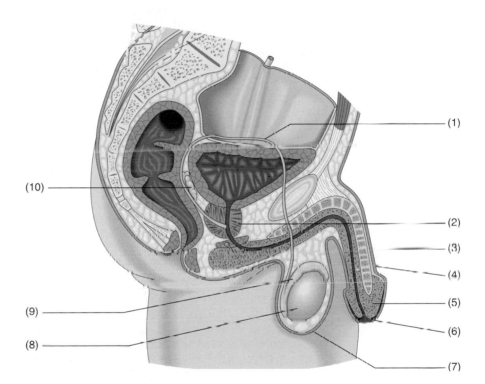

Figure 12-3 Male reproductive system labeling exercise

1. _____
2. _____
3. _____
4. _____
5. _____
6. _____
7. _____
8. _____
9. _____
10. _____

EXERCISE 5

Match the male reproductive system structures in Column 1 with the correct definition in Column 2.

COLUMN 1

_____ 1. Cowper's glands

_____ 2. epididymis

_____ 3. glans penis

_____ 4. penis

_____ 5. prepuce

_____ 6. prostate gland

_____ 7. scrotum

_____ 8. seminal vesicle

_____ 9. sperm

_____ 10. testes

_____ 11. vas deferens

COLUMN 2

a. assists in the ejaculation of semen

b. continuation of the epididymis

c. fold of retractable skin; foreskin

d. gonads; male sex glands

e. male sex cell

f. male sex organ

g. provides lubrication during intercourse

h. secretes seminal fluid

i. sac containing the testicles

j. tightly coiled tubules; sperm mature here

k. tip of the penis

Male Reproductive System Medical Terminology

Male reproductive system medical terms are organized into three main categories: (1) general medical terms; (2) disease and condition terms; and (3) diagnostic procedure, surgery, and laboratory test terms. The word roots *olig/o*, which means "few" or "diminished," and *varic/o*, which means "twisted veins," are used in a few male reproductive system medical terms. The roots, prefixes, and suffixes associated with the male reproductive system are listed in Table 12-2. Review these word parts and complete the related exercises.

TABLE 12-2   ROOTS, PREFIXES, AND SUFFIXES FOR MALE REPRODUCTIVE SYSTEM

Root	Meaning	Prefix	Meaning	Suffix	Meaning
cry/o	cold	a-	lack of; without	-cele	hernia; protrusion
olig/o	few; diminished	carcin-	cancer; malignant	-genesis	producing
				-oma	tumor
varic/o	twisted veins	epi-	upon; on	-pexy	surgical fixation
		hypo-	beneath; below		
				-plasty	surgical repair
				-(r)rhea	flow; discharge
				-trophy	growth; development

EXERCISE 6

Each term has either a prefix, suffix, or both. Write the prefix and suffix and its meaning on the spaces provided.

1. aspermia

   PREFIX: _____ MEANING: _____

   SUFFIX: _____ MEANING: _____

2. hypertrophy

   PREFIX: _____ MEANING: _____

   SUFFIX: _____ MEANING: _____

3. epispadias

   PREFIX: _____ MEANING: _____

   SUFFIX: _____ MEANING: _____

4. gonorrhea

   PREFIX: _____ MEANING: _____

   SUFFIX: _____ MEANING: _____

5. spermatocele

   PREFIX: _____ MEANING: _____

   SUFFIX: _____ MEANING: _____

6. spermatogenesis

   PREFIX: _____ MEANING: _____

   SUFFIX: _____ MEANING: _____

7. orchidopexy

   PREFIX: _____ MEANING: _____

   SUFFIX: _____ MEANING: _____

8. orchidoplasty

   PREFIX: _____ MEANING: _____

   SUFFIX: _____ MEANING: _____

Male Reproductive System General Medical Terms

Review the pronunciation and meaning of each term in Table 12-3. Complete the exercise for these terms.

TABLE 12–3 MALE REPRODUCTIVE SYSTEM GENERAL MEDICAL TERMS

Term with Pronunciation	Definition
ejaculation (ee-**jack**-yoo-**LAY**-shun)	expulsion of semen from the penis
genitalia (jen-ih-**TAY**-lee-ah)	male and female reproductive structures

(continues)

TABLE 12–3   MALE REPRODUCTIVE SYSTEM GENERAL MEDICAL TERMS (continued)

Term with Pronunciation	Definition
sexually transmitted disease (STD) sexually transmited infection (STI)	any disease that is spread from one person to another during any type of sexual contact
spermatogenesis (**sperm**-at-oh-**JEN**-eh-sis) spermat/o = sperm -genesis = formation	formation of mature sperm
testosterone (tess-**TOSS**-ter-ohn)	male hormone
urologist (yoor-**ALL**-oh-jist) ur/o = urine -(o)logist = specialist	physician who specializes in the study of the male reproductive and urinary systems

EXERCISE 7

Replace the italicized phrase with the correct medical term.

1. Chlamydia is classified as a *disease acquired as a result of sexual intercourse.*

   _____

2. Sperm are deposited in the vagina when *the expulsion of semen* occurs.

   _____

3. *The male hormone* is necessary for the development of male secondary sex characteristics.

   _____

4. After experiencing testicular pain, Roger made an appointment with a *physician specialist for the male reproductive system.*

   _____

5. Healthy *formation of mature sperm* is a necessary component of male fertility.

   _____

6. The *male reproductive structures* include both internal and external organs and glands.

   _____

Male Reproductive System Disease and Disorder Terms

Male reproductive system diseases and disorders include familiar problems such as prostate cancer as well as more complex and less familiar diagnoses such as priapism. Medical terms related specifically to the male reproductive system are discussed first. Sexually transmitted infections, which affect both male and female reproductive structures, are discussed second. In both cases, the terms are presented in alphabetical order in Table 12-4. Review the pronunciation and definition for each term and complete the exercises.

TABLE 12-4 MALE REPRODUCTIVE SYSTEM DISEASE AND
DISORDER TERMS

Term with Pronunciation	Definition
anorchism (an-**ORK**-izm) an- = without orch/i = testes -ism = condition	absence of one or both testes
aspermia (ah-**SPERM**-ee-ah) a- = lack of; without sperm/o = sperm -ia = condition	lack or absence of sperm
balanitis (bal-ah-**NIGH**-tis) balan/o = glans penis -itis = inflammation	inflammation of the glans penis
benign prostatic hypertrophy (BPH) (bee-**NIGHN** pross-**TAT**-ik high-**PER**-troh-fee) prostat/o = prostate -ic = pertaining to hyper- = excessive -trophy = growth; development	noncancerous enlargement of the prostate gland
cryptorchidism (kript-**OR**-kid-izm) crypt/o = hidden orchid/o = testes -ism = condition	undescended testicle; failure of one or both testes to descend into the scrotum
epididymitis (**ep**-ih-**did**-ih-**MIGH**-tis) epididym/o = epididymis -itis = inflammation	inflammation of the epididymis
epispadias (**ep**-ih-**SPAY**-dee-as)	congenital condition in which the urethra opens on the upper side of the penis (Figure 12-4)

(continues)

TABLE 12-4 MALE REPRODUCTIVE SYSTEM DISEASE AND DISORDER TERMS (continued)

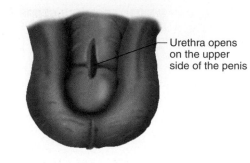

Urethra opens on the upper side of the penis

Urethra opens on the underside of the penis

Figure 12-4 Epispadias and hypospadias

Term with Pronunciation	Definition
erectile dysfunction	inability to achieve or maintain an erection; impotence
hydrocele (**HIGH**-droh-seel) hydr/o = water -cele = hernia; protrusion	accumulation of fluid in the scrotum or along the spermatic cord
hypospadias (**high**-poh-**SPAY**-dee-as)	congenital condition in which the urethra opens on the underside of the penis (Figure 12-4)
impotence (**IM**-poh-tens)	inability to achieve or maintain an erection; erectile dysfunction
indirect inguinal hernia (**ING**-gwih-nal **HER**-nee-ah)	protrusion of the intestine through the internal inguinal ring, possibly descending into the scrotum
oligospermia (**all**-ih-goh-**SPER**-mee-ah) olig/o = few; deficient sperm/o = sperm -ia = condition	deficient number of sperm present in semen
orchitis (or-**KIGH**-tis) orch/i = testes -itis = inflammation	inflammation of the testes
phimosis (fih-**MOH**-sis)	tightness of the prepuce, or foreskin, that prevents it from being pulled back from the glans penis
premature ejaculation	expulsion of semen before complete erection or immediately after vaginal penetration

(continues)

TABLE 12-4 MALE REPRODUCTIVE SYSTEM DISEASE AND DISORDER TERMS (continued)

Term with Pronunciation	Definition
priapism	abnormal, painful, and prolonged erection of the penis not related to sexual arousal
prostate cancer	malignant tumor or neoplasm of the prostate gland
prostatitis (**pross**-tah-**TIGH**-tis) prostat/o = prostate gland -itis = inflammation	Inflammation of the prostate gland
spermatolysis (sper-mah-**TALL**-ih-sis) spermat/o = sperm -lysis = destruction; break down	destruction, dissolution, or break down of sperm
testicular carcinoma (tess-**TICK**-yoo-lar **kar**-sin-**OH**-ma) testicul/o = testes; testicles -ar = pertaining to carcin- = cancer; malignant -oma = tumor	malignant tumor of one or both testes
varicocele (**VAIR**-ih-koh-seel) varic/o = enlarged; twisted veins -cele = hernia; protrusion	enlarged, twisted, and swollen veins of the spermatic cord

EXERCISE 8

Analyze each term by writing the prefix, root, combining vowel, and suffix separated by vertical slashes. Based on the meaning of the word parts, write a definition for each term. Check the definition in a medical dictionary. Note that some terms may have more than one root.

EXAMPLE: urologist:

	/ ur	/ o	/ logist
prefix	*root*	*combining vowel*	*suffix*

DEFINITION: specialist in the male reproductive and urinary system

1. anorchism

prefix	*root*	*combining vowel*	*suffix*

DEFINITION: _____

2. aspermia

prefix	*root*	*combining vowel*	*suffix*

DEFINITION: _____

3. balanitis

prefix	root	combining vowel	suffix

DEFINITION: _____

4. cryptorchidism

prefix	root	combining vowel	suffix

DEFINITION: _____

5. epididymitis

prefix	root	combining vowel	suffix

DEFINITION: _____

6. hydrocele

prefix	root	combining vowel	suffix

DEFINITION: _____

7. oligospermia

prefix	root	combining vowel	suffix

DEFINITION: _____

8. orchitis

prefix	root	combining vowel	suffix

DEFINITION: _____

9. prostatitis

prefix	root	combining vowel	suffix

DEFINITION: _____

10. spermatolysis

prefix	root	combining vowel	suffix

DEFINITION: _____

EXERCISE 9

Replace the italicized phrase with the correct medical term.

1. Calhoun's diagnosis was *noncancerous enlargement of the prostate gland.*

   _____

2. *Urethral opening on the underside of the penis* is a congenital condition that may require surgery.

   _____

3. The *inability to achieve or maintain an erection* may be caused by a physical or psychological condition.

   _____

4. Baby boy Smith was born with *a urethral opening on the upper side of the penis.*

   _____

5. A *protrusion of the intestine through the internal inguinal ring* can be corrected with surgery.

   _____

6. *Tightness of the foreskin* prevents proper cleansing of the penis.

   _____

7. Ziad sought treatment for *abnormal, painful, and prolonged erection of the penis.*

   _____

8. Surgical intervention or radiation may be used to treat *a malignant tumor of one or both testes.*

   _____

9. *Enlargement of the veins of the spermatic cord* may lead to male infertility.

   _____

EXERCISE 10

Match the medical terms in Column 1 with the descriptions in Column 2.

COLUMN 1	COLUMN 2
_____ 1. BPH	a. abnormal, prolonged, and painful penile erection
_____ 2. epispadias	b. accumulation of fluid in the scrotum or spermatic cord
_____ 3. hydrocele	
_____ 4. hypospadias	c. congenital condition; urethra on the underside of the penis
_____ 5. impotence	
_____ 6. phimosis	d. destruction or breakdown of sperm
_____ 7. priapism	e. enlarged veins of the spermatic cord
_____ 8. prostate cancer	f. erectile dysfunction
_____ 9. spermatolysis	g. malignant tumor of the prostate
_____ 10. varicocele	h. noncancerous tumor of the prostate
	i. tightness of the prepuce, or foreskin
	j. urethral opening on the upper side of the penis

Sexually Transmitted Infection Terms

Sexually transmitted infections (**STI**) are usually named for the bacteria or virus that cause the infection. Review the pronunciation and description for each term in Table 12-5 and complete the exercises. Note that symptoms might not be present, especially during the early stages of the infection. Because STIs affect men and women, the figures in this section include male and female genitalia.

TABLE 12–5   SEXUALLY TRANSMITTED INFECTION TERMS

Term with Pronunciation	Definition
chancre (**SHANG**-ker)	highly contagious pustule or lesion located on the penis, characteristic of primary syphilis (Figure 12-5)

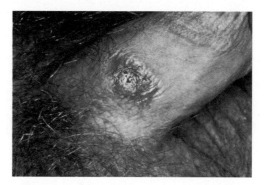

Figure 12-5   Chancre in primary syphilis/Center for Disease Control (Dr. Gavin Hart, Dr. N.J. Flumara)

chlamydia (klah-**MID**-ee-ah)	sexually transmitted infection caused by the bacteria *Chlamydia trachomatis*; symptoms are usually mild or absent and might include abnormal discharge from the penis or cervix, and a burning sensation during urination; bacteria can infect the urinary tract or cervix causing epididymitis in men and cervicitis in women (Figure 12-6)

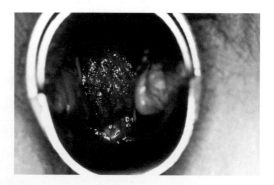

Figure 12-6   Chlamydia, cervix/Center for Disease Control (Dr. Lourdes Fraw, Jim Pledger)

(continues)

TABLE 12–5 SEXUALLY TRANSMITTED INFECTION TERMS (continued)

Term with Pronunciation	Definition
genital herpes (**JEN**-ih-tal **HER**-peez)	sexually transmitted infection caused by herpes simplex virus (HSV), type 2; symptoms are called *outbreaks*, which appear two weeks after infection; outbreaks are characterized by small blisters in the genital area, penis, cervix, vagina, or in the urethra; blisters rupture, leaving an ulceration (sore) that heals without leaving a scar; genital herpes can recur spontaneously once the virus has been acquired; also called venereal herpes (Figure 12-7)

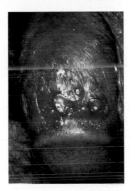

Figure 12-7 Genital herpes/Center for Disease Control (Dr. N.J. Flumara, Dr. Gavin Hart)

genital warts (**JEN**-ih-tal)	sexually transmitted infection caused by the human papillomavirus (HPV), characterized by small, cauliflower-like, fleshy growths usually seen along the penis and in or near the vagina or anus; also called venereal warts (Figure 12-8)

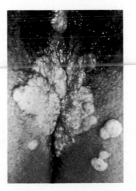

Figure 12-8 Genital warts/Center for Disease Control

TABLE 12–5 SEXUALLY TRANSMITTED INFECTION TERMS (continued)

Term with Pronunciation	Definition
gonorrhea (gon-oh-**REE**-ah)	sexually transmitted infection caused by bacteria (*Neisseria gonorrhoeae*) that infect male and female genitalia; symptoms, which typically appear within two to ten days after sexual contact with an infected individual, include yellow or bloody vaginal discharge; white, yellow, or green painful discharge from the penis; painful or burning sensations during urination; and swollen testicles; untreated, gonorrhea can lead to infection of the entire reproductive tract of both men and women
sexually transmitted infection (STI)	any disease that is spread from one person to another during any type of sexual contact
syphilis (**SIFF**-ih-lis)	sexually transmitted disease that has three distinct stages, each more serious than the previous stage; lesions may involve any organ or tissue
trichomoniasis (**trik**-oh-moh-**NIGH**-ah-sis)	sexually transmitted infection caused by the protozoa *Trichomonas vaginalis*; men are usually asymptomatic, but might experience dysuria, urinary frequency, or urethritis; symptoms in women include itching, burning, and a strong-smelling, frothy, greenish-yellow vaginal discharge (Figure 12-9 shows the "strawberry cervix" that is associated with trichomoniasis.)

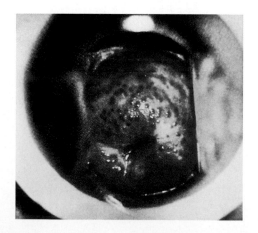

Figure 12-9 Trichomoniasis, strawberry cervix/Center for Disease Control

EXERCISE 11

Write the name of the sexually transmitted disease for each description.

1. cauliflower-like, fleshy growths _____

2. bacterial infection of genital
   mucous membranes _____

3. caused by herpes simplex virus type 2 _____

4. parasitic infection of the genitourinary tract _____

5. disease with three distinct stages _____

EXERCISE 12

Rewrite the misspelled terms.

1. shancre _____

2. chlamydia _____

3. gonnorrhea _____

4. syphillis _____

5. trichomoniasis _____

6. venerial herpes _____

Male Reproductive System Diagnostic and Treatment Terms

Review the pronunciation and definition of the diagnostic and treatment terms in Table 12-6 and complete the exercises.

TABLE 12-6 MALE REPRODUCTIVE SYSTEM DIAGNOSTIC AND TREATMENT TERMS

Term with Pronunciation	Definition
circumcision (sir-kum-**SIH**-shun)	surgical removal of the foreskin (prepuce) of the penis (Figure 12-10)

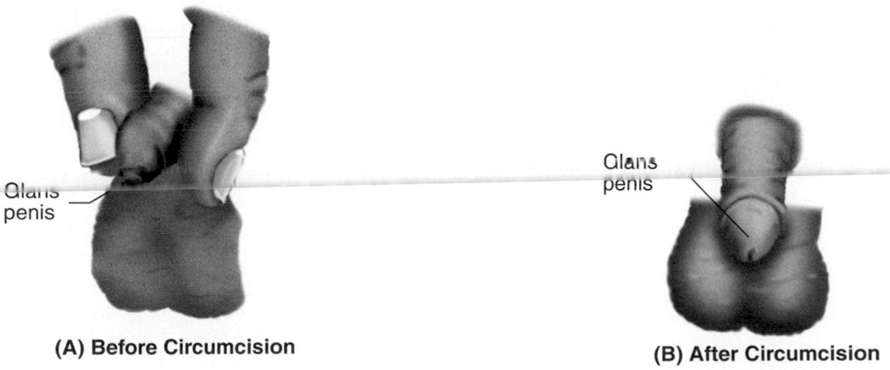

(A) Before Circumcision

Glans penis

Glans penis

(B) After Circumcision

Figure 12-10 Circumcision

(continues)

TABLE 12-6 MALE REPRODUCTIVE SYSTEM DIAGNOSTIC AND TREATMENT TERMS (continued)

Term with Pronunciation	Definition
epididymectomy (**ep**-ih-**did**-ih-**MEK**-toh-mee) epididym/o = epididymis -ectomy = surgical removal	surgical removal of the epididymis
orchidectomy (or-kid-**ECK**-toh-mee) orchid/o = testes -ectomy = surgical removal	surgical removal of one or both testes
orchidopexy; orchiopexy (**OR**-kid-oh-**pek**-see; **or**-kee-oh-**PEK**-see) orchid/o; orchi/o = testes -pexy = surgical fixation	surgical fixation of one or both testes
orchidoplasty; orchioplasty (**OR**-kid-oh-**plass**-tee; **OR**-kee-oh-**plass**-tee) orchid/o; orchi/o = testes -plasty = surgical repair or the testes	surgical repair of one or both testes; placement of undescended testes into the scrotum
prostatectomy (**pross**-tah-**TEK**-toh-mee) prostat/o = prostate gland -ectomy = surgical removal	surgical removal of all or part of the prostate
prostatic acid phosphatase (PAP) (pross-**STAT**-ic acid **FOSS**-fah-tays) prostat/o = prostate gland -ic = pertaining to	aboratory test that measures the level of acid phosphatase, an enzyme present in prostate cells and in the blood; elevated levels indicate prostate cancer
prostate-specific antigen (PSA) (**PROSS**-tayt specific **AN**-tih-jen) prostat/o = prostate gland -ic = pertaining to	laboratory test that measures the blood levels of PSA, a protein produced by the prostate gland; elevated PSA levels indicate benign prostatic hypertrophy or prostate cancer; a screening test for prostate cancer
semen analysis	laboratory analysis of the physical and chemical components of semen
sterilization	any procedure that renders a male incapable of producing sperm or impregnating a woman

(*continues*)

TABLE 12-6 MALE REPRODUCTIVE SYSTEM DIAGNOSTIC AND TREATMENT TERMS (continued)

Term with Pronunciation	Definition
suprapubic prostatectomy (**soo**-prah-**PYOO**-bic **pross**-tah-**TEK**-toh-mee) supra- = above pub/o = pubis, pubic bone -ic = pertaining to prostat/o = prostate gland -ectomy = surgical removal of	surgical removal of all or part of the prostate gland through an incision just above the pubic bone
transurethral resection of the prostate (TURP) (**tranz**-yoo-**REE**-thral) trans- = through urethr/o = urethra -al = pertaining to	surgical removal of all or part of the prostate gland by passing an instrument into and through the urethra (Figure 12–11)

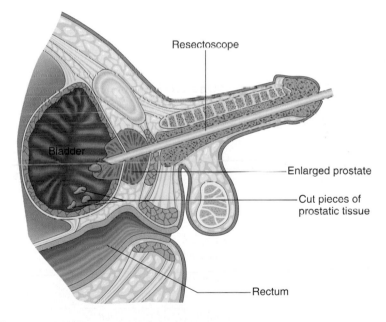

Resectoscope

Bladder

Enlarged prostate

Cut pieces of prostatic tissue

Rectum

Figure 12-11 Transurethral resection of the prostate

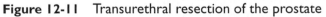

varicocelectomy (**vair**-ih-koh-see-**LEK**-toh-mee) varic/o = twisted veins -cele = hernia; protrusion -ectomy = surgical removal	surgical removal of a varicocele by excision of a portion of the scrotum and tying off (ligation) of the enlarged, twisted veins
vasectomy (vas-**EK**-toh-mee) vas/o = vas deferens -ectomy = surgical removal	surgical removal of all or a portion of the vas deferens (Figure 12-12)

(continues)

TABLE 12-6   MALE REPRODUCTIVE SYSTEM DIAGNOSTIC AND
TREATMENT TERMS (continued)

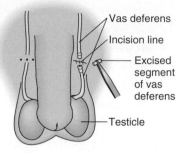

Vas deferens
Incision line
Excised
segment
of vas
deferens
Testicle

Figure 12-12   Vasectomy

EXERCISE 13

Analyze each term by writing the prefix, root, combining vowel, and suffix separated by vertical slashes. Based on the meaning of the word parts, write a definition for each term. Check the definition in a medical dictionary. Note that some terms might have more than one root.

1. epididymectomy

prefix	*root*	*combining vowel*	*suffix*

   DEFINITION: _____

2. orchidectomy

prefix	*root*	*combining vowel*	*suffix*

   DEFINITION: _____

3. orchidopexy

prefix	*root*	*combining vowel*	*suffix*

   DEFINITION: _____

4. orchioplasty

prefix	*root*	*combining vowel*	*suffix*

   DEFINITION: _____

5. prostatectomy

prefix	*root*	*combining vowel*	*suffix*

   DEFINITION: _____

6. suprapubic prostatectomy

prefix	root	combining vowel	suffix

prefix	root	combining vowel	suffix

DEFINITION: _____

7. varicocelectomy

prefix	root	combining vowel	suffix

DEFINITION: _____

EXERCISE 14

Replace the italicized phrase or abbreviation with the correct medical term.

1. Due to recurrent balanitis, Malcolm underwent *the removal of the foreskin.*

   _____

2. The *PAP test* is used to rule out prostate cancer.

   _____

3. The *PSA* laboratory blood test is a screening test for prostate cancer.

   _____

4. A *TURP* may result in an inability to achieve or sustain an erection.

   _____

5. *Surgical removal of all or part of the vas deferens* is a procedure for male sterilization.

   _____

Abbreviations

Review the male reproductive system abbreviations in Table 13-7. Practice writing out the meaning of each abbreviation.

TABLE 12–7 ABBREVIATIONS

Abbreviation	Meaning
BPH	benign prostatic hypertrophy
HPV	human papillomaviruo
HSV	herpes simplex virus
PAP	prostatic acid phosphatase
PSA	prostate specific antigen
STI	sexually transmitted infection
TURP	transurethral resection of the prostate

CHAPTER REVIEW

The Chapter Review can be used as a self-test. Go through each exercise and answer as many questions as you can without referring to previous exercises or earlier discussions within this chapter. Check your answers and fill in any blanks. Practice writing any terms you might have misspelled.

EXERCISE 15

Write the medical term for each definition.

1. expulsion of semen from the penis _____

2. formation or development of mature sperm _____

3. male hormone _____

4. physician who specializes in the study of the male reproductive system _____

5. lack or absence of sperm _____

6. undescended testicle(s) _____

7. inflammation of the epididymis _____

8. few, diminished, or deficient number of sperm present in semen _____

9. inflammation of the prostate gland _____

10. destruction or breakdown of sperm _____

11. enlargement of the veins of the spermatic cord _____

12. removal of one or both of the testes _____

13. surgical fixation of one or both of the testes _____

14. surgical repair of one or both of the testes _____

15. surgical removal of all or part of the prostate gland _____

EXERCISE 16

Read the following operative report and write a brief definition for each italicized medical term.

OPERATIVE REPORT
PREOPERATIVE DIAGNOSIS: (1) *Cryptorchidism.*
POSTOPERTIVE DIAGNOSIS: Cryptorchidism.
OPERATION: (2) *Orchiopexy.*
HISTORY: This 4-year-old Native American male presented with undescended (3) *testes*, nonresponsive to hormone treatment. His parents have consented to surgical intervention and were advised of the risks and benefits of the procedure.

PROCEDURE: After adequate general anesthesia, the patient was prepped and draped in the usual manner. He was placed in the supine position, and an incision was made in the inguinal canal. The testes were freed with sharp dissection. The (4) *spermatic cord* was stripped, and the (5) *vas deferens* and spermatic vessels were left intact. The testes were placed away from the operative site. A channel for each (6) *testis* was created from the inguinal incision to the bottom of the (7) *scrotum.* Each testis was delivered through the respective channels, and the scrotal wound was closed. Sponge and needle counts were reported as correct, and the patient was returned to the recovery room in good condition.

1. _____

2. _____

3. _____

4. _____

5. _____

6. _____

7. _____

EXERCISE 17

Match the medical term in Column 1 with the description in Column 2.

COLUMN 1

_____ 1. balanitis

_____ 2. chancre

_____ 3. circumcision

_____ 4. genital warts

_____ 5. genitalia

_____ 6. impotence

_____ 7. phimosis

_____ 8. priapism

_____ 9. semen analysis

_____ 10. syphilis

_____ 11. trichomoniasis

_____ 12. venereal herpes

COLUMN 2

a. abnormal, prolonged, painful erection

b. cauliflower-like, fleshy growths along the penis

c. disease with three distinct stages

d. highly contagious pustule or lesion on the penis

e. identifies the components of semen

f. inflammation of the glans penis

g. inability to achieve or sustain an erection

h. male and female reproductive structures

i. parasitic sexually transmitted infection

j. removal of the prepuce

k. STI caused by herpes simplex virus type 2

l. tightness of the foreskin

EXERCISE 18

Select the best answer to each statement or question.

1. Choose the term that means formation of mature sperm.
   a. spermatolysis
   b. spermatogenesis
   c. spermatosis
   d. spermatopoiesis

2. Which term means absence of one or both testes?
   a. aspermia
   b. anaorchidism
   c. anorchidism
   d. oligospermia

3. Select the term for urethral opening on the upper side of the penis.
   a. hypospadias
   b. perispadias
   c. hyperspadias
   d. epispadias

4. Choose the term for enlarged veins of the spermatic cord.
   a. varicocele
   b. spermatocele
   c. hydrocele
   d. inguinocele

5. Which term means surgical fixation of the testes?
   a. orchidoplasty
   b. orchidorrhaphy
   c. orchidopexy
   d. orchidodesis

6. Select the term for a procedure that results in male sterilization.
   a. epididymectomy
   b. prostatectomy
   c. orchidectomy
   d. vasectomy

7. Which term means undescended testicles?
   a. anorchism
   b. cryptorchidism
   c. orchidiasis
   d. orchiocele

8. Select the term for diminished number of sperm in the semen.
   a. oligospermia
   b. aspermia
   c. hypospermia
   d. spermatolysis

9. Which term means the placement of testes into the scrotum?
   a. orchidopexy
   b. orchidotomy
   c. orchidoplasty
   d. orchidectomy

10. Select the abbreviation that means a screening test for prostate cancer.
   a. PSA
   b. PAP
   c. TURP
   d. SPC

CHALLENGE EXERCISE

Human papillomavirus (HPV) is one of the most common causes of sexually transmitted infection (STI). Health experts believe there are more cases of genital HPV infection than any other STI in the United States. Approximately 5.5 million new cases of sexually transmitted HPV infections are reported every year. Search the Internet for information about HPV. Use the keywords human papillomavirus or HPV. Prepare a handout that answers these questions: What is the difference between high-risk and low-risk HPV? What role does a PAP smear play in identifying HPV infections? How does HPV affect pregnancy and childbirth? How can HPV infection be prevented? (Note: The National Institute of Allergy and Infectious Diseases (NAIAID), a division of the National Institutes of Health (NIH), maintains an excellent Web site at www.niaid.nih.gov.)

Pronunciation Review

Review the terms in the chapter. Pronounce each term using the following phonetic pronunciations. Check off the term when you are comfortable saying it.

TERM	PRONUNCIATION
☐ anorchidism	an-**ORK**-id-izm
☐ anorchism	an-**ORK**-izm
☐ aspermia	ah-**SPERM**-ee-ah
☐ balanitis	bal-ah-**NIGH**-tis
☐ benign prostatic hypertrophy	bee-**NIGHN** pross-**TAT**-ik high-**PER**-troh-fee
☐ chancre	**SHANG**-ker
☐ chlamydia	klah-**MID**-ee-ah
☐ circumcision	sir-kom-**SIH**-shun
☐ Cowper's gland	**COW**-perz gland
☐ cryptorchidism	kript-**OR**-kid-izm
☐ ejaculation	ee-**jack**-yoo-**LAY**-shun
☐ ejaculatory duct	ee-**JACK**-yoo-lah-**tor**-ee duct
☐ epididymectomy	ep-ih-**did**-ih-**MEK**-toh-me
☐ epididymis	ep-ih-**DID**-ih-miss
☐ epididymitis	ep-ih-**did**-ih-**MIGH**-tis
☐ epispadias	ep-ih-**SPAY**-dee-as
☐ genital herpes	**JEN**-ih-tal **HER**-peez
☐ genital warts	**JEN**-ih-tal warts
☐ genitalia	jen-ih-**TAY**-lee-ah

☐	glans penis	**GLANZ** penis
☐	gonorrhea	gon-oh-**REE**-ah
☐	hydrocele	**HIGH**-droh-seel
☐	hypospadias	high-poh-**SPAY**-dee-as
☐	impotence	**IM**-poh-tens
☐	indirect inguinal hernia	indirect **ING**-gwih-nal **HER**-nee-ah
☐	oligospermia	**all**-ih-goh-**SPER**-mee-ah
☐	orchidectomy	or-kid-**ECK**-toh-mee
☐	orchidopexy	**OR**-kid-oh-**pek**-see
☐	orchioplasty	**OR**-kee-oh-**plass**-tee
☐	orchitis	or-**KIGH**-tis
☐	penis	**PEE**-nis
☐	phimosis	fih-**MOH**-sis
☐	prepuce	**PREE**-pus
☐	priapism	**PRIGH**-ah-pizm
☐	prostate cancer	**PROSS**-tayt cancer
☐	prostate gland	**PROSS**-tayt gland
☐	prostate-specific antigen	**PROSS**-tayt-specific **AN**-tih-jen
☐	prostatectomy	pross-tah-**TEK**-toh-mee
☐	prostatitis	pross-tah-**TIGH**-tis
☐	scrotum	**SKROH**-tum
☐	semen	**SEE**-men
☐	semen analysis	**SEE**-men analysis
☐	seminal vesicle	**SEM**-ih-nall **VESS**-ih-kal
☐	seminiferous tubules	sem-ih-**NIH**-fer-us **TOO**-byools
☐	spermatic cord	sper-**MAT**-ik cord
☐	spermatogenesis	**sperm**-at-oh-**JEN**-eh-sis
☐	spermatolysis	sper-mah-**TALL**-ih-sis
☐	spermatozoa	sper-**mat**-oh-**ZOH**-ah
☐	suprapubic prostatectomy	**soo**-prah-**PYOO**-bik
		pross-tah-**TEK**-toh-mee
☐	syphilis	**SIFF**-ih-lis
☐	testes	**TESS**-teez
☐	testicular carcinoma	tess-**TICK**-yoo-lar **kar**-sin-**OH**-ma
☐	testosterone	tess-**TOSS**-ter-ohn
☐	transurethral resection of the	**tranz**-yoo-**REE**-thral resection of the
	prostate	prostate
☐	trichomoniasis	**trik**-oh-moh-**NIGH**-ah-sis
☐	urethra	yoo-**REE**-thrah
☐	urologist	yoor-**ALL**-oh-jist
☐	urology	yoor-**ALL**-oh-jee
☐	varicocele	**VAIR**-ih-koh-seel
☐	varicocelectomy	**vair**-ih-koh-see-**LEK**-toh-mee
☐	vas deferens	**VAZ DEFF**-er-enz
☐	vasectomy	vas-**EK**-toh-mee

Chapter 13
Female Reproductive System and Pregnancy

OBJECTIVES

At the completion of this chapter, the student should be able to:

1. Identify, define, and spell word roots associated with the female reproductive system and pregnancy.
2. Label the structures of the female reproductive system and structures relating to pregnancy.
3. Discuss the functions of the female reproductive system.
4. Provide the correct spelling of female reproductive system and pregnancy terms, given the definition of the terms.
5. Analyze female reproductive system and pregnancy terms by defining the roots, prefixes, and suffixes of those terms.
6. Identify, define, and spell disease, disorder, and procedure terms related to the female reproductive system and pregnancy.

OVERVIEW

The female reproductive system consists of external and internal genitalia (jen-ih-**TAY**-lee-ah). The internal genitalia function together to produce female hormones and provide an environment for the development and birth of a baby. The external genitalia function as a protective covering for internal female reproductive organs. General information about the female reproductive system is presented in the first section of this chapter. Specific information about the female reproductive system during pregnancy is presented in the second section of this chapter.

Female Reproductive System Word Roots

To understand and use female reproductive system medical terms, it is necessary to acquire a thorough knowledge of the associated word roots. The roots are listed with the combining vowel. Review the word roots in Table 13-1 and complete the exercises that follow.

TABLE 13-1 FEMALE REPRODUCTIVE SYSTEM WORD ROOTS

Word Root/Combining Form	Meaning
cervic/o	cervix
colp/o	vagina
epis/o	vulva
gyn/o; gynec/o	woman

(continues)

TABLE 14-1   FEMALE REPRODUCTIVE SYSTEM WORD ROOTS (continued)

Word Root/Combining Form	Meaning
hyster/o	uterus
mamm/o; mast/o	breast
men/o	menses; menstruation
metr/o; metr/i	uterus
oophor/o	ovary
ov/o	ovum; egg
ovari/o	ovary
salping/o	fallopian tubes; oviducts
uter/o	uterus
vagin/o	vagina
vulv/o	vulva

EXERCISE 1

Write the definitions of the following word roots.

1. uter/o   _____
2. men/o   _____
3. gynec/o   _____
4. colp/o   _____
5. cervic/o   _____
6. mast/o   _____
7. vagin/o   _____
8. oophor/o   _____
9. hyster/o   _____
10. mamm/o   _____

EXERCISE 2

Write the word root and its meaning.

1. dysmenorrhea

   ROOT:_____   MEANING: _____

2. mammography

   ROOT:_____   MEANING: _____

3. uterotomy

   ROOT:_____   MEANING: _____

4. oophoritis

   ROOT:_____   MEANING: _____

5. ovulation

   ROOT:_____   MEANING: _____

6. hysterectomy

ROOT:_____   MEANING: _____

7. mastectomy

ROOT:_____   MEANING: _____

8. endometriosis

ROOT:_____   MEANING: _____

9. salpingitis

ROOT:_____   MEANING: _____

10. menarche

ROOT:_____   MEANING: _____

EXERCISE 3

Write the correct word root(s) for the following definitions.

1. woman   _____

2. uterus   _____

3. ovary   _____

4. egg   _____

5. cervix   _____

6. menstruation   _____

7. fallopian tubes _____

8. vulva   _____

9. vagina   _____

External Genitalia

The external genitalia includes the (1) **mons pubis** (**MONS PYOO**-bis), (2) **labia majora** (**LAY**-bee-ah mah-**JOR**-ah), (3) **clitoris** (**KLIT**-oh-ris), (4) **labia minora** (min-**OR**-ah), (5) **vaginal orifice**, (6) **hymen**, **Bartholin's glands**, and (7) **perineum** (pair-ih-**NEE**-um). These structures, collectively called the *vulva*, are illustrated in Figure 13-1, with the exception of the Bartholin's glands. Refer to the figure as you learn about each structure.

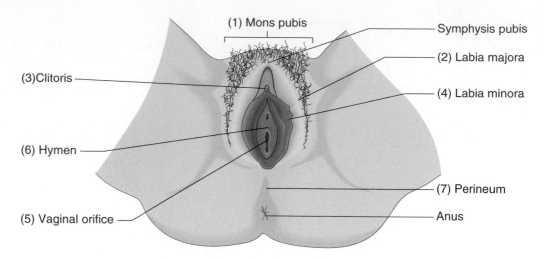

Figure 13-1   External genitalia, female reproductive system

The mons pubis, which is covered with hair in adult women, is a pad of fatty tissue that covers the symphysis pubis. The labia majora are two folds of fatty tissue, one on each side of the vaginal opening. The labia minora are two thinner folds of tissue that are located within the labia majora.

The clitoris, located above the urinary orifice, is made of highly sensitive, erectile tissue. The vaginal orifice, which is surrounded by a thin layer of elastic connective tissue called the *hymen*, is the opening to the vagina. Bartholin's glands, located on each side of the vaginal opening, secrete a mucous substance that lubricates the vagina. The perineum is the area between the vaginal orifice and the anus.

Internal Genitalia

The internal genitalia of the female reproductive system include the (1) **vagina**, (2) **uterus**, (3) **fallopian tubes**, and (4) **ovaries**. These structures are illustrated in Figure 13-2. Refer to the figure as you learn about the structures.

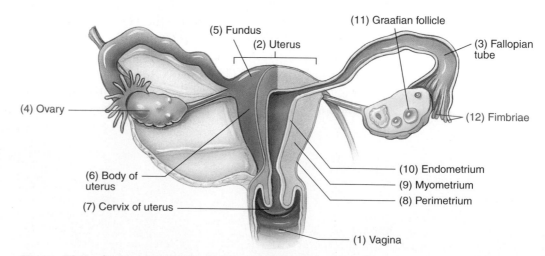

Figure 13-2   Internal genitalia, female reproductive system

Vagina

The vagina, commonly called the *birth canal,* is a muscular, elastic tube, about three inches long, that expands during childbirth. The vagina receives the penis during intercourse and is the outlet for the menstrual flow.

Uterus

The uterus is a hollow, pear-shaped, muscular organ commonly called the *womb.* It holds the fertilized ovum as it develops during pregnancy. The uterus has three distinct areas that are called the (5) **fundus**, the rounded upper section; the (6) **body**, the central section; and the (7) **cervix**, the lower end of the uterus. The walls of the uterus consist of the (8) **perimetrium** (pair-ih-**MEE**-tree-um), the outer layer; the (9) **myometrium** (my-oh-**MEE**-tree-um), the thick muscular layer; and the (10) **endometrium** (en-doh-**MEE**-tree-um), the inner layer or lining.

The endometrium thickens each month in preparation for implantation of a fertilized egg. When implantation does not occur, the endometrium is shed in a bloody discharge called **menses** (**MEN**-seez) or menstrual flow.

Ovaries and Fallopian Tubes

The ovaries are two small, almond-shaped organs located in the pelvic cavity on either side of the uterus. The fallopian tubes, also called *uterine tubes* and *oviducts,* are attached to the uterus and lie close to the ovaries. The ovaries and fallopian tubes are collectively known as the **adnexa** (add-**NECKS**-ah).

The ovaries are the female gonads and are responsible for producing mature **ovum**. Ova, commonly called *eggs,* are the female sex cells. Immature ova are stored in the microscopic sacs of the ovaries, called (11) **graafian follicles** (**GRAFF**-ee-an **FALL**-ih-kals). During the menstrual cycle, the ovum and graafian follicles mature. The graafian follicles move to the surface of the ovary and release the mature ovum. The release of a mature ovum is called **ovulation**.

The ovum is coaxed toward the (3) **fallopian tube** by the (12) **fimbriae** (**FIM**-bree-ay), fingerlike projections of the fallopian tubes that are very near the ovaries. The ovum travels through the fallopian tube and enters the uterus. If the ovum is not fertilized or does not implant in the endometrium, the ovum passes out of the body as part of the menstrual flow. The onset of menstruation is called **menarche** (men-**AR**-kee).

Mammary Glands

The mammary glands, or breasts, are responsible for the production of milk. This process is called **lactation** (lak-**TAY**-shun). Figure 13-3 illustrates the basic parts of the breast. Refer to this figure as you learn about the mammary glands.

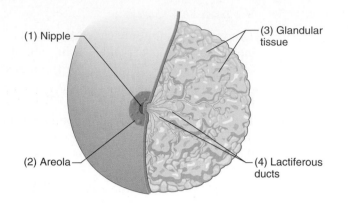

Figure 13-3 Structures of the breast

Each breast consists of a (1) **nipple** that is surrounded by a pigmented area called the (2) **areola** (air-ee-**OH**-lah). Areolar pigmentation can range from pink-flesh tones to a dark brown. The main internal structures of the breasts include the (3) **glandular tissue** and the (4) **lactiferous** (lak-**TIFF**-er-us) **ducts**. The glandular tissue produces milk that moves through the lactiferous ducts to the nipple.

EXERCISE 4

Write the name of the female reproductive system structures illustrated in Figure 13-4. Write your answer on the spaces provided.

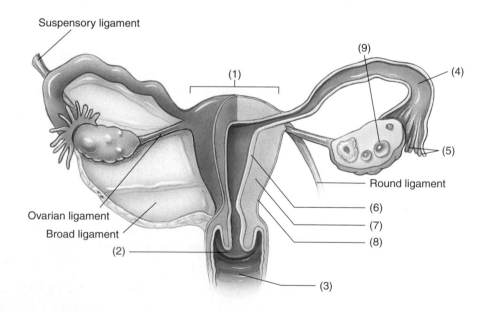

Figure 13-4 Labeling exercise

1. _____

2. _____

3. _____

4. _____

5. _____

6. _____

7. _____

8. _____

9. _____

EXERCISE 5

Write the name of the defined female reproductive system structure.

1. pad of fatty tissue; covers the symphysis pubis   _____

2. folds of fatty tissue surrounding the vaginal opening   _____

3. thinner folds of tissue around the vaginal opening   _____

4. highly sensitive erectile tissue   _____

5. secretes a lubricating substance   _____

6. produces ova   _____

7. storage sacs for the ova   _____

8. fingerlike projections   _____

9. near the ovaries and connected to the uterus   _____

Female Reproductive System Medical Terminology

Female reproductive system medical terms are organized into three main categories: (1) general medical terms; (2) disease and condition terms; and (3) diagnostic procedure, surgery, and laboratory test terms. The roots, prefixes, and suffixes associated with the female reproductive system are listed in Table 13-2. Review these word parts and complete the related exercises.

TABLE 13–2   ROOTS, PREFIXES, AND SUFFIXES FOR FEMALE REPRODUCTIVE SYSTEM TERMS

Root	Meaning	Prefix	Meaning	Suffix	Meaning
cry/o	cold	ante-	before; forward	-arche	beginning; onset
*cyst/o	cyst; **sac**	dys-	abnormal; painful; difficult	-cele	herniation, protrusion
fibr/o	fibrous tissue	endo-	within; inner	-ectomy	surgical removal
lapar/o	abdominal wall	pre-	before	-graphy	process of recording
olig/o	few; diminished	retro-	behind; backward; upward	-oma	tumor

(continues)

TABLE 13–2 ROOTS, PREFIXES, AND SUFFIXES FOR FEMALE REPRODUCTIVE SYSTEM TERMS (continued)

Root	Meaning	Prefix	Meaning	Suffix	Meaning
				-osis	condition
				-pexy	surgical fixation
				-(r)rhagia	hemorrhage
				-(r)rhea	flow; discharge
				-version	to turn

*cyst/o also means urinary bladder.

EXERCISE 6

Write the root, prefix, suffix, and their meanings for the following medical terms.

1. cryosurgery

ROOT: _____ MEANING: _____

PREFIX: _____ MEANING: _____

SUFFIX: _____ MEANING: _____

2. oligomenorrhea

ROOT: _____ MEANING: _____

PREFIX: _____ MEANING: _____

SUFFIX: _____ MEANING: _____

3. dysmenorrhea

ROOT: _____ MEANING: _____

PREFIX: _____ MEANING: _____

SUFFIX: _____ MEANING: _____

4. premenstrual

ROOT: _____ MEANING: _____

PREFIX: _____ MEANING: _____

SUFFIX: _____ MEANING: _____

5. laparoscopy

ROOT: _____ MEANING: _____

PREFIX: _____ MEANING: _____

SUFFIX: _____ MEANING: _____

6. fibrocystic

ROOT: _____ MEANING: _____

PREFIX: _____ MEANING: _____

SUFFIX: _____ MEANING: _____

7. anteflexion

ROOT: _____ MEANING: _____

PREFIX: _____ MEANING: _____

SUFFIX: _____ MEANING: _____

8. endocervical

ROOT: _____ MEANING: _____

PREFIX: _____ MEANING: _____

SUFFIX: _____ MEANING: _____

9. hysterectomy

ROOT: _____ MEANING: _____

PREFIX: _____ MEANING: _____

SUFFIX: _____ MEANING: _____

EXERCISE 7

Write the suffix for each word or phrase.

1. hemorrhage _____
2. condition _____
3. discharge, flow _____
4. herniation or protrusion _____
5. process of recording _____
6. surgical fixation _____
7. surgical removal _____
8. to turn _____
9. tumor _____

Female Reproductive System General Medical Terms

Review the pronunciation and meaning of each term in Table 13-3. Note that some terms are built from word parts and some are not. Complete the exercises for these terms.

TABLE 13-3 FEMALE REPRODUCTIVE SYSTEM GENERAL MEDICAL TERMS

Term with Pronunciation	Definition
gynecologist (gigh-neh-**KALL**-oh-jist, jin-eh-**KALL**-oh-jist) gynec/o = woman -(o)logist = specialist in the study of	physician who specializes in the study and treatment of diseases related the female reproductive system

(continues)

TABLE 13-3 FEMALE REPRODUCTIVE SYSTEM GENERAL MEDICAL TERMS (continued)

Term with Pronunciation	Definition
gynecology (gigh-neh-**KALL**-oh-jee, jin-eh-**KALL**-oh-jee) gynec/o = woman -(o)logy = study of	study of diseases and disorders related to the female reproductive system and breasts
menarche (men-**ARK**-ee) men/o = menses; menstruation -arche = onset; beginning	onset of menstruation, first menstrual cycle
menopause (**MEN**-oh-pawz) men/o = menses; menstruation	time frame that marks the permanent cessation of menstrual activity
menses (**MEN**-seez) men/o = menses; menstruation	bloody discharge associated with menstruation
menstruation (men-stroo-**AY**-shun) men/o = menses; menstruation	periodic flow of bloody fluid from the uterine lining
ovulation (ahv-yoo-**LAY**-shun) ov/o = ovum; egg	periodic release of a mature ovum from a graafian follicle

EXERCISE 8

Replace the italicized phrase with the correct medical term.

1. Rebecca was prepared for the *onset of menstruation.*

   _____

2. Shenesia completed a residency in the *study of the female reproductive system.*

   _____

3. *The periodic discharge from the uterine lining* begins during puberty.

   _____

4. *Permanent cessation of menstrual activity* may take several years.

   _____

5. Sanitary pads or tampons are needed to dispose of the *bloody discharge of menstruation.*

   _____

6. *A physician who specializes in the female reproductive system* is able to diagnose cervical cancer.

_____

7. *The periodic release of a mature ovum* usually occurs on a cyclical schedule.

_____

Female Reproductive System Disease and Disorder Terms

Female reproductive system, including the breast, diseases and disorders include familiar problems such as vaginitis as well as more complex and less familiar diagnoses such as endometriosis. The medical terms are presented in alphabetical order in Table 13-4. Review the pronunciation and definition for each term and complete the exercises.

TABLE 13-4   FEMALE REPRODUCTIVE SYSTEM DISEASE
AND DISORDER TERMS

Term with Pronunciation	Definition
amenorrhea (**ah**-men-oh-**REE**-ah) a- = lack of; without men/o = menses; menstrual flow -(r)rhea – flow; discharge	absence or lack of menstrual flow
anteflexion of the uterus (an-tee-**FLEK**-shun) ante – before; forward	forward displacement of the uterus
carcinoma of the breast (**kar**-sin-**OH**-mah)	malignant tumor of the breast tissue
cervical carcinoma (**SER**-vih-kal **kar**-sin-**OH**-mah) cervic/o = cervix -al = pertaining to carcin- = cancer; malignant -oma = tumor	malignant tumor of the cervix, also called cervical cancer (Figure 13-5)

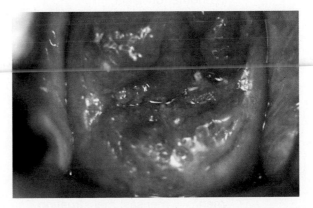

Figure 13-5   Cervical carcinoma/Center for Disease Control

(continues)

TABLE 13-4   FEMALE REPRODUCTIVE SYSTEM DISEASE AND DISORDER TERMS (continued)

Term with Pronunciation	Definition
cervicitis (ser-vih-**SIGH**-tis) cervic/o = cervix -itis = inflammation	inflammation of the cervix
cystocele (**SISS**-toh-seel) cyst/o = urinary bladder -cele = hernia; protrusion	herniation or downward protrusion of the urinary bladder into the wall of the vagina
dysmenorrhea (**diss**-men-oh-**REE**-ah) dys- = abnormal; painful; difficult men/o = menses; menstruation -(r)rhea = flow; discharge	painful menstrual flow
endometriosis (**en**-doh-**mee**-tree-**OH**-sis) endo- = inner metr/i = uterus -osis = condition	presence and growth of endometrial tissue in areas outside the uterus
fibrocystic breast disease (**figh**-broh-**SISS**-tik) fibr/o = fibrous tissue cyst/o = cyst; sac -ic = pertaining to	presence of single or multiple fluid-filled cysts in the breasts
genital warts	a sexually transmitted infection caused by the human papillomavirus virus (HPV); HPV is also responsible for a high percentage of cervical cancer; a vaccine is available to prevent HPV (Note: The vaccine **does not** prevent cervical cancer.)
menometrorrhagia (**men**-oh-**met**-roh-**RAY**-jee-ah) men/o = menses; menstruation metr/o = uterus -(r)rhagia = hemorrhage	excessive uterine bleeding during and the normal menstrual period
menorrhagia (men-oh-**RAY**-jee-ah) men/o = menses; menstruation -(r)rhagia = hemorrhage	excessive bleeding during the menstrual period
menorrhea (men-oh-**REE**-ah) men/o = menses; menstruation -(r)rhea = flow; discharge	normal menstrual flow

(continues)

TABLE 13-4 FEMALE REPRODUCTIVE SYSTEM DISEASE
AND DISORDER TERMS (continued)

Term with Pronunciation	Definition
metrorrhagia (meh-troh-**RAY**-jee-ah) metr/i = uterus -(r)rhagia = hemorrhage	excessive uterine bleeding at times other than during the menstrual period
oligomenorrhea (**oh**-lig-oh-**men**-oh-**REE**-ah) olig/o = few; diminished men/o = uterus -(r)rhea = flow; discharge	abnormally light or infrequent menstruation

EXERCISE 9

Analyze each term by writing the prefix, root, combining vowel, and suffix separated by vertical slashes. Based on the meaning of the word parts, write a definition for each term. Check the definition in a medical dictionary. Note that some terms might have more than one root.

EXAMPLE: gynecologist:

	/ gynec	/ o	/ logist
prefix	*root*	*combining vowel*	*suffix*

DEFINITION: specialist in the female reproductive system

1. amenorrhea

prefix	*root*	*combining vowel*	*suffix*

DEFINITION: _____

2. cervicitis

prefix	*root*	*combining vowel*	*suffix*

DEFINITION: _____

3. cystocele

prefix	*root*	*combining vowel*	*suffix*

DEFINITION: _____

4. dysmenorrhea

prefix	*root*	*combining vowel*	*suffix*

DEFINITION: _____

5. endometriosis

prefix	*root*	*combining vowel*	*suffix*

DEFINITION: _____

6. menorrhagia

prefix	root	combining vowel	suffix

DEFINITION: _____

7. metrorrhagia

prefix	root	combining vowel	suffix

DEFINITION: _____

8. menorrhea

prefix	root	combining vowel	suffix

DEFINITION: _____

9. oligomenorrhea

prefix	root	combining vowel	suffix

DEFINITION: _____

10. menometrorrhagia

prefix	root	combining vowel	suffix

DEFINITION: _____

EXERCISE 10

Replace the italicized phrase with the correct medical term.

1. The results of Maria's breast x-ray revealed *multiple fluid-filled cysts.*

   _____

2. After three abnormal evaluations, the final diagnosis was *a malignant tumor of the cervix.*

   _____

3. *Forward displacement* of the uterus might affect a woman's ability to become pregnant.

   _____

4. Athletes sometimes exhibit *abnormally light or infrequent menstruation.*

   _____

5. *Painful menstrual flow* might be alleviated with pain relievers.

   _____

6. *Excessive bleeding during the menstrual period* might be a symptom of uterine polyps.

   _____

7. Marlena informed her family physician that both her mother and sister had *malignant tumors of the breast* before they were 45 years of age.

    _____

8. *Normal menstrual flow* does not interfere with activities of daily living.

    _____

Review the pronunciation and definition for each term in Table 13-5 and complete the exercises.

TABLE 13-5 FEMALE REPRODUCTIVE SYSTEM DISEASE
AND DISORDER TERMS

Term with Pronunciation	Definition
oophoritis (oh-**off**-or-**EYE**-tis) oophor/o = ovary -itis = inflammation	inflammation of the ovaries
ovarian carcinoma (oh-**VAY**-ree-an **kar**-sin-**OH**-ma)	malignant tumor of the ovary
ovarian cyst (oh-**VAY**-ree-an **SIST**) ovari/o = ovary -an = pertaining to	fluid-filled, multichambered sac in the ovary
pelvic inflammatory disease (PID)	inflammation of the vagina, cervix, fallopian tubes, and broad ligament; often a result of untreated sexually transmitted infections such as chlamydia, gonorrhea, or genital herpes
premenstrual syndrome (PMS) (pre-**MEN**-stroo-al) pre- = before men/o = menstruation -al = pertaining to	a group of symptoms such as irritability, anxiety, mood changes, headaches, breast swelling, and water retention that begin several days before the onset of menstruation and end a short time after the onset of menstruation; PMS
prolapse of the uterus	protrusion of the uterus into the vaginal opening (Figure 13-6)

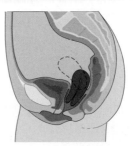

Figure 13-6 Prolapse of the uterus

(continues)

**TABLE 13-5   FEMALE REPRODUCTIVE SYSTEM DISEASE
AND DISORDER TERMS** (continued)

Term with Pronunciation	Definition
retroversion of the uterus (**reh**-troh-**VER**-shun) retro- = backward; toward the back -version = to turn	backward displacement of the uterus
salpingitis (**sal**-pin-**JIGH**-tis) salping/o = fallopian tube -itis = inflammation	inflammation of the fallopian tube
toxic shock syndrome (TSS)	a rare and sometimes fatal disease caused by an infection of the female reproductive organs associated with certain strains of *Staphylococcus aureus*
vaginitis (vaj-in-**EYE**-tis) vagin/o = vagina -itis = inflammation	inflammation of the vagina
vulvovaginitis (**vull**-voh-**vaj**-in-**EYE**-tis vulv/o = vulva vagin/o = vagina -itis = inflammation	inflammation of the vulva (external genitalia) and vagina

EXERCISE 11

Analyze each term by writing the prefix, root, combining vowel, and suffix separated by vertical slashes. Based on the meaning of the word parts, write a definition for each term. Check the definition in a medical dictionary. Note that some terms might have more than one root.

1. oophoritis

| *prefix* | *root* | *combining vowel* | *suffix* |

DEFINITION: _____

2. retroversion

| *prefix* | *root* | *combining vowel* | *suffix* |

DEFINITION: _____

3. salpingitis

| *prefix* | *root* | *combining vowel* | *suffix* |

DEFINITION: _____

4. vaginitis

_____

prefix   _root_   _combining vowel_   _suffix_

DEFINITION: _____

5. vulvovaginitis

_____

prefix   _root_   _combining vowel_   _suffix_

DEFINITION: _____

EXERCISE 12

Write the medical term for each definition or abbreviation.

1. malignant tumor of the ovary   _____

2. fluid-filled sac in the ovary   _____

3. PID   _____

4. PMS   _____

5. TSS   _____

6. displacement of the uterus
   into the vagina   _____

Female Reproductive System Diagnostic and Treatment Terms

Review the pronunciation and definition of the diagnostic and treatment terms in Table 13-6. Complete the exercises for each set of terms.

TABLE 13-6 FEMALE REPRODUCTIVE SYSTEM DIAGNOSTIC AND TREATMENT TERMS

Term with Pronunciation	Definition
colposcopy (kol-**POSS**-koh-pee) colp/o = vagina -scopy = examination with a scope	examination of vaginal and cervical tissue using a scope
conization (kon-ih-**ZAY**-shun)	surgical removal of a cone-shaped segment of the cervix for diagnosis or treatment; cone biopsy
cryosurgery (**krigh**-oh-**SER**-jer-ree) cry/o = cold	destruction and removal of tissue by rapid freezing
dilatation and curettage (D & C) (dill-ah-**TAY**-shun and koo-reh-**TAHZ**)	widening of the cervical canal followed by scraping of the uterine lining (Figure 13-7)

TABLE 13-6 FEMALE REPRODUCTIVE SYSTEM DIAGNOSTIC
AND TREATMENT TERMS (continued)

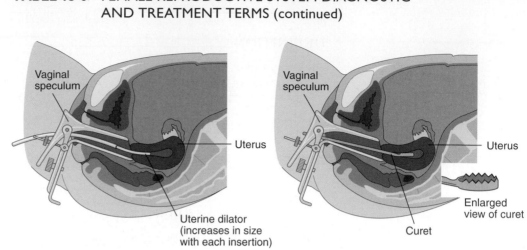

Figure 13-7 Dilatation of the cervix and curettage of the uterus

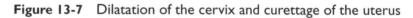

Term with Pronunciation	Definition
hysterectomy (**hiss**-ter-**EK**-toh-mee) hyster/o = uterus -ectomy = surgical removal	surgical removal of the uterus
hysterosalpingography (**hiss**-ter-oh-**sal**-pin-**GOG**-rah-fee) hyster/o = uterus salping/o = fallopian tubes -graphy = process of recording	x-ray of the uterus and fallopian tubes using a contrast medium
laparoscopy (lap-ar-**OSS**-koh-pee) lapar/o = abdominal wall -scopy = examination with a scope	examination of the contents of the abdominal and pelvic cavity using a scope
mammography (mam-**OG**-rah-fee) mamm/o = breast -graphy = process of recording	x-ray examination of the soft tissue of the breast (Figure 13-8)

(continues)

TABLE 13-6 FEMALE REPRODUCTIVE SYSTEM DIAGNOSTIC
AND TREATMENT TERMS (continued)

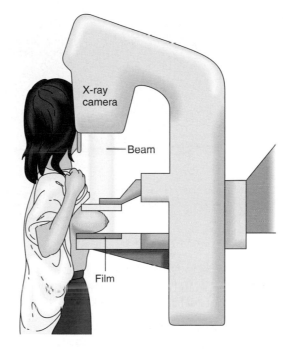

X-ray
camera

Beam

Film

Figure 13-8 Mammography

Term with Pronunciation	Definition
mastectomy (mass-TEK-toh-mee) mast/o = breast -ectomy = surgical removal	surgical removal of the breast and surrounding tissues
oophorectomy (oh-**off**-or-**EK**-toh-mee)	surgical removal of the ovary
oophoropexy (oh-**off**-or-oh-**PEK**-see) oophor/o = ovary -pexy = surgical fixation	surgical fixation of the ovary
ovariopexy (oh-**vay**-ree-oh-**PEK**-see) ovari/o = ovary -pexy = surgical fixation	surgical fixation of the ovary
Papanicolaou smear (pap-ah-**NIK**-oh-low)	microscopic examination of cervical cells; diagnostic test for cervical cancer; Pap smear, Pap test (Figure 13-9)

(continues)

TABLE 13-6 FEMALE REPRODUCTIVE SYSTEM DIAGNOSTIC AND TREATMENT TERMS (continued)

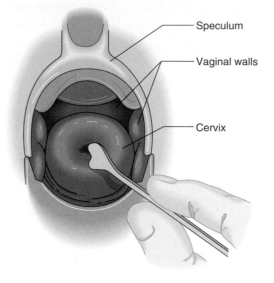

Figure 13-9 Pap smear

Term with Pronunciation	Definition
salpingo-oophorectomy (sal-ping-goh-oh-off-or-EK-toh-me) salping/o = fallopian tubes oophor/o = ovary -ectomy = surgical removal	surgical removal of the fallopian tubes and ovaries
tubal ligation (**TOO**-bal ligh-**GAY**-shun)	surgical cutting and tying of the fallopian tubes to prevent passage of the sperm and ova through the tube; female sterilization (Figure 13-10)

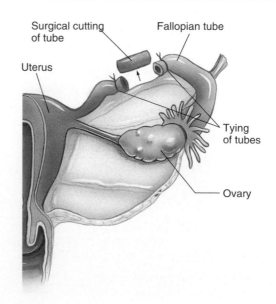

Figure 13-10 Tubal ligation

(continues)

TABLE 13-6   FEMALE REPRODUCTIVE SYSTEM DIAGNOSTIC AND TREATMENT TERMS (continued)

Term with Pronunciation	Definition
uteropexy (**YOO**-ter-oh-**pek**-see) uter/o = uterus -pexy = surgical fixation	surgical fixation of the uterus to the abdominal wall

EXERCISE 13

Analyze each term by writing the prefix, root, combining vowel, and suffix separated by vertical slashes. Based on the meaning of the word parts, write a definition for each term. Check the definition in a medical dictionary. Note that some terms might have more than one root.

1. colposcopy

prefix	root	combining vowel	suffix

DEFINITION: _____

2. hysterectomy

prefix	root	combining vowel	suffix

DEFINITION: _____

3. hysterosalpingography

prefix	root	combining vowel	suffix

DEFINITION: _____

4. laparoscopy

prefix	root	combining vowel	suffix

DEFINITION: _____

5. mammography

prefix	root	combining vowel	suffix

DEFINITION: _____

6. mastectomy

prefix	root	combining vowel	suffix

DEFINITION: _____

7. ovariopexy

prefix	root	combining vowel	suffix

DEFINITION: _____

8. oophoropexy

| prefix | root | combining vowel | suffix |

DEFINITION: _____

9. uteropexy

| prefix | root | combining vowel | suffix |

DEFINITION: _____

10. salpingo-oophorectomy

| prefix | root | combining vowel | suffix |

EXERCISE 14

Replace the italicized phrase with the correct medical term.

1. Carmen made every effort to have an annual *x-ray examination of her breasts.*

   _____

2. Melinda's initial *microscopic examination of cervical cells* was abnormal.

   _____

3. Helen chose *female sterilization* to prevent future pregnancies.

   _____

4. Irregular menstrual periods sometimes necessitate a *widening of the cervical canal and scraping of the uterine lining.*

   _____

5. After two abnormal cervical smears, the physician recommended a *surgical removal of cone-shaped segment of the cervix.*

   _____

6. *Rapid freezing, destruction, and removal of tissue* is a procedure for treating abnormal cervical tissue growth.

   _____

Abbreviations

Review the female reproductive system abbreviations in Table 13-7. Practice writing out the meaning of each abbreviation.

TABLE 13-7 ABBREVIATIONS

Abbreviation	Meaning
D&C	dilatation and curettage
GYN	gynecology
Pap smear	Papanicolaou smear
PID	pelvic inflammatory disease

(continues)

TABLE 13-7   ABBREVIATIONS (continued)

Abbreviation	Meaning
PMS	premenstrual syndrome
TAH	total abdominal hysterectomy
TSS	toxic shock syndrome
TVH	total vaginal hysterectomy

Pregnancy

This section of the chapter covers medical terms related to pregnancy. The generic medical term for male and female sex cells (ovum and sperm) is **gamete** (**GAM**-eet). Pregnancy occurs when an ovum has been fertilized by a sperm and is implanted into the endometrium. Fertilization usually takes place in the fallopian tube. The fertilized ovum is called a **zygote** (**ZIGH**-goht). From the second through the eighth week of pregnancy, the fertilized ovum is called an **embryo** (**EM**-bree-oh). For the remainder of the pregnancy, the fertilized ovum is called a **fetus** (**FEE**-tus). Pregnancy lasts 40 weeks or 280 days, which is about 9 calendar months or 10 lunar months. A lunar month is 4 weeks or 28 days.

Pregnancy is divided into trimesters; each trimester is about three months long. The time between fertilization, also known as conception, and labor is called **gestation** (JESS-**TAY**-shun), or the gestational period.

Pregnancy Word Roots

Word roots with the combining vowel are listed in Table 13-8. Review the word roots and complete the exercises that follow.

TABLE 13-8   PREGNANCY WORD ROOTS

Word Root/Combining Form	Meaning
amni/o; amnion/o	amnion
chori/o	chorion
embry/o	embryo
episi/o; vulv/o	vulva
fet/o; fet/i	fetus
gravid/o	pregnancy
lact/o	milk
nat/o	birth
par/o, part/o	bear; give birth to; labor; childbirth
pelv/i	pelvis
perine/o	perineum
puerper/o	childbirth
salping/o	fallopian tube
vagin/o	vagina

EXERCISE 15

Write the definitions of the following word roots.

1. fet/o _____

2. nat/o _____

3. par/o _____

4. amni/o _____

5. episi/o _____

6. salping/o _____

7. perine/o _____

8. pueper/o _____

9. pelv/i _____

10. lact/o _____

EXERCISE 16

Write the word root and its meanings on the spaces provided.

1. gravidarum

   ROOT:_____   MEANING: _____

2. perinatal

   ROOT:_____   MEANING: _____

3. salpingectomy

   ROOT:_____   MEANING: _____

4. fetoscope

   ROOT:_____   MEANING: _____

5. amniocentesis

   ROOT:_____   MEANING: _____

6. puerperium

   ROOT:_____   MEANING: _____

7. vaginal

   ROOT:_____   MEANING: _____

8. chorionitis

   ROOT:_____   MEANING: _____

9. lactorrhea

   ROOT:_____   MEANING: _____

10. episiotomy

    ROOT:_____   MEANING: _____

Structures Related to Pregnancy

In addition to the female reproductive organs already presented, the specific structures related to pregnancy include the **amniotic sac** (am-nee-**OT**-IK sac), (1) **placenta** (plah-**SEN**-tah), (2) **umbilicus** (um-**BILL**-ih-kus), and (3) **amniotic fluid** (am-nee-**OT**-ik fluid). Figure 13-11 illustrates these structures. Refer to this figure as you read about the structures.

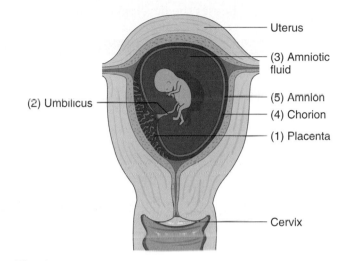

- Uterus
- (3) Amniotic fluid
- (5) Amnion
- (4) Chorion
- (1) Placenta
- (2) Umbilicus
- Cervix

Figure 13-11   The amniotic sac

The amniotic sac, also called the **fetal membrane**, houses the developing fetus. The sac is filled with amniotic fluid, which cushions and protects the fetus. The outer layer of the amniotic sac is the (4) **chorion** (**KOR**-ee-on), and the inner layer is the (5) **amnion** (**AM**-nee-on). Note that the umbilicus, also called the umbilical cord, connects the fetus to the placenta. The placenta, a temporary organ imbedded in the wall of the uterus, allows nutrients, oxygen, and waste to be exchanged between the mother and fetus. The placenta also produces several hormones necessary for a normal pregnancy.

EXERCISE 17

Write the medical term for each definition.

1. fertilized ovum   _____

2. fertilized ovum, ninth to fortieth week of pregnancy   _____

3. fertilized ovum, second to eighth week of pregnancy   _____

4. male and female sex cell   _____

5. period between fertilization and labor   _____

6. temporary organ embedded in the uterine wall   _____

7. structure that houses the developing fetus   _____

8. connects the fetus to the placenta _____

9. inner layer of the structure that houses the developing fetus _____

10. outer layer of the structure that houses the developing fetus _____

EXERCISE 18

Label the structures illustrated in Figure 13-12. Write your answers on the spaces provided.

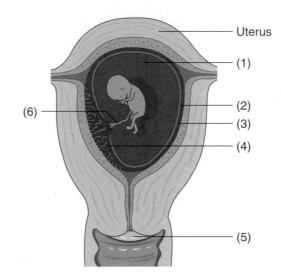

Uterus
(1)
(2)
(3)
(4)
(5)
(6)

Figure 13-12 Labeling exercise

1. _____
2. _____
3. _____
4. _____
5. _____
6. _____

Medical Terms Related to Pregnancy

Pregnancy medical terms are organized as: (1) general medical terms; (2) complications and disorders of pregnancy; and (3) diagnostic, surgical, and laboratory test terms. Prefixes and suffixes used in pregnancy terms are listed in Table 13-9. Review these word parts and complete the exercises that follow.

TABLE 13-9 PREFIXES AND SUFFIXES FOR PREGNANCY TERMS

Prefix	Meaning	Suffix	Meaning
ante-	before	-centesis	surgical puncture
micro-	small	-graphy	process of recording

(continues)

TABLE 13-9 PREFIXES AND SUFFIXES FOR PREGNANCY TERMS (continued)

Prefix	Meaning	Suffix	Meaning
multi-	many	-(o)logy	study of
nulli-	none	-metry	to measure
post-	after	-(o)tomy	incision into
primi-	first; one	-(r)rhexis	rupture
		-scopy	visualization with a scope
		-tocia	labor; birth

EXERCISE 19

Write the prefixes, suffixes, and their meanings in the spaces provided. Note that some terms have both a prefix and suffix, and some terms have only one or the other.

1. dystocia

   PREFIX: _____ MEANING: _____

   SUFFIX: _____ MEANING: _____

2. nullipara

   PREFIX: _____ MEANING: _____

   SUFFIX: _____ MEANING: _____

3. postpartum

   PREFIX: _____ MEANING: _____

   SUFFIX: _____ MEANING: _____

4. fetoscopy

   PREFIX: _____ MEANING: _____

   SUFFIX: _____ MEANING: _____

5. antepartum

   PREFIX: _____ MEANING: _____

   SUFFIX: _____ MEANING: _____

6. amniocentesis

   PREFIX: _____ MEANING: _____

   SUFFIX: _____ MEANING: _____

7. primigravida

   PREFIX: _____ MEANING: _____

   SUFFIX: _____ MEANING: _____

8. hysterorrhexis

   PREFIX: _____ MEANING: _____

   SUFFIX: _____ MEANING: _____

9. multigravida

PREFIX: _____ MEANING: _____

SUFFIX: _____ MEANING: _____

10. microscope

PREFIX: _____ MEANING: _____

SUFFIX: _____ MEANING: _____

EXERCISE 20

Write the prefix or suffix for each definition.

1. after _____

2. before _____

3. first _____

4. labor; birth _____

5. many _____

6. none _____

7. process of recording _____

8. rupture _____

9. surgical puncture _____

10. visualization with a scope _____

Pregnancy General Medical Terms

Review the pronunciation and meaning for each term in Table 13-10. Note that some terms are built from word parts and some are not. Complete the exercises for these terms.

TABLE 13-10 PREGNANCY GENERAL MEDICAL TERMS

Term with Pronunciation	Definition
antepartum (an-tee-**PAR**-tum) ante- = before part/o = giving birth; labor -um = noun ending	before the onset of labor; before giving birth
Braxton Hicks contraction	irregular and nonproductive contractions of the uterus that might occur throughout pregnancy
effacement (eh-**FACE**-ment)	normal thinning and shortening of the cervix during the birth process
embryologist (em-bree-**ALL**-oh-jist) embry/o = embryo -(o)logist = specialist in the study of	physician who specializes in the study and treatment of the growth and development of the human organism

(continues)

TABLE 13-10   PREGNANCY GENERAL MEDICAL TERMS (continued)

Term with Pronunciation	Definition
embryology (em-bree-**ALL**-oh-jist) embry/o = embryo -(o)logy = study of	study and treatment of the growth and development of the human organism
lochia (**LOH**-kee-ah)	vaginal discharge from the uterus that occurs for the first week or two after childbirth
meconium (meh-**KOH**-nee-um)	first feces of a newborn
multigravida (mull-tee-**GRAV**-ih-dah) multi- — many gravid/o = pregnancy	having been pregnant more than two times
multipara (mull-**TIP**-ah-rah) multi- = many par/o = giving birth to -a = noun ending	having given birth two or more times to a viable fetus
nulligravida (null-ee-**GRAV**-ih-dah) nulli- — none gravid/o = pregnancy -a = noun ending	never having been pregnant
nullipara (null-**IP**-ah-rah) nulli- = none par/o = giving birth to -a = noun ending	never having given birth to a viable fetus
obstetrician (**ob**-steh-**TRISH**-an)	physician who specializes in the study and treatment of pregnancy and deliver
obstetrics (ob-**STEH**-triks)	medical specialty related to pregnancy and delivery
parturition (par-too-**RISH**-un)	act of giving birth; childbirth; delivery
postpartum (post-**PAR**-tum) post- = after part/o = giving birth to -um = noun ending	occurring after childbirth

(continues)

TABLE 13-10   PREGNANCY GENERAL MEDICAL TERMS (continued)

Term with Pronunciation	Definition
primigravida (prigh-mih-**GRAV**-ih-dah) primi- = first gravid/o = pregnancy -a = noun ending	first pregnancy
primipara (prigh-**MIP**-ah-rah) primi- = first par/o = giving birth to -a = noun ending	giving birth for the first time following 20 or more weeks of gestation
puerperium (pyoo-er-**PEER**-ee-um) puerper/o = childbirth -um = noun ending	three- to six-week time period following childbirth

EXERCISE 21

Analyze each term by writing the prefix, root, combining vowel, and suffix separated by vertical slashes. Based on the meaning of the word parts, write a definition for each term. Check the definition in a medical dictionary. Note that some terms might have more than one root

EXAMPLE: gynecologist

	/ gynec	/ o	/ logist
prefix	*root*	*combining vowel*	*suffix*

DEFINITION: specialist in the female reproductive system

1. antepartum

prefix	*root*	*combining vowel*	*suffix*

DEFINITION: _____

2. embryologist

prefix	*root*	*combining vowel*	*suffix*

DEFINITION: _____

3. embryology

prefix	*root*	*combining vowel*	*suffix*

DEFINITION: _____

4. multigravida

prefix	*root*	*combining vowel*	*suffix*

DEFINITION: _____

5. multipara

prefix	root	combining vowel	suffix

DEFINITION: _____

6. nulligravida

prefix	root	combining vowel	suffix

DEFINITION: _____

7. ullipara

prefix	root	combining vowel	suffix

DEFINITION: _____

8. postpartum

prefix	root	combining vowel	suffix

DEFINITION: _____

9. primigravida

prefix	root	combining vowel	suffix

DEFINITION: _____

10. primipara

prefix	root	combining vowel	suffix

DEFINITION: _____

EXERCISE 21

Write the medical term for each definition.

1. childbirth _____

2. first childbirth after 20 weeks of gestation _____

3. first feces of a newborn _____

4. irregular, nonproductive contractions at any time during pregnancy _____

5. medical specialty related to pregnancy and delivery _____

6. more than one pregnancy _____

7. thinning and shortening of the cervix during the birth process _____

8. physician who specializes in pregnancy and delivery _____

9. specialty related to the growth and development of humans _____

10. three to six weeks following childbirth _____

11. vaginal discharge lasting a few weeks
    after childbirth _____

Pregnancy Complication and Disorder Terms

Complications and disorders associated with pregnancy and delivery include familiar problems such as ectopic, or tubal, pregnancy as well as more serious complications such as abruptio placentae (ah-**BRUP**-shee-oh plah-**SEN**-tee). Review the medical terms, pronunciations, and definitions in Table 13-11 and complete the exercises.

TABLE 13-11   PREGNANCY COMPLICATION AND DISORDER TERMS

Term with Pronunciation	Definition
abortion (ah-**BOR**-shun)	spontaneous or induced termination of a pregnancy; a spontaneous abortion is commonly called a *miscarriage*
abruptio placentae (ah-**BRUP**-shee-oh plah-**SEN**-tee)	premature separation of the placenta from the uterine wall
amnionitis (**am**-nee-oh-**NIGH**-tis) amni/o = amnion -itis = inflammation	inflammation of the amnion
amniorrhea (**am**-nee-oh-**REE**-ah) amni/o = amnion -(r)rhea =flow; discharge	discharge of amniotic fluid from the amniotic sac; leaking of amniotic fluid
breech birth	delivery presentation with the buttocks appearing first
dystocia (diss-**TOH**-see-ah) dys- = abnormal; painful; difficult -tocia = labor; birth	difficult or painful labor
eclampsia (ee-**KLAMP**-see-ah)	most severe form of gestational hypertension characterized by seizures
ectopic pregnancy (ek-**TOP**-ik)	abnormal implantation of a fertilized ovum outside the uterus; also called a *tubal pregnancy*
gestational diabetes (jess-**TAY**-shun-al digh-ah-**BEE**-teez)	diabetes that develops during pregnancy and that usually resolves after pregnancy
gestational hypertension (jess-**TAY**-shun-al high-per-**TEN**-shun)	hypertension that develops during pregnancy and that usually resolves after pregnancy; also called *pregnancy induced hypertension* (PIH)

(continues)

TABLE 13-11   PREGNANCY COMPLICATION AND DISORDER TERMS (continued)

Term with Pronunciation	Definition
hydatidiform mole (**high**-dah-**TID**-ih-form)	a cystic mass resembling a cluster of grapes that develops in place of a placenta and fetus; also called a *molar pregnancy*
hyperemesis gravidarum (**high**-per-**EM**-eh-sis **grav**-ih-**DAR**-um) hyper- = excessive -emesis = vomiting gravid/o = pregnancy -um = noun ending	condition characterized by excessive and severe vomiting that results in maternal dehydration and weight loss
hysterorrhexis (**hiss**-ter-oh-**REKS**-iss) hyster/o = uterus -(r)rhexis = rupture	rupture of the uterus
incompetent cervix	inability of the cervix to retain the contents of the pregnant uterus that results in a spontaneous abortion
placenta previa (plah-**SEN**-tah **PREE** vee-ah)	condition in which the placenta is implanted in a lower part of the uterus and precedes the fetus during delivery (Figure 13-13)

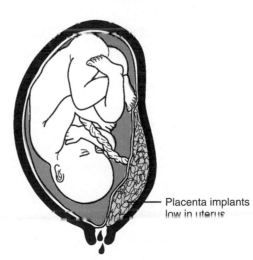

Placenta implants low in uterus

Figure 13-13   Placenta previa

pre-eclampsia (**pre**-ee-**KLAMP**-see-ah)	gestational hypertension characterized by edema and proteinuria, the presence of protein in the urine

(continues)

TABLE 13-11 PREGNANCY COMPLICATION AND DISORDER TERMS (continued)

Term with Pronunciation	Definition
Rh incompatibility	reaction between Rh negative (Rh–) blood and the Rh positive (Rh+) fetal blood of a first pregnancy that the immune system of the mother to develop antibodies against Rh+ blood cells; in subsequent pregnancies, the antibodies will attack Rh+ fetal blood cells
tubal pregnancy	implantation of a fertilized ovum in the wall of a fallopian tube; also called *ectopic pregnancy*

EXERCISE 23

Analyze each term by writing the prefix, root, combining vowel, and suffix separated by vertical slashes. Based on the meaning of the word parts, write a definition for each term. Check the definitions in a medical dictionary. Note that some terms might have more than one root.

1. amnionitis

| *prefix* | *root* | *combining vowel* | *suffix* |

DEFINITION: _____

2. amniorrhea

| *prefix* | *root* | *combining vowel* | *suffix* |

DEFINITION: _____

3. dystocia

| *prefix* | *root* | *combining vowel* | *suffix* |

DEFINITION: _____

4. hyperemesis gravidarum

| *prefix* | *root* | *combining vowel* | *suffix* |

| *prefix* | *root* | *combining vowel* | *suffix* |

DEFINITION: _____

5. hysterorrhexis

| *prefix* | *root* | *combining vowel* | *suffix* |

DEFINITION: _____

EXERCISE 24

Replace the italicized phrase with the correct medical term.

1. At 12 weeks gestation, Marcia had a spontaneous *termination of pregnancy*.

   _____

2. *Premature separation of the placenta* is a life-threatening condition for both mother and child.

   _____

3. Cheryl experienced *diabetes during pregnancy* for each of her pregnancies.

   _____

4. Due to an *implantation of a fertilized ovum outside the uterus*, Sara underwent removal of a fallopian tube.

   _____

5. Melinda's labor was prolonged due to a *delivery presentation with buttocks appearing first*.

   _____

EXERCISE 25

Match the condition in Column 1 with the correct definition in Column 2.

COLUMN 1

_____ 1. abruptio placentae
_____ 2. breech birth
_____ 3. dystocia
_____ 4. eclampsia
_____ 5. hydatidiform mole
_____ 6. hysterorrhexis
_____ 7. incompetent cervix
_____ 8. PIH
_____ 9. placenta previa
_____ 10. pre-eclampsia
_____ 11. Rh incompatibility
_____ 12. tubal pregnancy

COLUMN 2

a. rupture of the uterus

b. reaction between maternal and fetal blood

c. premature separation of the placenta

d. placenta precedes the fetus during delivery

e. most severe form of gestational hypertension

f. inability of the cervix to retain contents of pregnant uterus

g. gestational hypertension with edema and proteinuria

h. ectopic pregnancy

i. development of hypertension during pregnancy

j. difficult or painful labor

k. delivery presentation with buttocks appearing first

l. cystic mass that develops in place of a placenta and fetus

**Pregnancy
Diagnostic,
Treatment, and
Surgical Terms**

Review the pronunciation and definition for the terms listed in Table 13-12 and complete the exercises.

TABLE 13-12 PREGNANCY DIAGNOSTIC, TREATMENT, AND
SURGICAL TERMS

Term with Pronunciation	Definition
amniocentesis (**am**-nee-oh-sen-**TEE**-sis) amni/o = amnion -centesis = surgical puncture to remove fluid	surgical puncture into the amniotic sac to remove fluid for analysis to identify genetic disorders of the fetus; usually performed during the 15th week of pregnancy or later (Figure 13-14)

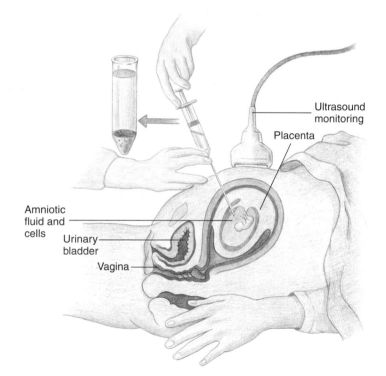

Figure 13-14 Amniocentesis

amniography (**am**-nee-**OG**-rah-fee) amni/o = amnion -graphy = process of recording	process of taking an x-ray of the amniotic sac using a contrast medium
amnioscopy (**am**-nee-**OSS**-koh-pee) amni/o = amnion -scopy = visualization with a scope	visualization of the fetus with a scope that enters the amniotic cavity through the abdominal wall
amniotomy (**am**-nee-**OT**-oh-mee) amni/o = amnion -(o)tomy = incision into	incision into or rupture of the amniotic membranes to induce labor; also called "breaking the water"

(continues)

TABLE 13-12 PREGNANCY DIAGNOSTIC, TREATMENT, AND
SURGICAL TERMS (continued)

Term with Pronunciation	Definition
cerclage (ser-**KLOZH**)	suturing the cervical opening to prevent spontaneous abortion; treatment for a history of incompetent cervix
cesarean section (see-**SAYR**-ee-an) (C-section)	incision into the abdominal wall and uterus to deliver a baby
chorionic villus sampling (**kor**-ee-**ON**-ik **VILL**-us) (CVS) chori/o = chorion -ic = pertaining to	removal of a small sample of the placenta by inserting a catheter or needle through the cervix and withdrawing placental tissue for analysis to identify genetic disorders of the fetus; usually performed between the 10th and 12th weeks of pregnancy
contraction stress test (CST)	introduction of a diluted intravenous (IV) solution containing the hormone oxytocin to stimulate uterine contractions to evaluate whether the fetus can tolerate the stress of labor and delivery; also called the *oxytocin challenge test*
electronic fetal monitoring	application and use of an internal or external electronic device to monitor fetal heart rate and maternal uterine contractions; such monitoring can assess the quality of the uterine contractions and the effects of labor on the fetus
episiotomy (eh-**pihz**-ee-**OT**-oh-mee) episi/o = vulva -(o)tomy = incision into	incision into the perineum to facilitate delivery and prevent perineal laceration or tearing
fetal ultrasonography (**ull**-trah-soh-**NOG**-rah-fee)	noninvasive examination of the fetus in utero using high-frequency sound waves (Figure 13-15)

(continues)

TABLE 13-12 PREGNANCY DIAGNOSTIC, TREATMENT, AND SURGICAL TERMS (continued)

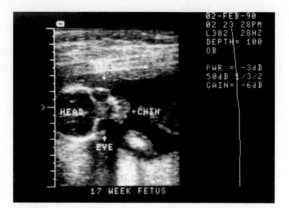

Figure 13-15   Fetal ultrasound

Term with Pronunciation	Definition
fetometry (fee-**TOM**-eh-tree) fet/o = fetus -metry = process of measuring	measuring or estimating the size of the fetus or the fetal head before delivery
pelvimetry (pell-**VIM**-eh-tree) pelv/i = pelvis -metry = process of measuring	measuring the pelvic outlet to determine if its size is adequate for childbirth
pregnancy test	laboratory blood and urine tests to determine pregnancy

EXERCISE 26

Analyze each term by writing the root, combining vowel, and suffix separated by vertical slashes. Based on the meaning of the word parts, write a definition for each term. Check the definition in a medical dictionary.

1. amniocentesis

   _____
   prefix   *root*   *combining vowel*   *suffix*
   DEFINITION: _____

2. amniography

   _____
   prefix   *root*   *combining vowel*   *suffix*
   DEFINITION: _____

3. amnioscopy

   _____
   prefix   *root*   *combining vowel*   *suffix*
   DEFINITION: _____

4. amniotomy

prefix	root	combining vowel	suffix

DEFINITION: _____

5. episiotomy

prefix	root	combining vowel	suffix

DEFINITION: _____

6. fetography

prefix	root	combining vowel	suffix

DEFINITION: _____

7. fetometry

prefix	root	combining vowel	suffix

DEFINITION: _____

8. pelvimetry

prefix	root	combining vowel	suffix

DEFINITION: _____

EXERCISE 27

Circle the medical term that best fits the description.

DESCRIPTION	CIRCLE ONE ITEM
1. surgical puncture to remove fluid	*amniotomy* OR *amniocentesis*
2. estimating fetal size before delivery	*fetometry* OR *fetography*
3. x-ray examination of the fetus	*fetography* OR *fetoscopy*
4. incision into the perineum	*cerclage* OR *episiotomy*
5. endoscopic visualization of the fetus	*fetal ultrasound* OR *amnioscopy*
6. measuring the pelvic outlet	*pelvimetry* OR *CST*
7. rupture of the amniotic membranes	*amniotomy* OR *C-section*
8. suturing the cervical opening	*CVS* OR *cerclage*
9. labor and delivery fetal stress test	*electronic fetal monitoring* OR *CST*
10. incision to deliver a baby	*cesarean section* OR *amniotomy*

Abbreviations

Review the abbreviations in Table 13-13. Practice writing out the meaning of each abbreviation.

TABLE 13-13   ABBREVIATIONS

Abbreviation	Meaning
C-section	cesarean section
CST	contraction stimulation test
CVS	chorionic villus sampling
EDB	expected date of birth
EDC	expected or estimated date of confinement
EDD	expected date of delivery
FHR	fetal heart rate
L & D	labor and delivery
LMP	last menstrual period
NSD	normal spontaneous delivery
OB	obstetrics
PIH	pregnancy induced hypertension
SVD	spontaneous vaginal delivery

CHAPTER REVIEW

The Chapter Review can be used as a self-test. Go through each exercise and answer as many questions as you can without referring to previous exercises or earlier discussions within this chapter. Check your answers and fill in any blanks. Practice writing any terms you might have misspelled.

EXERCISE 28

Write the medical term for each definition.

1. physician who specializes in the female reproductive system _____

2. study of the female reproductive system _____

3. absence or lack of menstrual flow _____

4. painful or difficult menstrual flow _____

5. excessive bleeding during the menstrual period _____

6. excessive uterine bleeding at times other than the menstrual period _____

7. excessive uterine bleeding during and between the regular menstrual period _____

8. diminished menstrual flow _____

9. inflammation of the ovaries _____

10. inflammation of the fallopian tubes _____

11. examination of the vagina with a scope _____

12. process of recording an x-ray of the uterus and fallopian tubes

_____

13. process of recording an x-ray of the breasts

_____

14. surgical removal of the breast

_____

15. surgical fixation of the ovaries

_____

16. surgical removal of the uterus

_____

17. surgical removal of the fallopian tubes and ovaries

_____

18. surgical fixation of the uterus to the abdominal wall

_____

19. inflammation of the vagina

_____

20. inflammation of the vulva and vagina

_____

EXERCISE 29

Read the following operative report and write a brief definition for each italicized medical term on the spaces provided.

OPERATIVE REPORT

PREOPERATIVE DIAGNOSIS: (1) _Menometrorrhagia_ and (2) _cervical_ stenosis.

POSTOPERATIVE DIAGNOSIS: Menometrorrhagia and cervical stenosis.

OPERATION: Diagnostic (3) _hysteroscopy_ and (4) _dilatation and curettage_ of the uterus.

DESCRIPTION OF PROCEDURE: Under adequate general anesthesia, the patient was prepped and draped in the low lithotomy position. Bimanual examination revealed the (5) _uterus_ to be 6-weeks' size and midline. A speculum was placed in the (6) _vagina_, and the (7) _cervix_ was grasped with a single-toothed tenaculum. It was very stenotic, and we started with the smallest dilator available and dilated up to a No. 9 Pratt. An Olympus fiberoptic (8) _hysteroscope_ was then inserted, and inspection was carried out. There was extensive glandular- and abnormal-appearing tissue along the entire posterior wall of the uterus that appeared to be hyperplastic. The hysteroscope was removed from the uterus, and the cervix was then dilated. (9) _Endometrial_ curettage was performed, with removal of a very large amount of glandular-appearing tissue. The patient tolerated the procedure well and left the operating room in good condition.

1. _____

2. _____

3. _____

4. _____

5. _____

6. _____

7. _____

8. _____

9. _____

EXERCISE 30

Write out the abbreviations and provide a brief description of the disease or procedure.

1. D&C   _____

   DEFINITION: _____

2. PID   _____

   DEFINITION: _____

3. PMS   _____

   DEFINITION: _____

4. TAH   _____

   DEFINITION: _____

5. TSS   _____

   DEFINITION: _____

EXERCISE 31

Select the best answer for each statement or question.

1. Which structures coax the ovum into the fallopian tubes?
   a. villi
   b. fimbriae
   c. vulva
   d. adnexa

2. Which term means the outer layer of the uterus?
   a. endometrium
   b. epimetrium
   c. perimetrium
   d. myometrium

3. Select the medical term for the external genitalia.
   a. fimbriae
   b. vulva
   c. adnexa
   d. villi

4. Which term is used to describe the fallopian tubes and ovaries?
   a. fimbriae
   b. vulva
   c. adnexa
   d. villi

5. Select the term for the ovarian structures where ova mature.
   a. graafian follicles
   b. ovarian cyst
   c. adnexa
   d. ovarial follicles

6. Select the medical term for the muscle layer of the uterus.
   a. endometrium
   b. perimetrium
   c. myometrium
   d. musculometrium

7. Which female reproductive structure is commonly called the womb?
   a. vulva
   b. uterus
   c. adnexa
   d. vagina

8. Select the medical term for the onset of menstruation.
   a. menarche
   b. menses
   c. menopause
   d. menstrual period

9. Which term means the inner layer of the uterus?
   a. perimetrium
   b. endometrium
   c. myometrium
   d. endometriosis

10. Select the term for the periodic release of ovum.
    a. menstruation
    b. menses
    c. menarche
    d. ovulation

EXERCISE 32

Write the medical term for each definition.

1. physician who specializes in the growth and development of the human organism   _____

2. has been pregnant many times   _____

3. occurring after childbirth   _____

4. first pregnancy   _____

5. discharge or leaking of amniotic fluid   _____

6. never has been pregnant   _____

7. difficult or painful labor   _____

8. inflammation of the amnion   _____

9. excessive and severe vomiting during pregnancy   _____

10. uterine rupture   _____

11. incision into the amniotic membranes   _____

12. surgical puncture into the amniotic sac
to remove fluid   _____

13. incision into the perineum to
facilitate delivery   _____

14. measuring the size of the fetus
before delivery   _____

15. study of the growth and development of
the human organism   _____

16. physician who specializes in pregnancy
and delivery   _____

17. act of giving birth   _____

18. three- to six- week time period following childbirth   _____

19. delivery presentation with buttocks appearing first   _____

20. most severe form of gestational hypertension
characterized by seizures   _____

EXERCISE 33

Match the medical terms in Column 1 with the correct definition in Column 2.

COLUMN 1

_____ 1. abruptio placentae

_____ 2. Braxton Hicks contractions

_____ 3. cerclage

_____ 4. effacement

_____ 5. hydatidiform mole

_____ 6. lochia

_____ 7. meconium

_____ 8. nullipara

_____ 9. obstetrics

_____ 10. placenta previa

_____ 11. pre-eclampsia

_____ 12. Rh incompatibility

_____ 13. tubal pregnancy

_____ 14. eclampsia

COLUMN 2

a. cystic grapelike mass in the uterus

b. severe gestational hypertension

c. ectopic pregnancy

d. first feces of a newborn

e. gestational hypertension with proteinuria

f. implantation of the placenta toward the
cervix

g. reaction between maternal and fetal
blood

h. irregular, nonproductive contractions

i. medical specialty related to pregnancy

j. normal thinning of the cervix during
childbirth

k. never having given birth to a viable fetus

l. premature separation of the placenta

m. suturing of the cervical opening

n. vaginal discharge from the uterus

EXERCISE 34

Read the following progress note and write the meaning of the italicized terms.

PROGRESS NOTE

The patient was admitted to the (1) *obstetrical* unit with contractions 5 minutes apart. According to her history, she is (2) *multigravida* and (3) *nullipara*. She has had two miscarriages and (4) *cerclage* was done at 8 weeks gestation, due to (5) *incompetent cervix*. She presents at 39 weeks gestation with (6) *amniorrhea* that is negative for (7) *meconium*. (8) *Effacement* was noted during her (9) *prenatal* visit last Friday. The patient states that she is comfortable with her current pain level. Prenatal (10) *pelvimetry* supported her decision for (11) *SVD*. However, given her history (12) *electronic fetal monitoring* is appropriate and the patient has signed a consent for a (13) *C-section*, should that be necessary.

1. _____
2. _____
3. _____
4. _____
5. _____
6. _____
7. _____
8. _____
9. _____
10. _____
11. _____
12. _____
13. _____

CHALLENGE EXERCISE

1. *Endometriosis is a painful, chronic disease that affects 5.5 million females in the United States and Canada alone. Access the Endometriosis Association's (EA) Web site at www.endometriosisassn.org to learn more about this condition. Prepare a handout that answers these questions: What are the symptoms, causes, and treatments for endometriosis? What languages are available for EA brochures? Does the site provide links for additional information about endometriosis? What startling discovery was made regarding toxic chemicals such as dioxin?*

2. *Amniocentesis and chorionic villus sampling (CVS) are tests that help identify fetal genetic disorders before birth. Access the American Academy of Family Physician's (AAFP) Web site at www.familydoctor.org to learn more about these tests. After reviewing the information, answer the following questions. What is the difference between amniocentesis and CVS? Who should consider having these tests? What are the risks involved with these tests?*

Pronunciation Review

Review the terms in the chapter. Pronounce each term using the following phonetic pronunciations. Check off the term when you are comfortable saying it.

TERM	PRONUNCIATION
☐ abortion	ah-**BOR**-shun
☐ abruptio placentae	ah-**BRUP**-shee-oh plah-**SEN**-tee
☐ amenorrhea	**ah**-men-oh-**REE**-ah
☐ amniocentesis	**am**-nee-oh-sen-**TEE**-sis
☐ amniography	**am**-nee-**OG**-rah-fee
☐ amnionitis	**am**-nee-oh-**NIGH**-tis
☐ amniorrhea	**am**-nee-oh-**REE**-ah
☐ amnioscopy	**am**-nee-**OSS**-koh-pee
☐ amniotic sac	**am**-nee-**OT**-ik sac
☐ anteflexion	an-tee-**FLEX**-shun
☐ antepartum	an-tee-**PAR**-tum
☐ Braxton Hicks contraction	**BRACKS**-ton Hicks contraction
☐ carcinoma of the breast	kar-sin-**OH**-mah of the breast
☐ cerclage	sar-**KLOZH**
☐ cervical carcinoma	**SER**-vih-kal **kar**-sin-**OH**-mah
☐ cervicitis	serv-vih-**SIGH**-tis
☐ cesarean section (C-section)	see-**SAYR**-ee-an section
☐ colposcopy	kol-**POSS**-koh-pee
☐ cone biopsy	cone **BIGH**-op-see
☐ conization	kon-ih-**ZAY**-shun
☐ cryosurgery	**krigh**-oh-**SER**-jer-ree
☐ cystocele	**SISS**-toh-seel
☐ dilatation and curettage	dill-ah-**TAY**-shun and koo-reh-**TAHZ**
☐ dysmenorrhea	**diss**-men-oh-**REE**-ah
☐ dystocia	diss-**TOH**-see-ah
☐ eclampsia	ee-**KLAMP**-see-ah
☐ ectopic pregnancy	ek-**TOP**-ik pregnancy
☐ effacement	eh-**FACE**-ment
☐ embryo	**EM**-bree-oh
☐ embryologist	em-bree-**ALL**-oh-jist
☐ embryology	em-bree-**ALL**-oh-jee
☐ endometriosis	**en**-doh-**mee**-tree-**OH**-sis
☐ episiotomy	eh-**pihz**-ee-**OT**-oh-mee
☐ fetal ultrasonography	**FEE**-tal **ull**-trah-soh-**NOG**-rah-fee
☐ fetometry	fee-**TOM**-eh-tree
☐ fetus	**FEE**-tus
☐ fibrocystic breast disease	**figh**-broh-**SIS**-tik breast disease
☐ gamete	**GAM**-eet
☐ gestation	jess-**TAY**-shun
☐ gestational diabetes	jess-**TAY**-shun-al digh-ah-**BEE**-teez
☐ gestational hypertension	jess-**TAY**-shun-al high-per-**TEN**-shun
☐ gynecologist	gigh-neh-**KALL**-oh-jist OR jin-eh-**KALL**-oh-jist
☐ gynecology	gigh-neh-**KALL**-oh-jee OR jin-eh-**KALL**-oh-jee
☐ hydatidiform mole	**high**-dah-**TID**-ih-form mole
☐ hyperemesis gravidarum	**high**-per-**EM**-eh-sis **grav**-ih-**DAR**-um

☐ hysterectomy   **hiss**-ter-**EK**-toh-mee

☐ hysterorrhexis   **hiss**-teh-roh-**EK**-sis

☐ hysterosalpingography   **hiss**-ter-oh-**sal**-pin-**GOG**-rah-fee

☐ laparoscopy   lap-ah-**ROSS**-koh-pee

☐ lochia   **LOH**-kee-ah

☐ mammography   mam-**OG**-rah-fee

☐ mastectomy   mass-**TEK**-toh-mee

☐ meconium   meh-**KOH**-nee-um

☐ menometrorrhagia   **men**-oh-**met**-roh-**RAY**-jee-ah

☐ menopause   **MEN**-oh-pawz

☐ menorrhagia   men-oh-**RAY**-jee-ah

☐ menorrhea   men-oh-**REE**-ah

☐ metrorrhagia   meh-troh-**RAY**-jee-ah

☐ multigravida   mull-tee-**GRAV**-ih-dah

☐ multipara   mull-**TIP**-ah-rah

☐ nulligravida   null-ee-**GRAV**-ih-dah

☐ nullipara   null-**IP**-ah-rah

☐ obstetrician   **ob**-steh-**TRISH**-an

☐ obstetrics   ob-**STEH**-triks

☐ oligomenorrhea   **oh**-lig-oh-**men**-oh-**REE**-ah

☐ oophorectomy   oh-**off**-or-**EK**-toh-mee

☐ oophoritis   oh-**off**-or-**EYE**-tis

☐ oophoropexy   oh-**off**-or-**PEK**-see

☐ ovarian carcinoma   oh-**VAY**-ree-an **kar**-sin-**OH**-mah

☐ ovarian cyst   oh-**VAY**-ree-an **SIST**

☐ ovariopexy   oh-**vay**-ree-oh-**PEK**-see

☐ ovary   **OH**-vah-ree

☐ Papanicolaou smear   pap-ah-**NIK**-oh-loh smear

☐ parturition   par-too-**RISH**-un

☐ pelvimetry   pell-**VIM**-eh-tree

☐ placenta   plah-**SEN**-tah

☐ placenta previa   plah-**SEN**-tah **PREE**-vee-ah

☐ postpartum   post-**PAR**-tum

☐ pre-eclampsia   **pree**-ee-**KLAM**-see-ah

☐ premenstrual syndrome   pree-**MEN**-strool syndrome

☐ primigravida   prigh-mih-**GRAV**-ih-dah

☐ primipara   prigh-**MIP**-ah-rah

☐ puerperium   pyoo-er-**PEE**-ree-um

☐ retroversion of the uterus   **reh**-troh-**VER**-shun of the uterus

☐ salpingitis   **sal**-pin-**JIGH**-tis

☐ salpingo-oophorectomy   sal-**ping**-oh-**oh**-off-or-**EK**-toh-mee

☐ tubal ligation   **TOO**-bal ligh-**GAY**-shun

☐ tubal pregnancy   **TOO**-bal pregnancy

☐ umbilicus   um-**BILL**-ih-kus

☐ vaginitis   vaj-in-**EYE**-tis

☐ vulvovaginitis   **vull**-voh-**vaj**-in-**EYE**-tis

☐ zygote   **ZIGH**-goht

Chapter 14
Nervous System

OBJECTIVES

At the completion of this chapter, the student should be able to:

1. Identify, define, and spell word roots associated with the nervous system.
2. Label the basic structures of the nervous system.
3. Discuss the functions of the nervous system.
4. Provide the correct spelling of nervous system terms, given the definition of the terms.
5. Analyze nervous system terms by defining the roots, prefixes, and suffixes of these terms.
6. Identify, define, and spell disease, disorder, and procedure terms related to the nervous system.

OVERVIEW

The nervous system includes nerve cells, the brain, the spinal cord, 12 pairs of cranial nerves, and 31 pairs of spinal nerves. The brain and spinal cord are known as the **central nervous system (CNS)**. The cranial and spinal nerves are known as the **peripheral** (peh-**RIF**-er-al) **nervous system (PNS)**. Spinal nerves are also called the *peripheral* nerves. Figure 14-1 illustrates the divisions of the nervous system.

The structures of the nervous system function together to (1) regulate all activities of the body, (2) control consciousness, (3) detect environmental stimuli, (4) respond to environmental stimuli, (5) process and store sensory and motor information, and (6) transmit sensory and motor impulses between the brain and all parts of the body.

Nervous System Word Roots

To understand and use nervous system medical terms, it is necessary to acquire a thorough knowledge of the associated word roots. These word roots are listed with the combining vowel in Table 14-1. Review the word roots and complete the exercises that follow.

TABLE 14-1 NERVOUS SYSTEM WORD ROOTS

Word Root/Combining Form	Meaning
cephal/o	head
cerebell/o	cerebellum
cerebr/o	cerebrum
crani/o	cranium; skull

(continues)

TABLE 14-1 NERVOUS SYSTEM WORD ROOTS (continued)

Word Root/Combining Form	Meaning
dendr/o	branching
encephal/o	brain
gli/o	neuroglia; nerve cell
mening/o	meninges
myel/o	spinal cord (also bone marrow)
neur/o	nerve
olig/o	few; diminished amount
thec/o	sheath
ventricul/o	ventricle

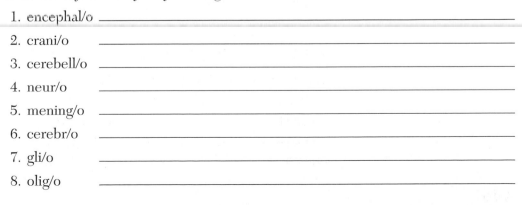

Figure 14-1 Divisions of the nervous system

EXERCISE 1

Write the definitions of the following word roots.

1. encephal/o _____

2. crani/o _____

3. cerebell/o _____

4. neur/o _____

5. mening/o _____

6. cerebr/o _____

7. gli/o _____

8. olig/o _____

9. dendr/o _____

10. myel/o _____

EXERCISE 2

Write the nervous system word root(s) and meanings for each term.

1. craniotomy

   ROOT: _____   MEANING: _____

2. neuropathy

   ROOT: _____   MEANING: _____

3. intrathecal

   ROOT: _____   MEANING: _____

4. cephalalgia

   ROOT: _____   MEANING: _____

5. cerebrovascular

   ROOT: _____   MEANING: _____

6. meningitis

   ROOT: _____   MEANING: _____

7. glioma

   ROOT: _____   MEANING: _____

8. myeloma

   ROOT: _____   MEANING: _____

9. oligodendroglia

   ROOT: _____   MEANING: _____

   ROOT: _____   MEANING: _____

10. ventriculitis

   ROOT: _____   MEANING: _____

EXERCISE 3

Write the correct word root(s) for the following definitions.

1. brain _____

2. cerebellum _____

3. cerebrum _____

4. cranium _____

5. head _____

6. meninges _____

7. nerve _____

8. nerve cell   _____

9. sheath   _____

10. spinal cord   _____

11. ventricle   _____

Cells of the Nervous System

Nerve cells are the basic structure or unit of the nervous system. There are two general categories of nerve cells: **neurons** (**NOO**-ronz), which transmit nerve impulses from the body to the brain and back to the body, and **neuroglia** (noo-**ROG**-lee-ah), the nerve cells that support the nervous system.

Neurons consist of a (1) **cell body** that contains the cell nucleus; (2) **dendrites** (**DEN**-drights), which are branchlike structures that receive impulses and send them to the cell body; an (3) **axon** (**ACKS**-on), which sends impulses away from the cell body; (4) **myelin** (**MIGH**-eh-lin), a white fatty tissue that covers the axon; and (5) **terminal end fibers**, branching fibers that lead the impulse away from the axon. The space between neurons or a neuron and an organ is called a (6) **synapse** (**SIN**-apps). Figure 14-2 illustrates a neuron.

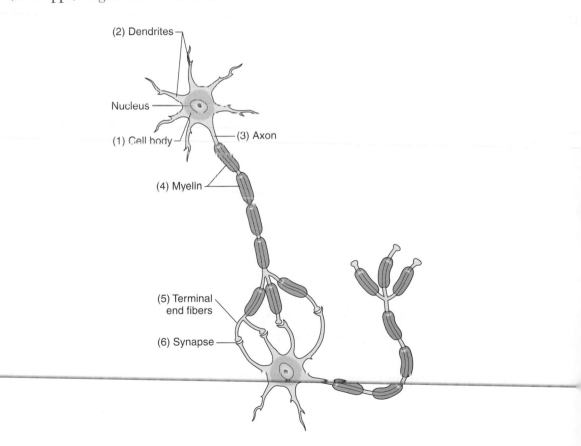

Figure 14-2 Structures of a neuron

Neuroglia are the supportive and connective cells of the nervous system and do not conduct impulses. There are three types of neuroglial cells: (1) **astrocytes** (**ASS**-troh-sights), (2) **microglia** (my-**KROG**-lee-ah), and (3) **oligodendroglia** (**all**-ih-goh-den-**DROG**-lee-ah). Figure 14-3 illustrates the neuroglia.

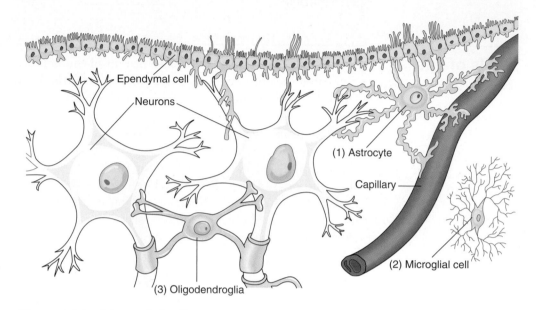

Figure 14-3 Neuroglial cells

EXERCISE 4

Label the parts of the neuron shown in Figure 14-4. Write your answers in the spaces provided.

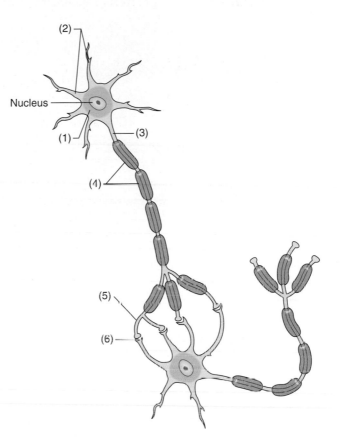

Nucleus

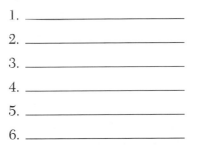

Figure 14-4   Labeling exercise

1. _____

2. _____

3. _____

4. _____

5. _____

6. _____

Brain and Spinal Cord

As previously stated, the brain and spinal cord are known as the *central nervous system.* The brain weighs about three pounds and controls almost every physical and mental activity of the body. The spinal cord transmits nerve impulses to and from the brain to all parts of the body. Refer to Figure 14-1 for an illustration of the spinal cord. The parts of the brain are illustrated in Figure 14-5. Refer to this figure as you learn about these structures.

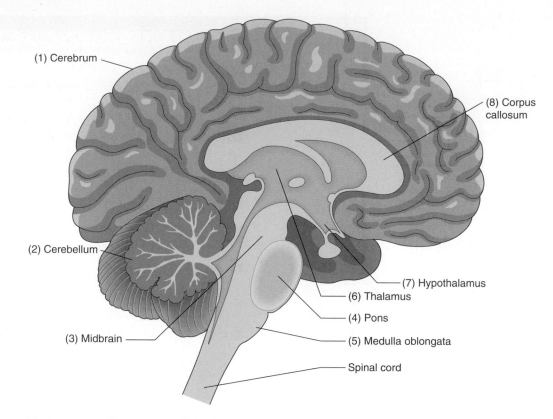

Figure 14-5 Structures of the brain

Major structures of the brain include the (1) **cerebrum** (seh-**REE**-brum), (2) **cerebellum** (ser-eh-**BELL**-um), (3) **midbrain**, (4) **pons** (PONZ), (5) **medulla oblongata** (meh-**DULL**-ah ob-long-**AH**-tah), (6) **thalamus** (**THAL**-ah-mus), (7) **hypothalamus** (**high**-poh-**THAL**-ah-mus), and (8) **corpus callosum** (**KOR**-pus kal-**OH**-sum). The midbrain, pons, and medulla oblongata are collectively known as the **brainstem**. Table 14-2 lists the parts of the brain and describes their functions.

TABLE 14-2 PARTS OF THE BRAIN WITH DESCRIPTIONS

Parts of the Brain	Description
cerebrum	largest section of the brain; controls consciousness, memory, sensations, emotions, and voluntary movement
cerebellum	attaches the brain to the brainstem; maintains muscle tone, movement, and balance
midbrain	area of the brain that provides nerve-conduction pathways to and from the brain
pons	literally means "bridge"; nerve cells cross from one side of the brain to control the opposite side of the body
medulla oblongata	lowest section of the brainstem; controls the muscles of respiration, heart rate, and blood pressure
thalamus	relays nerve impulses to and from the cerebral cortex and the sense organs of the body

(continues)

TABLE 14-2 PARTS OF THE BRAIN WITH DESCRIPTIONS (continued)

Parts of the Brain	Description
hypothalamus	regulates heart rate, blood pressure, respiratory rate, digestive activities, emotional responses, behavior, body temperature, water balance and thirst, sleep-wake cycles, hunger sensations, and endocrine system activities; often called the "thermostat" of the body
corpus callosum	structure that connects the two hemispheres of the brain

The cerebrum is divided into right and left hemispheres. The **cerebral cortex** (seh-**REE**-bral **KOR**-teks) is the outer layer of the cerebrum; it is characterized by folds and grooves. The cerebral cortex folds are called **gyri** (**JIGH**-righ), and the grooves are called **sulci** (**SULL**-kigh), or fissures. A single fold is a gyrus, and a single groove is a sulcus. Each hemisphere of the cerebrum has four distinct lobes, which are illustrated in Figure 14-6.

The (1) **frontal lobe** is responsible for motor function. The (2) **temporal** (**TEM**-por-al) **lobe** is responsible for hearing and smell. The (3) **occipital** (ok-**SIP**-ih-tal) **lobe** is responsible for sight. The (4) **parietal** (pah-**RIGH**-eh-tal) **lobe** receives and interprets nerve impulses from the sensory receptors located throughout the body.

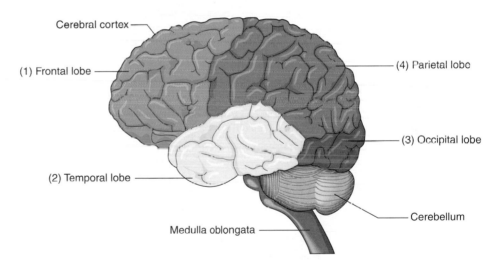

Cerebral cortex
(1) Frontal lobe
(4) Parietal lobe
(3) Occipital lobe
(2) Temporal lobe
Cerebellum
Medulla oblongata

Figure 14-6 Lobes of the cerebrum

Label the structures of the brain shown in Figure 14-7. Write your answers on the spaces provided.

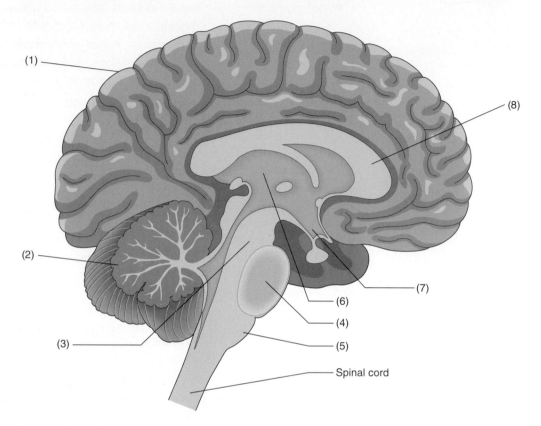

Figure 14-7 Labeling exercise

1. _____
2. _____
3. _____
4. _____
5. _____
6. _____
7. _____
8. _____

EXERCISE 6

Match the medical term in Column 1 with the correct definition in Column 2.

COLUMN 1

_____ 1. cerebellum

_____ 2. cerebral cortex

_____ 3. cerebrum

_____ 4. corpus callosum

_____ 5. frontal lobe

_____ 6. gyri

_____ 7. hypothalamus

_____ 8. medulla oblongata

_____ 9. occipital lobe

_____ 10. pons

_____ 11. sulci

_____ 12. temporal lobe

_____ 13. thalamus

COLUMN 2

a. attaches the brain to the brainstem

b. connects the two hemispheres of the brain

c. folds of the cerebral cortex

d. grooves of the cerebral cortex

e. largest section of the brain

f. literally means "bridge"

g. lowest section of the brainstem

h. outer layer of the cerebrum

i. relays impulses between the cerebral cortex and sense organs

j. responsible for hearing and smell

k. responsible for motor function

l. responsible for sight

m. "thermostat" of the body

Meninges and Cerebrospinal Fluid

The **meninges** (men-**IN**-jeez) are three layers of membranes that surround and protect the brain and spinal cord. The outer membrane layer is the **dura mater** (**DOO**-rah **MAY**-ter), which is a tough, white connective tissue just beneath the skull. The middle layer is the **arachnoid** (ah **RAK**-noyd) **membrane**, a web-like tissue with several strands that attach to the inner membrane layer. The inner membrane layer is the **pia mater** (**PEE**-ah **MAY**-ter), which is attached directly to the surface of the brain and spinal cord.

   Cerebrospinal (seh-**ree**-broh-**SPIGH**-nal) **fluid (CSF)** flows in and around the brain and spinal cord. CSF cushions the brain and spinal cord and also provides some nutrition to those structures.

Cranial and Spinal Nerves

As stated previously, the twelve pairs of cranial nerves and thirty-one pairs of spinal nerve are known as the *peripheral nervous system* (PNS). The peripheral nervous system transmits information from all parts of the body to the brain and back to the body. **Afferent**, or **sensory**, nerves carry impulses from the body to the brain, and **efferent**, or **motor**, nerves carry impulses from the brain to the appropriate body structure.

   The peripheral nervous system is further classified as the **somatic** (soh-**MAT**-ik) **nervous system (SNS)** and the **autonomic** (ot-oh-**NOM**-ik) **nervous system (ANS)**. The somatic nervous system is responsible for voluntary movements and also for responses such as walking, talking, and swimming. The autonomic nervous system is responsible for involuntary movement and responses such as hormone secretion, heart rate, blood flow, and digestive system functions. Figure 14-8 illustrates the body areas and functions that are controlled by the autonomic nervous system.

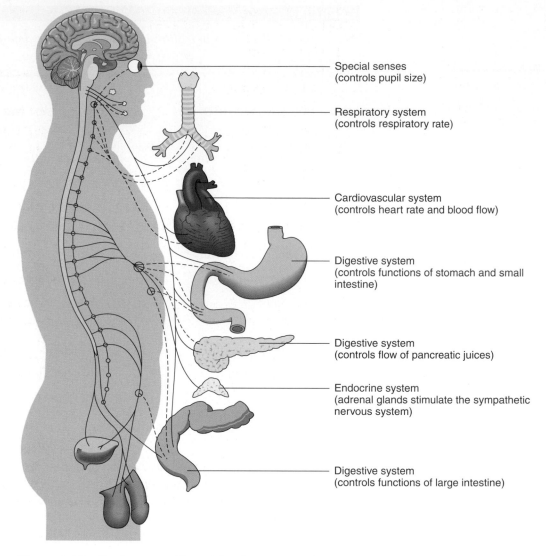

Special senses
(controls pupil size)

Respiratory system
(controls respiratory rate)

Cardiovascular system
(controls heart rate and blood flow)

Digestive system
(controls functions of stomach and small
intestine)

Digestive system
(controls flow of pancreatic juices)

Endocrine system
(adrenal glands stimulate the sympathetic
nervous system)

Digestive system
(controls functions of large intestine)

Figure 14-8 Body areas affected by the autonomic nervous system

The cranial nerves are numbered from one to 12, using Roman numerals. Table 14-3 lists the cranial nerves and provides a brief description of their functions. Figure 14-9 illustrates the body areas affected by the 12 pairs of cranial nerves.

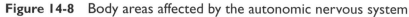

TABLE 14-3   CRANIAL NERVES

	Cranial Nerves	Description
I	olfactory nerve (ohl-**FAK**-tor-ee)	transmits sensory impulses necessary for the sense of smell
II	optic nerve (**OP**-tik)	transmits sensory impulses necessary for sight
III	oculomotor nerve (**ok**-yoo-loh-**MOH**-tor)	transmits impulses necessary for eye movement
IV	trochlear nerve (**TROK**-lee-ar)	transmits impulses necessary for eye movement and eye muscle sensations

(continues)

TABLE 14-3 CRANIAL NERVES (continued)

Cranial Nerves	Description
V trigeminal nerve (trigh-**JEM**-ih-nal)	transmits impulses necessary for chewing and facial sensations
VI abducens nerve (ab-**DOO**-senz)	transmits impulses necessary to turn the eyeball outward or away from the midline
VII facial nerve (**FAY**-shee-al)	transmits impulses to the scalp, forehead, eyelids, cheek, jaw, and other facial muscles
VIII acoustic nerve (ah **KOO**-stik)	transmits impulses necessary for hearing and balance; also called the *auditory nerve*
IX glossopharyngeal (**gloss**-oh-fair-in-**JEE**-al)	transmits impulses necessary for taste, some sensations from the viscera, and secretions from some glands
X vagus nerve (**VAY**-gus)	transmits impulses necessary for speech, swallowing, as well as the activity of cardiac muscle, smooth, and glands and ducts of the respiratory system
XI accessory nerve	transmits impulses necessary for speech, swallowing, and some head and shoulder movements
XII hypoglossal nerve (**high**-poh-**GLOSS**-al)	transmits impulses necessary for swallowing and moving the tongue

The 31 pairs of spinal or peripheral nerves transmit impulses to all parts of the body. The spinal nerves are attached to the spinal cord and exit the vertebral column through openings in the vertebrae. These nerves have many branches that eventually reach every part of the body.

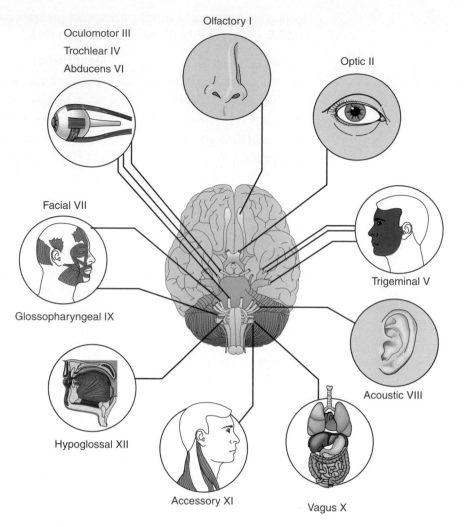

Figure 14-9   Body areas affected by the cranial nerves

Write the medical term for each definition.

1. membranes that surround and protect the brain and spinal cord

   _____

2. weblike membrane located between the outer and inner membrane

   _____

3. outer membrane just beneath the skull

   _____

4. inner membrane attached directly to the surface of the brain

   _____

5. fluid that flows around the brain and spinal cord

   _____

6. nerves that carry impulses from the body to the brain

   _____

7. nerves that carry impulses from the brain to the body structures

   _____

8. twelve pairs of nerves that are identified by name and number

   _____

9. thirty-one pairs of nerves that are also called peripheral nerves

   _____

Write out the following abbreviations.

1. ANS _____
2. CSF _____
3. PNS _____
4. SNS _____

Nervous System Medical Terminology

Nervous system medical terms are organized into three main categories: (1) general medical terms; (2) disease and condition terms; and (3) diagnostic procedure, surgery, and laboratory test terms. The roots, prefixes, and suffixes associated with the nervous system are listed in Table 14-4. Review these word parts and complete the related exercises.

TABLE 14-4 ROOTS, PREFIXES, AND SUFFIXES FOR NERVOUS SYSTEM TERMS

Root	Meaning	Prefix	Meaning	Suffix	Meaning
arachn/o	spider	an-; a-	lack of; without	-algia	pain
electr/o	electricity	dura-	hard	-cele	hernia; protrusion
hemat/o	blood	echo-	sound	-gram	picture; record
hydr/o	water; fluid	epi-	above; upon	-graphy	process of recording
quadr/i	four	hemi-	half	-itis	inflammation
thromb/o	clot	poly-	many	-malacia	softening
		sub-	beneath; below	-oma	tumor
				-osis	condition
				-(o)tomy	incision into
				-paresis	partial paralysis
				-pathy	disease
				-plegia	paralysis

EXERCISE 9

Write and define the root(s), prefix, and suffix for each medical term. Note: Anencephaly has the noun ending -y as a suffix. Based on the meaning of the word parts, write a definition for each term. Check the definition in a medical dictionary.

1. anencephaly

    ROOT: _____ MEANING: _____

    PREFIX: _____ MEANING: _____

    SUFFIX: _____ MEANING: _____

    DEFINITION: _____

2. cephalagia

    ROOT: _____ MEANING: _____

    PREFIX: _____ MEANING: _____

    SUFFIX: _____ MEANING: _____

    DEFINITION: _____

3. cerebromalacia

    ROOT: _____ MEANING: _____

    PREFIX: _____ MEANING: _____

    SUFFIX: _____ MEANING: _____

    DEFINITION: _____

4. electromyelography

    ROOT: _____ MEANING: _____

    PREFIX: _____ MEANING: _____

    SUFFIX: _____ MEANING: _____

    DEFINITION: _____

5. epidural

    ROOT: _____ MEANING: _____

    PREFIX: _____ MEANING: _____

    SUFFIX: _____ MEANING: _____

    DEFINITION: _____

6. hematoma

    ROOT: _____ MEANING: _____

    PREFIX: _____ MEANING: _____

    SUFFIX: _____ MEANING: _____

    DEFINITION: _____

7. hydrocephalus

ROOT: _____ MEANING: _____

PREFIX: _____ MEANING: _____

SUFFIX: _____ MEANING: _____

DEFINITION: _____

8. meningocele

ROOT: _____ MEANING: _____

PREFIX: _____ MEANING: _____

SUFFIX: _____ MEANING: _____

DEFINITION: _____

9. neuritis

ROOT: _____ MEANING: _____

PREFIX: _____ MEANING: _____

SUFFIX: _____ MEANING: _____

DEFINITION: _____

10. thrombosis

ROOT: _____ MEANING: _____

PREFIX: _____ MEANING: _____

SUFFIX: _____ MEANING: _____

DEFINITION: _____

Nervous System General Medical Terms

Review the pronunciation and meaning of each term in Table 14-5. Note that some terms are built from word parts and some are not. Complete the exercises for these terms.

TABLE 14-5 NERVOUS SYSTEM GENERAL MEDICAL TERMS

Term with Pronunciation	Definition
afferent nerves (**AFF**-er-ent)	nerves that carry impulses toward the brain
cauda equina (**KAW**-dah ee-**KWIGH**-nah)	lower end of the spinal cord and spinal nerve roots; resembles a horse's tail
cerebral (seh-**REE**-bral) cerebr/o = cerebrum -al = pertaining to	pertaining to the cerebrum
craniocerebral (**kray**-nee-oh-seh-**REE**-bral) crani/o = skull; cranium cerebr/o = cerebrum -al = pertaining to	pertaining to the cranium or skull and cerebrum

(continues)

TABLE 14-5 NERVOUS SYSTEM GENERAL MEDICAL TERMS (continued)

Term with Pronunciation	Definition
efferent nerves (**EE**-fair-ent)	nerves that carry impulses away from the brain
epidural (ep-ih-**DOO**-ral) epi- = above; over dura- = hard -al = pertaining to	above or over the dura mater
neurologist (noo-**RALL**-oh-jist) neur/o = nerve -(o)logist = specialist	physician who specializes in nervous system diseases
neurology (noo-**RALL**-oh-jee) neur/o = nerve -(o)logy = study of	medical specialty related to diseases and disorders of the nervous system
neurosurgeon (**noo**-roh-**SER**-jun) neur/o = nerve	surgeon who specializes in surgical techniques related to the nervous system
neurosurgery (**noo**-roh-**SER**-jer-ree) neur/o = nerve	surgical specialty related to diseases and disorders of the nervous system; any nervous system surgery
plexus (**PLECKS**-us)	network of interwoven nerves
subarachnoid (sub-ah-**RAK**-noyd) sub- = beneath; below arachn/o = spider -oid = like; resembling	beneath or below the arachnoid membrane
subdural (sub-**DOO**-ral) sub- = beneath; below dura- = hard -al = pertaining to	beneath or below the dura mater
ventricle (**VEN**-trih-kal)	small hollow or space within the brain that is filled with cerebrospinal fluid

EXERCISE 10

Analyze each term by writing the prefix, root, combining vowel, and suffix separated by vertical slashes. Based on the meaning of the word parts, write a definition for each term. Check the definition in a medical dictionary. Note that some terms might have more than one root.

EXAMPLE: cerebromalacia

	/ cerebr	/ o	/ malacia
prefix	*root*	*combining vowel*	*suffix*

DEFINITION: softening of the cerebrum

1. craniocerebral

prefix	*root*	*combining vowel*	*suffix*

DEFINITION: _____

2. epidural

prefix	*root*	*combining vowel*	*suffix*

DEFINITION: _____

3. neurologist

prefix	*root*	*combining vowel*	*suffix*

DEFINITION: _____

4. neurology

prefix	*root*	*combining vowel*	*suffix*

DEFINITION: _____

5. subarachnoid

prefix	*root*	*combining vowel*	*suffix*

DEFINITION: _____

6. subdural

prefix	*root*	*combining vowel*	*suffix*

DEFINITION: _____

7. cerebral

prefix	*root*	*combining vowel*	*suffix*

DEFINITION: _____

EXERCISE 11

Write the medical term for each definition.

1. carrying impulses away from the brain   _____

2. carrying impulses toward the brain   _____

3. lower end of the spinal cord   _____

4. network of interwoven nerves   _____

5. any nervous system surgery   _____

6. space or hollow within the brain   _____

7. specialist in nervous system surgery   _____

Nervous System Disease and Disorder Terms

Nervous system diseases and disorders include familiar problems such as headaches as well as more complex and less familiar diagnoses such as encephalomalacia. The medical terms are presented in alphabetical order in Table 14-6. Review the pronunciation and definition for each term and complete the exercises.

TABLE 14-6 NERVOUS SYSTEM DISEASE AND DISORDER TERMS

Term with Pronunciation	Definition
Alzheimer's disease (**ALTS**-high-merz)	progressive, extremely debilitating deterioration of an individual's intellectual functioning
amyotrophic lateral sclerosis (ALS) (ah-**migh**-oh-**TROFF**-ik **LAT**-er-al skleh-**ROH**-sis)	severe weakening and wasting of various muscle groups due to loss of motor neuron function in the brainstem and spinal cord
anencephaly (an-en-**SEFF**-ah-lee) an- = lack of; absence encephal/o = brain -y = noun ending	congenital absence of the brain and, in some cases, the spinal cord
ataxia (ah-**TAK**-see-ah)	lacking muscular coordination, especially voluntary muscle movement
Bell's palsy (Bell's **PALL**-zee)	weakness or paralysis of the muscles of one side of the face
cephalalgia (seff-al-**AL**-jee-ah) cephal/o = head -algia = pain	pain in the head; headache
cerebral aneurysm (seh-**REE**-bral **AN**-yoo-rizm)	dilatation of a cerebral artery that might put pressure on cerebral tissue and interfere with cerebral function
cerebral hemorrhage (seh-**REE**-bral **HEM**-oh-rij) hem/o = blood -(r)rhage = bursting forth	bursting forth of blood into cerebral tissue due to rupture of a cerebral vessel (Figure 14-10)

(continues)

TABLE 14-6 NERVOUS SYSTEM DISEASE AND DISORDER TERMS (continued)

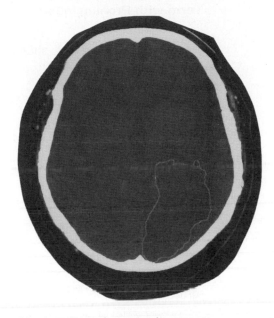

Figure 14-10 Cerebral hemorrhage, lower right area

Term with Pronunciation	Definition
cerebral palsy (CP) (seh-**REE**-bral **PALL**-zee)	lack of voluntary muscle control and/or coordination caused by a lack of oxygen to the brain at or near the time of birth
cerebral thrombosis (seh-**REE**-bral throm-**BOH**-sis) . thromb/o = clot -osis = condition	presence of an atherosclerotic clot in a cerebral blood vessel that causes death of a specific portion of brain tissue
cerebrovascular accident (CVA) (seh-**REE**-broh-**VASS**-kyoo-lar) cerebr/o = brain vascul/o = vessel -al = pertaining to	occlusion or rupture of a cerebral blood vessel resulting in decreased blood flow to the affected area and death of a specific portion of brain tissue; a *stroke*
concussion (kon-**KUSH**-on)	violent jarring, shaking, or other blunt nonpenetrating injury to the brain; may or may not involve loss of consciousness
contusion (kon-**TOO**-zhun)	small venous hemorrhages in the brain caused by the brain striking the cranium; also called a bruise
dementia (deh-**MEN**-shee-ah)	progressive, irreversible deterioration of memory, judgment, and other thought processes
encephalitis (**en**-seff-ah-**LIGH**-tis) encephal/o = brain -itis = inflammation	inflammation of the brain

(*continues*)

TABLE 14-6 NERVOUS SYSTEM DISEASE AND DISORDER TERMS (continued)

Term with Pronunciation	Definition
encephalomalacia (**en**-seff-ah-loh-mah-**LAY**-shee-ah) encephal/o = brain -malacia = softening	softening of brain tissue
encephalopathy (**en**-seff-ah-**LOP**-ah-thee) encephal/o = brain -pathy = disease	any disease of the brain
epidural hematoma (ep-ih-**DOO**-ral **hee**-mah-**TOH**-mah) epi- = above dura- = dura mater -al = pertaining to hemat/o = blood -oma = tumor	a swelling or mass of blood between the cranium and dura mater that applies pressure on the brain tissue in the affected area (Figure 14-11)

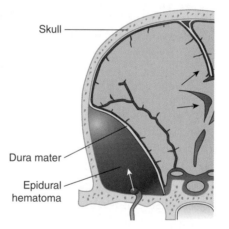

Skull

Dura mater

Epidural hematoma

Figure 14-11 Epidural hematoma

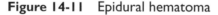

EXERCISE 12

Analyze each term by writing the prefix, root, combining vowel, and suffix separated by vertical slashes. Based on the meaning of the word parts, write a definition for each term. Check the definition in a medical dictionary.

1. anencephaly

prefix	*root*	*combining vowel*	*suffix*

DEFINITION: _____

2. cephalalgia

prefix	*root*	*combining vowel*	*suffix*

DEFINITION: _____

3. encephalitis

prefix	root	combining vowel	suffix

DEFINITION: _____

4. encephalomalacia

prefix	root	combining vowel	suffix

DEFINITION: _____

5. encephalopathy

prefix	root	combining vowel	suffix

DEFINITION: _____

EXERCISE 13

Replace the italicized phrase or abbreviation with the correct medical term.

1. The computed tomography (CT) scan revealed a *dilatation of a cerebral artery.*

   _____

2. Erik sustained a *blunt nonpenetrating injury to the brain* as a result of being struck with a baseball.

   _____

3. Shayna's diagnosis of *facial muscle paralysis* was established by her family physician.

   _____

4. After a *stroke*, Victoria was paralyzed on her left side.

   _____

5. An *atherosclerotic clot* resulted in temporal lobe brain tissue death.

   _____

6. *ALS* is also called Lou Gehrig's disease, after the famous baseball player who had this condition.

   _____

7. Bridget was diagnosed with *CP* as a result of a lack of oxygen during delivery.

   _____

Review the pronunciation and definition for each term in Table 14-7 and complete the exercises.

TABLE 14-7 NERVOUS SYSTEM DISEASE AND DISORDER TERMS

Term with Pronunciation	Definition
epilepsy (**EP**-ih-lep-see)	recurring episodes of excessive or irregular electrical activity of the central nervous system; commonly called *seizures*
glioma (gligh-**OH**-mah) gli/o = neuroglia; nerve cell -oma = tumor	malignant tumor of neuroglial cells
Guillain-Barré syndrome (**GEE**-yon bah-**RAY SIN**-drohm)	acute inflammation of several nerves of the peripheral nervous system
hemiparesis (**hem**-ee-pah-**REE**-sis) hemi- = half -paresis = partial paralysis	partial paralysis of one side of the body
hemiplegia (**hem**-ee-**PLEE**-jee-ah) hemi- = half -plegia = paralysis	paralysis of one side of the body
Huntington's disease (HD)	genetic disorder characterized by progressive, irreversible degeneration of cerebral neurons that results in uncontrolled movements, loss of intellectual capabilities, and emotional disturbances; also called *Huntington's chorea*
hydrocephalus (**high**-droh-**SEFF**-ah-lus) hydr/o = water; fluid cephal/o = head -us = noun ending	abnormal accumulation of cerebrospinal fluid around the brain, often causing swelling of the head; commonly called "water on the brain"
meningioma (men-**in**-jee-**OH**-mah) mening/o = meninges -oma = tumor	slow-growth tumor of the meninges of the brain, primarily from the arachnoid membrane
meningitis (**men**-in-**JIGH**-tis) mening/o = meninges -itis = inflammation	infection or inflammation of the membranes covering the brain or spinal cord (meninges); may be bacterial or viral and is characterized by severe headache, vomiting, and pain and stiffness in the neck (Figure 14-12)
meningocele (men-**IN**-goh-seel) mening/o = meninges -cele = hernia; protrusion	herniation of the meninges through a hole in the skull or vertebral column

(continues)

TABLE 14-7 NERVOUS SYSTEM DISEASE AND DISORDER TERMS (continued)

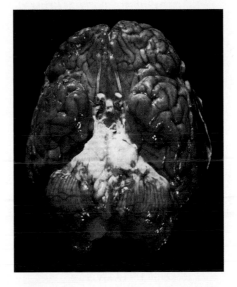

Figure 14-12 Meningitis cerebral tissue damage (Centers for Disease Control)

Term with Pronunciation	Definition
meningomyelocele (men-**in**-goh-my-**ELL**-oh-seel) mening/o = meninges myel/o = spinal cord -cele = hernia; protrusion	herniation of the spinal cord and meninges through a defect in the vertebral column
multiple sclerosis (MS) (sklair-**OH**-sis)	degenerative inflammatory disease of the central nervous system that attacks the myelin sheath of the spinal cord and brain, resulting in hardening and scarring
myelomalacia (**migh**-eh-loh-mah-**LAY**-shee-ah) myel/o = spinal cord -malacia = softening	abnormal softening of the spinal cord
neuralgia (noo-**RAL**-jee-ah) neur/o = nerve -algia = pain	severe sharp pain of a nerve or along the course of a nerve
neuritis (noo-**RIGH**-tis) neur/o = nerve -itis = inflammation	inflammation of nerve or nerves

EXERCISE 14

Analyze each term by writing the prefix, root, combining vowel, and suffix separated by vertical slashes. Based on the meaning of the word parts, write a definition for each term. Check the definition in a medical dictionary.

1. glioma

prefix	root	combining vowel	suffix

   DEFINITION: _____

2. hemiplegia

prefix	root	combining vowel	suffix

   DEFINITION: _____

3. hydrocephalus

prefix	root	combining vowel	suffix

   DEFINITION: _____

4. meningioma

prefix	root	combining vowel	suffix

   DEFINITION: _____

5. meningitis

prefix	root	combining vowel	suffix

   DEFINITION: _____

6. meningocele

prefix	root	combining vowel	suffix

   DEFINITION: _____

7. meningomyelocele

prefix	root	combining vowel	suffix

   DEFINITION: _____

8. neuralgia

prefix	root	combining vowel	suffix

   DEFINITION: _____

9. neuritis

prefix	root	combining vowel	suffix

   DEFINITION: _____

EXERCISE 15

Replace the italicized phrase or abbreviation with the correct medical term.

1. Lillian's diagnosis was a *malignant tumor of neuroglial cells*.

   _____

2. *MS* is a debilitating disease that often strikes young adults.

   _____

3. Armando's *seizure disorder* was successfully treated with medication.

   _____

4. *Inflammation of the meninges* can result in severe brain damage.

   _____

5. The cause of *an acute inflammation of many nerves of the peripheral nervous system* is unknown.

   _____

6. *Paralysis of one side of the body* can be the result of a stroke.

   _____

7. Belinda's *abnormal accumulation of cerebrospinal fluid around the brain* was relieved by the placement of a shunt.

   _____

Review the pronunciation and definition for each term in Table 14-8 and complete the exercises.

TABLE 14-8   NERVOUS SYSTEM DISEASE AND DISORDER TERMS

Term with Pronunciation	Definition
neuroblastoma (**noo**-roh-blast-**OH**-mah) neur/o = nerve blast/o = embryonic state of development -oma = tumor	highly malignant tumor composed of cells derived from embryonic neural tissue; usually occurrs in young children
neuropathy (noo-**ROP**-ah-thee) neur/o = nerve -pathy = disease	any disease of the nerves
paraplegia (**pair**-ah-**PLEE**-jee-ah) para- = around -plegia = paralysis	paralysis of the lower half of the body, including the legs
Parkinson's disease	chronic, progressive nervous disease characterized by tremor, muscular weakness, and rigidity

(continues)

TABLE 14-8 NERVOUS SYSTEM DISEASE AND DISORDER TERMS (continued)

Term with Pronunciation	Definition
poliomyelitis (**poh**-lee-oh-**migh**-eh-**LIGH**-tis)	infectious viral disease that affects the motor (efferent) neurons of the brain and spinal cord, resulting in muscle paralysis and wasting
polyneuritis (**pall**-ee-noo-**RIGH**-tis) poly- = many neur/o = nerve -itis = inflammation	inflammation of many nerves or nerve fibers
postpolio syndrome (post-**POH**-lee-oh **SIN**-drom)	slow, progressive weakening of muscles that occurs in approximately 25% of poliomyelitis survivors 20–30 years after the initial illness
quadriplegia (**kwad**-rih-**PLEE**-jee-ah) quadr/i = four -plegia = paralysis	paralysis of all four limbs, usually resulting from spinal cord injury
Reye's syndrome (**RIGH's SIN**-drohm)	acute encephalopathy following an acute viral infection
sciatica (sigh-**AT**-ih-kah)	severe pain along the course of the sciatic nerve, from the back of the thigh and down the inside of the leg
seizure (**SEE**-zhoor)	excessive irregular electrical activity of the central nervous system associated with epilepsy
shingles; herpes zoster (**HER**-peez **ZOSS**-ter)	acute viral infection characterized by an inflammation of a spinal or cranial nerve pathway that produces painful vesicular eruptions on the skin (Figure 14-13)

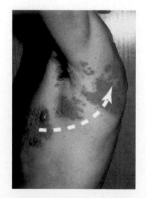

Figure 14-13 Shingles (Photo courtesy of Robert A. Silverman, MD, Pediatric Dermatology, Georgetown University)

(continues)

TABLE 14-8 NERVOUS SYSTEM DISEASE AND DISORDER TERMS (continued)

Term with Pronunciation	Definition
subdural hematoma (sub-**DOO**-ral **hee**-mah-**TOH**-mah) sub- = beneath; below dura- = hard -al = pertaining to hemat/o = blood -oma = tumor	collection of blood below the dura mater and above the arachnoid membrane, usually the result of a closed head injury (Figure 14-14)

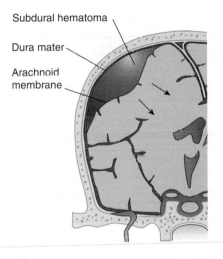

Subdural hematoma

Dura mater

Arachnoid membrane

Figure 14-14 Subdural hematoma

syncope (**SIN**-koh-pee)	loss of consciousness due to a lack of blood supply to the brain; fainting
transient ischemic attack (TIA) (iss-**KEE**-mik)	temporary interference or interruption of the blood supply to a portion of the brain
trigeminal neuralgia; tic douloureaux (trigh-**JEM**-ih-nal noo-**RAL**-jee-ah; **TIK DOO**-loh-roo)	severe pain that radiates along the fifth cranial nerve and usually affects one side of the head and face

EXERCISE 16

Write the medical term for each definition.

1. any disease of the nerves _____

2. paralysis of the lower half of the body _____

3. inflammation of many nerves _____

4. paralysis of all four limbs _____

5. severe pain along the sciatic nerve _____

6. fainting _____

EXERCISE 17

Match the medical term in Column 1 with the definition in Column 2.

COLUMN 1

_____ 1. neuropathy

_____ 2. paraplegia

_____ 3. Parkinson's disease

_____ 4. poliomyelitis

_____ 5. polyneuritis

_____ 6. quadriplegia

_____ 7. Reye's syndrome

_____ 8. shingles

_____ 9. syncope

_____ 10. transient ischemic
         attack

_____ 11. trigeminal neuralgia

COLUMN 2

a. acute encephalopathy following an acute
   viral infection

b. any disease of the nerves

c. chronic progressive nerve disease with tremors

d. fainting

e. infectious viral disease of the motor neurons

f. inflammation of many nerves

g. inflammation of a nerve pathway with skin
   eruptions

h. paralysis of all four limbs

i. paralysis of the lower half of the body,
   including the legs

j. severe pain along the fifth cranial nerve

k. temporary interruption of the blood supply to
   the brain

Nervous System Diagnostic and Treatment Terms

Review the pronunciation and definition of the diagnostic and treatment terms in Table 14-9. Complete the exercises for each set of terms.

TABLE 14-9 NERVOUS SYSTEM DIAGNOSTIC AND TREATMENT TERMS

Term with Pronunciation	Definition
cerebrospinal fluid analysis (seh-**ree**-broh-**SPIGH**-nal) cerebr/o = cerebrum spin/o = spine -al = pertaining to	laboratory analysis of cerebrospinal fluid (CSF) to detect the presence of bacteria, blood, and malignant cells, and to measure glucose and protein content
craniotomy (**kray**-nee-**OT**-oh-me) crani/o = skull -(o)tomy = incision into	incision into the skull to provide access to the brain
echoencephalography (EEG) (**ek**-oh-en-**seff**-ah-**LOG**-rah-fee) echo- = sound encephal/o = brain -graphy = process of recording	process of recording a picture of the structures of the brain using sound waves

(continues)

TABLE 14-9 NERVOUS SYSTEM DIAGNOSTIC AND TREATMENT TERMS (continued)

Term with Pronunciation	Definition
electroencephalogram (ee-**lek**-troh-en-**SEFF**-ah-loh-gram) electr/o = electricity encephal/o = brain -gram = record of	graphic record of the electrical activity of the brain
electroencephalography (ee-**lek**-troh-en-**seff**-ah-**LOG**-rah-fee) electr/o = electricity encephal/o = brain -graphy = process of recording	process of recording the electrical activity of the brain
evoked potential studies (ee-**VOHKT**)	electroencephalographic test that measures the brain activity in response to various types of electrical stimulation
lumbar puncture (LP) (**LUM**-bar)	insertion of a needle into the subarachnoid space, usually between the third and fourth lumbar vertebrae, to withdraw cerebrospinal fluid; also called *spinal tap* (Figure 14-15)

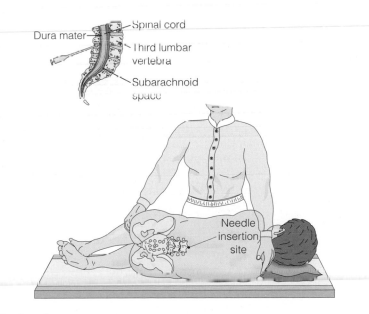

Figure 14-15 Lumbar puncture

myelography (**migh**-eh-**LOG**-rah-fee) myel/o = spinal cord -graphy = process of recording	process of recording an x-ray picture of the spinal cord and spinal cavity

(continues)

TABLE 14-9 NERVOUS SYSTEM DIAGNOSTIC AND TREATMENT TERMS
(continued)

Term with Pronunciation	Definition
myelogram (**MIGH**-eh-loh-gram) myel/o = spinal cord -gram = record of	x-ray record of the spinal cord and spinal cavity
neurectomy (noo-**REK**-toh-me) neur/o = nerve -ectomy = surgical removal	surgical excision of a nerve or nerve fibers
pneumoencephalography (noo-moh-en-**seff**-ah-**LOG**-rah-fee) pneum/o = air encephal/o = brain -graph = process of recording	process of recording an x-ray picture of the ventricles and other fluid-filled cavities of the central nervous system; air or another type of gas is used as the contrast medium
Romberg test (**ROM**-berg)	technique used to assess and evaluate cerebellar function and balance
transcutaneous electrical nerve stimulation (TENS) (**tranz**-kyoo-**TAY**-nee-us) trans- = across, through cutane/o = skin -ous = pertaining to	pain-relief treatment during which electrical impulses are delivered through the skin to nerve endings near the pain site; the impulses prevent the transmission of pain signals to the brain

EXERCISE 18

Analyze each term by writing the prefix, root, combining vowel, and suffix separated by vertical slashes. Based on the meaning of the word parts, write a definition for each term. Check the definition in a medical dictionary. Note that some terms have more than one root.

1. craniotomy

    prefix   *root*   *combining vowel*   *suffix*

    DEFINITION: _____

2. electroencephalogram

    prefix   *root*   *combining vowel*   *suffix*

    DEFINITION: _____

3. electroencephalography

    prefix   *root*   *combining vowel*   *suffix*

    DEFINITION: _____

4. myelogram

| prefix | root | combining vowel | suffix |

DEFINITION: _____

5. neurectomy

| prefix | root | combining vowel | suffix |

DEFINITION: _____

EXERCISE 19

Match the medical term in Column 1 with the definition in Column 2.

COLUMN 1

_____ 1. cerebrospinal fluid analysis
_____ 2. craniotomy
_____ 3. echoencephalography
_____ 4. electroencephalogram
_____ 5. electroencephalography
_____ 6. evoked potential studies
_____ 7. lumbar puncture
_____ 8. myelogram
_____ 9. neurectomy
_____ 10. Romberg test

COLUMN 2

a. excision of a nerve or nerve fibers
b. graphic record of the electrical activity of the brain
c. incision into the skull
d. laboratory test of CSF
e. recording the electrical activity of the brain
f. spinal tap
g. technique for assessing cerebellar function and balance
h. ultrasound analysis of the structures of the brain
i. x-ray record of the spinal cord and spinal cavity
j. measure the brain's response to electrical stimulation

Abbreviations

Review the nervous system abbreviations in Table 14-10. Practice writing out the meaning of each abbreviation.

TABLE 14-10   ABBREVIATIONS

Abbreviation	Meaning
ALS	amyotrophic lateral sclerosis
ANS	autonomic nervous system
CNS	central nervous system
CP	cerebral palsy

(continues)

TABLE 14-10   ABBREVIATIONS (continued)

Abbreviation	Meaning
CSF	cerebrospinal fluid
CVA	cerebrovascular accident
EEG	electroencephalography
HD	Huntington's disease
ICP	intracranial pressure
LP	lumbar puncture
MS	multiple sclerosis
PEG	pneumoencephalogram
PNS	peripheral nervous system
PPS	postpolio syndrome
SNS	somatic nervous system
TENS	transcutaneous electrical nerve stimulation
TIA	transient ischemic attack

CHAPTER REVIEW

The Chapter Review can be used as a self-test. Go through each exercise and answer as many questions as you can without referring to previous exercises or earlier discussions within this chapter. Check your answers and fill in any blanks. Practice writing any terms you might have misspelled.

EXERCISE 20

Write the medical term for each definition.

1. pertaining to the cranium and cerebrum   _____

2. above the dura mater   _____

3. physician who specializes in the nervous system   _____

4. study of the nervous system   _____

5. below the arachnoid membrane   _____

6. congenital absence of the brain   _____

7. pain in the head; headache   _____

8. inflammation of the brain   _____

9. malignant tumor of the neuroglial cells   _____

10. inflammation of the meninges   _____

11. herniation of the meninges through a hole in the skull or vertebral column   _____

12. sharp pain along the course of a nerve   _____

13. paralysis of the lower half of the body, including the legs   _____

14. inflammation of many nerves or nerve fibers   _____

15. paralysis of all four limbs   _____

16. incision into the skull   _____

17. recording the electrical activity of the brain   _____

18. excision of a nerve or nerve fibers   _____

19. partial paralysis of one side of the body   _____

20. any disease of the brain   _____

EXERCISE 21

Replace the italicized phrase or abbreviation with the correct medical term.

1. Vaneesha was accepted into a residency program for *surgery related to the nervous system.*

   _____

2. After receiving a blow to the head, Patrick had *below the dura mater* bleeding.

   _____

3. A *blunt, nonpenetrating injury to the brain can be caused* by violent jarring or shaking.

   _____

4. A closed head injury can result in a *collection of blood below the dura mater.*

   _____

5. Marko underwent *an incision into the skull* to relieve the pressure on his brain.

   _____

6. Dr. Rodriguez ordered an *LP* to obtain a sample of cerebrospinal fluid.

   _____

7. The *ANS* is responsible for involuntary movements, including hormone secretion.

   _____

8. *Lack of muscular coordination* is associated with several neuromuscular diseases.

   _____

9. A *dilatation of a cerebral artery* puts the patient at risk for a stroke.

   _____

10. *Irregular electrical activity of the central nervous system* can be congenital or caused by trauma.

    _____

EXERCISE 22

Read the discharge summary and write a brief definition for each italicized medical term or phrase.

DISCHARGE SUMMARY

FINAL DIAGNOSIS: (1) *Subarachnoid* hemorrhage. (2) *Hydrocephalus.* Anterior communicating artery aneurysm and (3) *cerebral* failure.

PROCEDURES: CT head scans. (4) *Cerebral angiography.*

HOSPITAL COURSE: The patient was admitted in a comatose condition and was intubated. CT head scans revealed blood in the subarachnoid space and demyelination patterns consistent with (5) *MS.* There was excessive blood in the (6) *ventricular* space. Due to the extensive nature of the subarachnoid hemorrhage, the patient's comatose state, and the fact that surgery was not an option, the patient's comfort was maintained. The (7) *EEG* done on the third day of hospitalization showed no brain wave activity. Mechanical life support was discontinued, per the patient's advance directive.

1. _____
2. _____
3. _____
4. _____
5. _____
6. _____
7. _____

EXERCISE 23

Write out the abbreviation and provide a brief definition for the abbreviation.

EXAMPLE: EEG = electroencephalogram
DEFINITION: record of the electrical activity of the brain

1. ALS _____
   DEFINITION: _____
2. ANS _____
   DEFINITION: _____
3. CNS _____
   DEFINITION: _____
4. CVA _____
   DEFINITION: _____
5. ICP _____
   DEFINITION: _____
6. LP _____
   DEFINITION: _____
7. MS _____
   DEFINITION: _____

8. PNS _____

DEFINITION: _____

9. SNS _____

DEFINITION: _____

10. TIA _____

DEFINITION: _____

EXERCISE 24

Match the cranial nerve in Column 1 with the description in Column 2. Note: Each cranial nerve is also identified by its Roman numeral, which is the number in the parentheses.

COLUMN 1

_____ 1. olfactory nerve (I)

_____ 2. optic nerve (II)

_____ 3. oculomotor nerve (III)

_____ 4. trochlear nerve (IV)

_____ 5. trigeminal nerve (V)

_____ 6. abducens nerve (VI)

_____ 7. facial nerve (VII)

_____ 8. acoustic nerve (VIII)

_____ 9. glossopharyngeal
nerve (IX)

_____ 10. vagus nerve (X)

_____ 11. accessory nerve (XI)

_____ 12. hypoglossal nerve (XII)

COLUMN 2

a. chewing and facial sensations

b. eye movement

c. eye movement and eye muscle sensations

d. hearing and balance

e. innervates the scalp, forehead, eyelids, cheek, and jaw

f. sense of smell

g. speech and swallowing

h. speech, swallowing, and head and shoulder movements

i. swallowing and moving the tongue

j. taste, visceral sensations, and glandular secretions

k. transmits impulses necessary for sight

l. turning the eyeball outward

EXERCISE 25

Select the best answer for each question or statement.

1. Which part of the brain is often called the thermostat?
   a. thalamus
   b. pons
   c. midbrain
   d. hypothalamus

2. Select the correct term for the part of the brain that literally means bridge.
   a. thalamus
   b. pons
   c. midbrain
   d. hypothalamus

3. Which part of the brain is responsible for maintaining muscle tone, movement, and balance?
   a. cerebrum
   b. midbrain
   c. cerebellum
   d. medulla oblongata

4. Select the type of nerves that carry impulses toward the brain.
   a. efferent
   b. cauda equina
   c. afferent
   d. neuroglia

5. Which type of nerves carry impulses away from the brain?
   a. efferent
   b. cauda equina
   c. afferent
   d. neuroglia

6. Select the term that means a network of interwoven nerves.
   a. cauda equina
   b. plexus
   c. nerve fiber
   d. neuroglia

7. Which term describes a progressive and debilitating deterioration of intellectual functioning?
   a. amyotrophic lateral sclerosis
   b. multiple sclerosis
   c. cerebral palsy
   d. Alzheimer's disease

8. Select the term that describes a weakness or paralysis of the muscles of one side of the face.
   a. cerebrovascular accident
   b. Bell's palsy
   c. cerebral palsy
   d. multiple sclerosis

9. Which term best describes a swelling or mass of blood between the cranium and dura mater?
   a. epidural hematoma
   b. subdural hematoma
   c. subarachnoid hematoma
   d. concussion

10. Select the term for an acute polyneuritis of the peripheral nervous system.
    a. amyotrophic lateral sclerosis
    b. multiple sclerosis
    c. Guillain-Barré syndrome
    d. Bell's palsy

11. Which term best describes a hardening and scarring of the myelin sheath of the brain and spinal cord?
    a. cerebral palsy
    b. multiple sclerosis
    c. amyotrophic lateral sclerosis
    d. Guillain-Barré syndrome

12. Select the term for a chronic and progressive condition of tremors, muscular rigidity, and weakness.
    a. Bell's palsy
    b. Guillain-Barré syndrome
    c. Reye's syndrome
    d. Parkinson's disease

13. Which term best describes an acute encephalopathy that follows an acute viral infection?
    a. Bell's palsy
    b. Guillain-Barré syndrome
    c. Reye's syndrome
    d. Parkinson's disease

14. Select the term that means the process of recording the electrical activity of the brain.
    a. electroencephalography
    b. electroencephalogram
    c. evoked potential studies
    d. echoencephalography

15. Which test or procedure is used to assess and evaluate cerebellar function?
    a. electroencephalography
    b. evoked potential studies
    c. cerebrospinal fluid analysis
    d. Romberg test

CHALLENGE EXERCISE

Alzheimer's disease is a debilitating disease for the patient and presents many challenges to family and friends. Using current medical references, research the effects this disease has on the brain and the behaviors of the affected individual.

Pronunciation Review

Review the terms in the chapter. Pronounce each term using the following phonetic pronunciations. Check off the term when you are comfortable saying it.

MEDICAL TERM	PRONUNCIATION
☐ afferent nerves	**AFF**-er-ent nerves
☐ Alzheimer's disease	**ALTS**-high-merz disease
☐ amyotrophic lateral sclerosis (ALS)	ah-**migh**-oh-**TROFF**-ik **LAT**-er-al skleh-**ROH**-sis
☐ anencephaly	an-en-**SEFF**-ah-lee
☐ arachnoid membrane	ah-**RAK**-noyd membrane
☐ astrocyte	**ASS**-troh-sight
☐ ataxia	ah-**TAK**-see-ah
☐ autonomic nervous system	ot-oh-**NOM**-ik nervous system
☐ axon	**ACKS**-on
☐ Bell's palsy	Bell's **PALL**-zee
☐ cauda equina	**KAW**-dah ee-**KWIGH**-nah
☐ cephalalgia	seff-al-**AL**-jee-ah
☐ cerebellum	ser-eh-**BELL**-um
☐ cerebral	seh-**REE**-bral
☐ cerebral aneurysm	seh-**REE**-bral **AN**-yoo-rizm
☐ cerebral cortex	seh-**REE**-bral **KOR**-teks
☐ cerebral palsy (CP)	seh-**REE**-bral **PALL**-zee
☐ cerebral thrombosis	seh-**REE**-bral throm-**BOH**-sis
☐ cerebrospinal fluid (CSF)	seh-**ree**-broh-**SPIGH**-nal fluid
☐ cerebrospinal fluid analysis	seh-**ree**-broh-**SPIGH**-nal fluid analysis
☐ cerebrovascular accident (CVA)	seh-**REE**-broh-**VASS**-kyoo-lar accident
☐ cerebrum	seh-**REE**-brum
☐ contusion	kon-**TOO**-zhun
☐ concussion	kon-**KUSH**-on
☐ corpus callosum	**KOR**-pus kal-**OH**-sum
☐ craniocerebral	**kray**-nee-oh-seh-**REE**-bral
☐ craniotomy	**kray**-nee-**OT**-oh-me
☐ dementia	deh-**MEN**-shee-ah
☐ dendrite	**DEN**-dright
☐ dura mater	**DOO**-rah **MAY**-ter
☐ echoencephalography	**ek**-oh-en-**seff**-ah-**LOG**-rah-fee
☐ efferent nerves	**EE**-fair-ent nerves
☐ electroencephalogram	ee-**lek**-troh-en-**SEFF**-ah-loh-gram
☐ electroencephalography	ee-**lek**-troh-en-**seff**-ah-**LOG**-rah-fee
☐ encephalitis	**en**-seff-ah-**LIGH**-tis
☐ encephalopathy	**en**-seff-ah-**LOP**-ah-thee
☐ epidural	ep-ih-**DOO**-ral
☐ epidural hematoma	ep-ih-**DOO**-ral **hee**-mah-**TOH**-mah
☐ epilepsy	**EP**-ih-lep-see
☐ evoked potential studies	ee-**VOHKT** potential studies
☐ glioma	gligh-**OH**-mah
☐ Guillain-Barré syndrome	**GEE**-yon bah-**RAY SIN**-drohm
☐ gyrus; gyri (pl.)	**JIGH**-rus; **JIGH**-righ
☐ hemiparesis	**hem**-ee-pah-**REE**-sis
☐ hemiplegia	**hem**-ee-**PLEE**-jee-ah
☐ hydrocephalus	**high**-droh-**SEFF**-ah-lus

☐ hypothalamus	**high**-poh-**THAL**-ah-mus
☐ lumbar puncture (LP)	**LUM**-bar puncture
☐ medulla oblongata	meh-**DULL**-ah ob-long-**AH**-tah
☐ meninges	men-**IN**-jeez
☐ meningitis	**men**-in-**JIGH**-tis
☐ meningioma	men-**in**-jee-**OH**-mah
☐ meningitis	**men**-in-**JIGH**-tis
☐ meningocele	men-**IN**-goh-seel
☐ meningomyelocele	men-**in**-goh-my-**ELL**-oh-seel
☐ microglia	my-**KROG**-lee-ah
☐ multiple sclerosis (MS)	multiple sklair-**OH**-sis
☐ myelin	**MIGH**-ch-lin
☐ myelogram	**MIGH**-eh-loh-gram
☐ myelography	**migh**-ch-**LOG**-rah-fee
☐ myelomalacia	**migh**-eh-loh-mah-**LAY**-shee-ah
☐ neuralgia	noo-**RAL**-jee-ah
☐ neurectomy	noo-**REK**-toh-me
☐ neuritis	noo-**RIGH**-tis
☐ neuroblastoma	**noo**-roh-blast-**OH**-mah
☐ neuroglia	noo-**ROG**-lee-ah
☐ neurologist	noo-**RALL**-oh-jist
☐ neurology	noo-**RALL**-oh-jee
☐ neurons	**NOO**-ronz
☐ neuropathy	noo-**ROP**-ah-thee
☐ neurosurgeon	**noo** roh **SER**-jun
☐ neurosurgery	**noo**-roh-**SER**-jer-ree
☐ occipital lobe	ok-**SIP**-ih-tal lobe
☐ oligodendroglia	**all**-ih-goh-den-**DROG**-lee-ah
☐ paraplegia	**pair** ah-**PLEE**-jee-ah
☐ parietal lobe	pah-**RIGH**-eh-tal lobe
☐ peripheral nervous system (PNS)	peh-**RIF**-er-al nervous system
☐ pia mater	**PEE**-ah **MAY**-ter
☐ plexus	**PLECKS**-us
☐ pneumonencephalography	noo-moh-en-**seff**-ah-**LOG**-rah-fee
☐ poliomyelitis	**poh**-lee-oh-**migh**-eh-**LIGH**-tis
☐ polyneuritis	**pall**-ee-noo-**RIGH**-tis
☐ pons	PONZ
☐ postpolio syndrome	post-**POH**-lee-oh **SIN**-drom
☐ quadriplegia	**kwad**-rih-**PLEE**-jee-ah
☐ Reye's syndrome	**RIGH**'s **SIN**-drohm
☐ Romberg test	**ROM**-berg test
☐ sciatica	sigh-**AT**-ih-kah
☐ seizure	**SEE**-zhoor
☐ shingles; herpes zoster	shingles; **HER**-peez **ZOSS**-ter
☐ somatic nervous system	soh-**MAT**-ik nervous system
☐ subarachnoid	sub-ah-**RAK**-noyd
☐ subdural	sub-**DOO**-ral
☐ subdural hematoma	sub-**DOO**-ral **hee**-mah-**TOH**-mah
☐ sulcus; sulci (pl.)	**SULL**-kus; **SULL**-kigh
☐ syncope	**SIN**-koh-pee
☐ temporal lobe	**TEM**-por-al lobe

☐ thalamus — **THAL**-ah-mus

☐ transcutaneous electrical nerve stimulation — **tranz**-kyoo-**TAY**-nee-us electrical nerve stimulation

☐ trigeminal neuralgia; tic douloureux — trigh-**JEM**-ih-nal noo-**RAL**-jee-ah; **TIK DOO**-loh-roo

☐ ventricle — **VEN**-trih-kal

Chapter 15

Sensory System: Vision and Hearing

OBJECTIVES

At the completion of this chapter, the student should be able to:

1. Identify, define, and spell word roots associated with the eyes and ears.
2. Label the basic structures of the eyes and ears.
3. Discuss the functions of the eyes and ears.
4. Provide the correct spelling of eye and ear terms, given the definition of the terms.
5. Analyze the eye and ear terms by defining the roots, prefixes, and suffixes of these terms.
6. Identify, define, and spell disease, disorder, and procedure terms related to the eyes and ears.

OVERVIEW

The eyes and ears are primary sense organs that capture information through sight and sound. The information is transmitted via the nervous system to areas of the brain responsible for vision and hearing. This chapter presents information about the structures, functions, diseases, procedures, and tests related to these important organs.

The Eye

The eyes are located in the bony orbits at the front of the skull. The structures of the eyes are arranged in three layers, also called tunics. The eyes receive light rays; bend, or **refract**, those rays; and transmit the nerve impulses generated by the light rays to the occipital lobe of the brain. After the impulses reach the occipital lobe, they are interpreted as images and we are able to "see." Our vision is dependent on the health of our eyes, our sight-related nerves, and our brain.

Word Roots Related to the Eyes

To understand and use the medical terms related to the eyes, it is necessary to acquire a thorough knowledge of the associated word roots and combining forms. Review the word roots in Table 15-1 and complete the exercises that follow.

TABLE 15-1 WORD ROOTS RELATED TO THE EYES

Word Root/Combining Form	Meaning
aque/o	watery
blephar/o	eyelid

(continues)

TABLE 15-1   WORD ROOTS RELATED TO THE EYES (continued)

Word Root/Combining Form	Meaning
conjunctiv/o	conjunctiva
corne/o	cornea
dacry/o	tears
dacryocyst/o	tear sac
glauc/o	silver; gray
ir/o; irid/o	iris
kerat/o	cornea
lacrim/o	tears
ocul/o	eye
ophthalm/o	eye
opt/o	eye; vision
palpebr/o	eyelid
phac/o; phak/o	lens
phot/o	light
pupill/o	pupil
retin/o	retina
scler/o	sclera; hard
uve/o	uvea
vitre/o	glassy; jelly-like

EXERCISE 1

Write the definitions of the following word roots.

1. corne/o _____

2. dacry/o _____

3. retin/o _____

4. scler/o _____

5. ocul/o _____

6. irid/o _____

7. glauc/o _____

8. ir/o _____

9. aque/o _____

10. conjunctiv/o _____

11. dacryocyst/o _____

12. vitre/o _____

13. opt/o _____

14. phac/o _____

15. lacrim/o _____

16. ophthalm/o _____

17. kerat/o _____

18. blephar/o _____

19. phak/o _____

20. pupill/o _____

EXERCISE 2

Write the combining form of the word root and its meaning for each of the listed terms.

1. aqueous

   ROOT: _____ MEANING: _____

2. blepharoptosis

   ROOT: _____ MEANING: _____

3. conjunctivitis

   ROOT: _____ MEANING: _____

4. corneitis

   ROOT: _____ MEANING: _____

5. glaucoma

   ROOT: _____ MEANING: _____

6. keratotomy

   ROOT: _____ MEANING: _____

7. lacrimal

   ROOT: _____ MEANING: _____

8. oculomotor

   ROOT: _____ MEANING: _____

9. ophthalmoscope

   ROOT: _____ MEANING: _____

10. optic

    ROOT: _____ MEANING: _____

11. palpebral

    ROOT: _____ MEANING: _____

12. photophobia

    ROOT: _____ MEANING: _____

13. pupillary

    ROOT: _____ MEANING: _____

14. retinitis

    ROOT: _____ MEANING: _____

15. vitreous

    ROOT: _____ MEANING: _____

EXERCISE 3

Write the correct word root(s) with the combining form for the following definitions.

1. cornea _____
2. eye _____
3. eyelid _____
4. tears _____
5. glassy _____
6. sclera _____
7. lens _____
8. light _____
9. pupil _____
10. retina _____
11. silver _____
12. tear sac _____
13. watery _____

Structures of the Eye

As stated previously, the structures of the eye are arranged in three layers, or tunics. The outer layer is the **sclera** (**SKLAIR**-ah), the middle layer is the **choroid** (**KOH**-royd), and the inner layer is the **retina** (**RET**-ih-nah). Each layer consists of additional structures and provides specific functions related to sight. Figure 15-1 illustrates the structures of the eye. Refer to this figure as you learn about each layer and its structures.

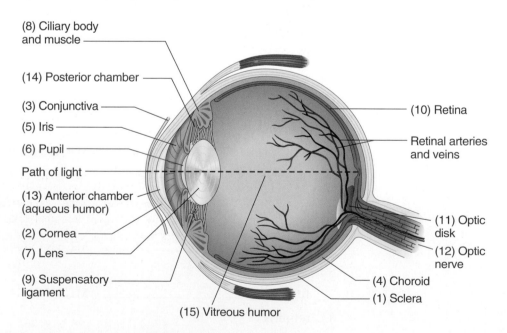

(8) Ciliary body and muscle
(14) Posterior chamber
(3) Conjunctiva
(5) Iris
(6) Pupil
Path of light
(13) Anterior chamber (aqueous humor)
(2) Cornea
(7) Lens
(9) Suspensatory ligament
(15) Vitreous humor
(10) Retina
Retinal arteries and veins
(11) Optic disk
(12) Optic nerve
(4) Choroid
(1) Sclera

Figure 15-1 Structures of the eye

Outer Layer

The outer layer of the eye consists of the sclera, cornea, and conjunctiva. The (1) **sclera** is a tough or fibrous tissue that maintains the shape of the eyeball and serves as its protective covering. The sclera is commonly called the "white of the eyes." The (2) **cornea** (**KOR**-nee-ah) is the transparent anterior portion of the sclera that covers the iris. The (3) **conjunctiva** (kon-junk-**TIGH**-vah) is a mucous membrane that lines the outer surface of the eye and the inside of the eyelid.

Middle Layer

The middle layer of the eye includes the choroid, iris, pupil, lens, and ciliary body. The (4) **choroid** is a layer of tissue beneath the sclera that contains blood vessels that supply oxygen and nutrients to the eye. The (5) **iris**, which gives our eyes their unique color, is a muscular ring that surrounds the (6) **pupil**. The iris adjusts the opening of the pupil to control the amount of light that enters the eye. The (7) **lens**, also called the **crystalline** (**KRIS**-tah-lin) **lens**, is connected to the choroid by the (8) **ciliary** (**SILL**-ee-air-ee) **body** and the (9) **suspensatory** (suh-**SPEN**-sah-tor-ee) **ligaments**. The choroid, iris, and ciliary body are collectively known as the **uvea** (**YOO**-vee-ah).

The ciliary body and suspensatory ligaments adjust the shape of the lens to help focus light rays on the retina. When an object is near, the lens is shortened and becomes thicker; when an object is distant, the lens is lengthened and becomes thinner.

Inner Layer

The inner layer of the eye includes the retina, nerve cells, and optic disk. The (10) **retina** is the sensory nerve tissue that coats the inside of the eye. It contains nerve cells called **rods** and **cones**, which convert light rays into nerve impulses. Rods are responsible for vision in dim light and also peripheral vision. Cones are responsible for the vision in bright light, central vision, and color vision. The (11) **optic disk**, located at the back of the eye, is the area where the nerve endings of the retina come together to form the (12) **optic nerve**. The optic nerve transmits impulses to the occipital lobe of the brain.

Cavities of the Eye

The interior of the eye has two cavities: the anterior cavity and the posterior cavity. The anterior cavity consists of the (13) **anterior chamber**, the area in the front of the lens; and the (14) **posterior chamber**, the area behind the lens. These chambers are filled with a watery fluid called **aqueous** (**AY**-kwee-us) **humor**; this fluid maintains the proper pressure within the eye.

The posterior cavity is filled with a clear, jelly-like substance called (15) **vitreous** (**VIH**-tree-us) **humor**; this fluid gives the eyeball its shape. Vitreous humor is necessary for sight. If the eyeball is injured and vitreous humor escapes, blindness can result. Both aqueous and vitreous humor help bend light rays as they pass through the eye and focus on the retina.

EXERCISE 4

Write the name of the labeled structures in Figure 15-2 on the spaces provided.

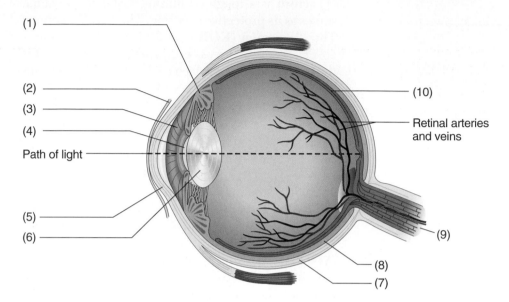

Figure 15-2 Labeling exercise

1. _____
2. _____
3. _____
4. _____
5. _____
6. _____
7. _____
8. _____
9. _____
10. _____

EXERCISE 5

Match the medical term in Column 1 with the definition in Column 2.

COLUMN 1

_____ 1. choroid

_____ 2. ciliary body

_____ 3. conjunctiva

_____ 4. cornea

_____ 5. iris

_____ 6. lens

_____ 7. optic disk

_____ 8. optic nerve

_____ 9. pupil

COLUMN 2

a. adjusts to focus light rays on the retina

b. area where retinal nerve endings come together

c. clear jelly-like substance necessary for sight

d. colorful muscular ring that adjusts the pupil

e. fibrous outer layer of the eye; white of the eye

f. helps adjust the shape of the lens

g. membrane that lines the outer surface of the eye

h. opening or hole in the eye

i. sensory nerve tissue; inner layer of the eye

_____ 10. retina   j. tissue containing the blood vessels of the eye

_____ 11. sclera   k. transmits impulses to the brain

_____ 12. vitreous humor   l. transparent, anterior portion of the sclera

---

Accessory Structures of the Eye

Accessory structures of the eye include the orbit; eyebrows; eyelashes; oil glands; and lacrimal glands, fluid, sacs, and ducts. The purpose of the accessory structures is to protect the eye from disease and injury. Refer to Figure 15-3 as you learn about these structures.

The **orbit**, also called the **eye socket**, is the bony cavity of the skull that houses and protects the eyeball. The (1) **upper** and (2) **lower eyelids** and (3) **eyelashes**, along with the (4) **eyebrows**, prevent foreign matter from reaching the eyes. The **meibomian** (migh-**BOH**-mee-an) **glands**, located between the conjunctiva and the tissue of the upper and lower eyelids, are small oil glands that lubricate the eyes. These glands are not visible unless they become obstructed. The (5) **lacrimal** (**LAK**-rih-mal) **glands**, located above the outer corner of each eye, produce **lacrimal fluid** (tears) that moisten the anterior surface of the eyeball. The (6) **lacrimal ducts** drain lacrimal fluid away from the eye and into the nose via the (7) **nasolacrimal duct**. The upper expanded portion of the lacrimal duct is called the (8) **lacrimal sac**.

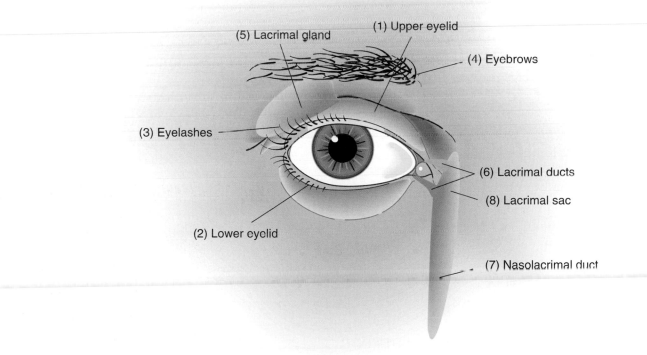

Figure 15-3 Accessory structures of the eye

Write the name of the accessory structure of the eye.

1. bony cavity of the skull; houses the eyes   _____

2. oil glands; lubricate the eye   _____

3. drain tears away from the eye   _____

4. tears   _____

5. produce tears   _____

Medical Terms Related to the Eye

Medical terms related to the eye are organized into three main categories: (1) general medical terms; (2) disease and condition terms; and (3) diagnostic procedure, surgery, and laboratory test terms. The roots, prefixes, and suffixes associated with the eye are listed in Table 15-2. Review these word parts and complete the exercises.

TABLE 15-2 ROOTS, PREFIXES, AND SUFFIXES FOR THE EYE

Root	Meaning	Prefix	Meaning	Suffix	Meaning
blast/o	immature	ect-	outside; out	-ectomy	surgical removal
dipl/o	two; double	en-; eso-	in; inward	-ist	specialist
fund/o	fundus; base	ex-	out; outward	-itis	inflammation
nas/o	nose	intra-	within	-metry	to measure
		presby-	old	-opia	vision
				-(o)tomy	incision into
				-pathy	disease
				-plasty	surgical repair
				-ptosis	drooping
				-scope	instrument for viewing
				-tropia; -tropio	to turn; turning

Write the root, prefix, suffix, and their meanings on the spaces provided. Based on these meanings, write a brief definition for each term.

1. blepharoplasty

     ROOT: _____   MEANING: _____

     PREFIX: _____   MEANING: _____

     SUFFIX: _____   MEANING: _____

     DEFINITION: _____

2. blepharoptosis

ROOT: _____ MEANING: _____

PREFIX: _____ MEANING: _____

SUFFIX: _____ MEANING: _____

DEFINITION: _____

3. conjunctivitis

ROOT: _____ MEANING: _____

PREFIX: _____ MEANING: _____

SUFFIX: _____ MEANING: _____

DEFINITION: _____

4. diplopia

ROOT: _____ MEANING: _____

PREFIX: _____ MEANING: _____

SUFFIX: _____ MEANING: _____

DEFINITION: _____

5. exophthalmia

ROOT: _____ MEANING: _____

PREFIX: _____ MEANING: _____

SUFFIX: _____ MEANING: _____

DEFINITION: _____

6. exotropia

ROOT: _____ MEANING: _____

PREFIX: _____ MEANING: _____

SUFFIX: _____ MEANING: _____

DEFINITION: _____

7. intraocular

ROOT: _____ MEANING: _____

PREFIX: _____ MEANING: _____

SUFFIX: _____ MEANING: _____

DEFINITION: _____

8. iridectomy

ROOT: _____ MEANING: _____

PREFIX: _____ MEANING: _____

SUFFIX: _____ MEANING: _____

DEFINITION: _____

9. keratotomy

ROOT: _____ MEANING: _____

PREFIX: _____ MEANING: _____

SUFFIX: _____ MEANING: _____

DEFINITION: _____

10. nasolacrimal

ROOT: _____ MEANING: _____

PREFIX: _____ MEANING: _____

SUFFIX: _____ MEANING: _____

DEFINITION: _____

11. ophthalmoscope

ROOT: _____ MEANING: _____

PREFIX: _____ MEANING: _____

SUFFIX: _____ MEANING: _____

DEFINITION: _____

12. presbyopia

ROOT: _____ MEANING: _____

PREFIX: _____ MEANING: _____

SUFFIX: _____ MEANING: _____

DEFINITION: _____

13. retinopathy

ROOT: _____ MEANING: _____

PREFIX: _____ MEANING: _____

SUFFIX: _____ MEANING: _____

DEFINITION: _____

General Medical Terms of the Eye

Review the pronunciation and meaning of each term in Table 15-3. Note that some terms are built from word parts and some are not. Complete the exercises for these terms.

TABLE 15-3   GENERAL MEDICAL TERMS OF THE EYE

Term with Pronunciation	Definition
intraocular (**in**-trah-**OK**-yoo-lar) intra- = within ocul/o = eye -ar = pertaining to	pertaining to within the eye

(continues)

TABLE 15-3   GENERAL MEDICAL TERMS OF THE EYE (continued)

Term with Pronunciation	Definition
lacrimal (**LAK**-rih-mal) lacrim/o = tears -al = pertaining to	pertaining to tears
miotic (my-**OT**-ik)	pertaining to constricting the pupil; agent that constricts the pupil
mydriatic (mid-ree-**AT**-ik)	pertaining to dilating the pupil; agent that dilates the pupil
nasolacrimal (**nay**-zoh-**LAK**-rih-mal) nas/o = nose lacrim/o = tears -al = pertaining to	pertaining to the nose and tear duct
ophthalmologist (**off**-thall-**MALL**-oh-jist) ophthalm/o = eye -(o)logist = specialist	physician who specializes in diseases, disorders, and treatments of the eye
ophthalmology (**off**-thall-**MALL**-oh-jee) ophthalm/o = eye -(o)logy = study of	medical specialty related to the study of diseases, disorders, and treatments of the eye
optician (op-**TIH**-shun)	individual who measures and fits eyeglasses
optometrist (op **TOM**-eh-trist) opt/o = eye -metr = to measure; measurement -ist = specialist	doctor of optometry; health-care provider who measures visual acuity, prescribes corrective lenses, and might diagnose and treat some eye problems
optometry (op-**TOM**-eh-tree) opt/o = eye -metr = to measure; measurement -y = noun ending	measuring and testing the eyes for visual acuity and corrective lenses
visual acuity (**VIZH**-yoo-al an-**KYOO**-ih-tee)	sharpness or clearness of vision in one or both eyes

Analyze each term by writing the prefix, root, combining vowel, and suffix separated by vertical slashes. Based on the meaning of the word parts, write a definition for each term. Check the definition in a medical dictionary. Note that some terms might have more than one root.

EXAMPLE: retinopathy

	/ retin	/ o	/ pathy
prefix	*root*	*combining vowel*	*suffix*

DEFINITION: disease of the retina

1. intraocular

prefix	*root*	*combining vowel*	*suffix*

DEFINITION: _____

2. nasolacrimal

prefix	*root*	*combining vowel*	*suffix*

DEFINITION: _____

3. ophthalmologist

prefix	*root*	*combining vowel*	*suffix*

DEFINITION: _____

4. ophthalmology

prefix	*root*	*combining vowel*	*suffix*

DEFINITION: _____

5. optometrist

prefix	*root*	*combining vowel*	*suffix*

DEFINITION: _____

6. optometry

prefix	*root*	*combining vowel*	*suffix*

DEFINITION: _____

Write the medical term for each definition.

1. agent that constricts the pupil _____
2. agent that dilates the pupil _____
3. sharpness or clearness of vision _____
4. pertaining to tears _____
5. individual who measures and fits eyeglasses _____

Disease and Disorder Terms of the Eye

Eye diseases and disorders include familiar problems such as cataract as well as more complex and less familiar diagnoses such as retinitis pigmentosa. The medical terms are presented in alphabetic order in Table 15-4. Review the pronunciation and definition for each term and complete the exercises.

TABLE 15-4 DISEASE AND DISORDER TERMS OF THE EYE

Term with Pronunciation	Definition
astigmatism (ah-**STIG**-mah-tizm)	a refractive error causing light rays to be focused irregularly on the retina due to an abnormally shaped cornea
blepharitis (**bleh**-fah-**RIGH**-tis) blephar/o = eyelids -itis = inflammation	inflammation of the eyelids
blepharoptosis (**bleh**-fah-roh-**TOH**-sis) blephar/o = eyelid -ptosis = drooping	drooping of an eyelid
cataract (**KAT**-ah-rakt)	progressive cloudiness of the crystalline lens (Figure 15-4)

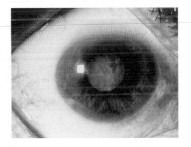

Figure 15-4 Cataract (Courtesy of the National Eye Institute, NIH)

chalazion (kah-**LAY**-zee-on)	cyst or nodule on the eyelid as a result of an obstructed meibomian gland (Figure 15-5)

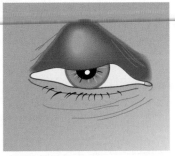

Figure 15-5 Chalazion

(continues)

TABLE 15-4 DISEASE AND DISORDER TERMS OF THE EYE (continued)

Term with Pronunciation	Definition
color blindness	inability to recognize or "see" certain colors
conjunctivitis (kon-**junk**-tih-**VIGH**-tis) conjunctiv/o = conjunctiva -itis = inflammation	inflammation of the conjunctiva; commonly called pinkeye
dacryocystitis (**dak**-ree-oh-sis-**TIGH**-tis) dacryocyst/o = tear sac -itis = inflammation	inflammation of the tear sac or lacrimal sac
detached retina	separation of the retina from the choroid layer of the eye
diabetic retinopathy (**digh**-ah-**BEH**-tik **reh**-tin-**OP**-ah-thee) retin/o = retina -pathy = disease	disease of the retina and its capillaries caused by long-standing and usually poorly controlled diabetes mellitus (Figure 15-6)

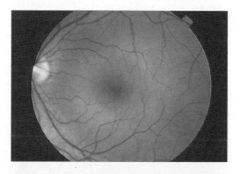

(A)

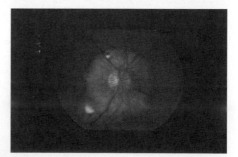

(B)

Figure 15-6 A. Normal retina; B. diabetic retinopathy, proliferative (Courtesy of the National Eye Institute, NIH)

diplopia (dih-**PLOH**-pee-ah) dipl/o = two; double -opia = vision	double vision; may be in one or both eyes

(continues)

TABLE 15-4   DISEASE AND DISORDER TERMS OF THE EYE (continued)

Term with Pronunciation	Definition
ectropion (ek-**TROH**-pee-on) ect- = outside; out -tropion = turning	turning outward of the eyelash margins, usually affects the lower eyelid (Figure 15-7)

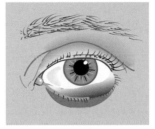

Figure 15-7   Ectropion

entropion (en-**TROH**-pee-on) en- = in; Inward -tropion = turning	turning inward of the eyelash margins, usually affects the lower eyelid
esotropia (ess-oh-**TROH**-pee-ah) eso- = in; inward -tropia = turning	inward turning of the eyes; also known as *convergent strabismus;* commonly called *cross-eyed*
exophthalmia (**ecks**-off-**THAL**-mee-ah) ex- = out; outward ophthalm/o – eye -ia = noun ending	abnormal protrusion of the eyeball(s)
exotropia (**ecks**-oh-**TROH**-pee-ah) ex- = out; outward -tropia = turning	outward turning of the eyes; also known as *divergent strabismus;* commonly called *walleyed*
glaucoma (glaw-**KOH**-mah)	increased intraocular pressure

EXERCISE 10

Analyze each term by writing the prefix, root, combining vowel, and suffix separated by vertical slashes. Based on the meaning of the word parts, write a definition for each term. Check the definition in a medical dictionary. Note that some terms might have more than one root.

   1. blepharitis

_____

prefix   *root*   *combining vowel*   *suffix*

DEFINITION: _____

2. blepharoptosis

prefix	root	combining vowel	suffix

DEFINITION: _____

3. conjunctivitis

prefix	root	combining vowel	suffix

DEFINITION: _____

4. dacryocystitis

prefix	root	combining vowel	suffix

DEFINITION: _____

5. exophthalmia

prefix	root	combining vowel	suffix

DEFINITION: _____

6. diplopia

prefix	root	combining vowel	suffix

DEFINITION: _____

7. entropion

prefix	root	combining vowel	suffix

DEFINITION: _____

8. esotropia

prefix	root	combining vowel	suffix

DEFINITION: _____

9. exotropia

prefix	root	combining vowel	suffix

DEFINITION: _____

EXERCISE 11

Replace the italicized phrase with the correct medical term.

1. *Cloudiness of the crystalline lens* is a common problem associated with aging.

   _____

2. *A refractive error of irregularly focused light rays* can be corrected with glasses.

   _____

3. Trauma to the eye can result in *double vision*.

   _____

4. Surgical intervention might be needed to correct *convergent strabismus.*

   _____

5. A thorough eye examination includes an assessment for *increased intraocular pressure.*

   _____

6. *Walleye* is often caused by a problem with the muscles of the eye.

   _____

7. An obstructed meibomian gland is a common cause of a *cyst on the eyelid.*

   _____

8. *Abnormal protrusion of the eyeballs* is often seen in severe hyperthyroidism.

   _____

9. *Turning outward of the eyelash margin* usually affects the lower eyelid.

   _____

10. *Turning inward of the eyelash margin* might cause irritation of the eye.

    _____

Review the pronunciation and definition for each term in Table 15-5 and complete the exercises.

TABLE 15-5 DISEASE AND DISORDER TERMS OF THE EYE

Term with Pronunciation	Definition
hordeolum (hor-**DEE**-oh-lum)	bacterial infection of an eyelash follicle or sebaceous gland; commonly called a *sty*
hyperopia (**high**-per-**OH**-pee-ah) hyper- = increased; excessive -opia = vision	impaired vision of close objects; light rays focus beyond the retina; commonly called *farsightedness* (Figure 15-8)

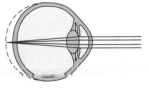

Hyperopia (farsightedness)
Light rays focus behind the retina

Figure 15-8 Hyperopia

iritis (ir-**RIGH**-tis) ir/o = iris -itis = inflammation	inflammation of the iris

(continues)

TABLE 15-5   DISEASE AND DISORDER TERMS OF THE EYE (continued)

Term with Pronunciation	Definition
keratitis (**kair**-ah-**TIGH**-tis) kerat/o = cornea -itis = inflammation	inflammation of the cornea
myopia (my-**OH**-pee-ah)	impaired vision of distant objects; light rays focus in front of the retina; commonly called *nearsightedness* (Figure 15-9)

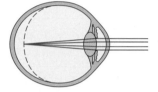

Myopia (nearsightedness)
Light rays focus in front of the retina

Figure 15-9   Myopia

nyctalopia (**nik**-tah-**LOH**-pee-ah)	impaired or inadequate vision at night; commonly called *night blindness*
nystagmus (niss-**TAG**-mus)	involuntary movements of the eye(s), which may or may not be apparent to the individual
ophthalmia neonatorum (off-**THAL**-mee-ah nee-oh-nay-**TOR**-um) ophthalm/o = eye -ia = condition neo- = new nat/o = birth	inflammation of the conjunctiva of a newborn caused by irritation, a blocked tear duct, or a bacterial or viral infection contracted as the infant passes through the birth canal; bacterial infections include chlamydia, and viral infections include genital herpes; also called *newborn* or *neonatal conjunctivitis* (Figure15-10)

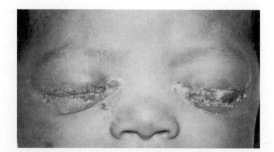

Figure 15-10   Bacterial ophthalmia neonatorum (Centers for Disease Control/ J. Pledger)

(*continues*)

TABLE 15-5 DISEASE AND DISORDER TERMS OF THE EYE (continued)

Term with Pronunciation	Definition
photophobia (foh-toh-**FOH**-bee-ah) phot/o = light -phobia = fear	abnormal sensitivity to light
photoretinitis (**foh**-toh-reh-tih-**NIGH**-tis) phot/o = light retin/o = retina -itis = inflammation	damage or inflammation of the retina due to excessive exposure to light
presbyopia (prez-bee-**OH**-pee-ah) presby- = old -opia = vision	impaired vision due to aging
pterygium (ter-**IJ**-ee-um)	irregular growth and thickening of the conjunctiva on the nasal side of the cornea
retinitis pigmentosa (**reh**-tih-**NIGH**-tis **pig**-men-**TOH**-sah) retin/o = retina -itis – inflammation	degenerative disease of the retina without inflammation that results in defective night vision and a decreased field of vision
retinoblastoma (**reh**-tih-noh-blass-**TOH**-mah) retin/o = retina blast/o = immature cell -oma = tumor	malignant tumor of the retina
retinopathy (**reh**-tih-**NOP**-ah-thee) retin/o = retina -pathy = disease	any disease or disorder of the retina
sclerokeratitis (**sklair**-oh-**kair**-ah-**TIGH**-tis) scler/o = sclera kerat/o = cornea -itis = inflammation	inflammation of the sclera and cornea
strabismus (strah-**BIZ**-mus)	inability of the eyes to gaze in the same direction because of weakness of the eye muscles
trachoma (tray-**KOH**-mah)	chronic, contagious form of conjunctivitis characterized by hypertrophy of the conjunctiva
uveitis (yoo-vee-**EYE**-tis) uve/o = uvea -itis = inflammation	inflammation of the iris, ciliary body, and choroid

EXERCISE 12

Analyze each term by writing the prefix, root, combining vowel, and suffix separated by vertical slashes. Based on the meaning of the word parts, write a definition for each term. Check the definition in a medical dictionary. Note that some terms might have more than one root.

1. hyperopia

prefix	*root*	*combining vowel*	*suffix*

   DEFINITION: _____

2. iritis

prefix	*root*	*combining vowel*	*suffix*

   DEFINITION: _____

3. keratitis

prefix	*root*	*combining vowel*	*suffix*

   DEFINITION: _____

4. photophobia

prefix	*root*	*combining vowel*	*suffix*

   DEFINITION: _____

5. photoretinitis

prefix	*root*	*combining vowel*	*suffix*

   DEFINITION: _____

6. presbyopia

prefix	*root*	*combining vowel*	*suffix*

   DEFINITION: _____

7. retinoblastoma

prefix	*root*	*combining vowel*	*suffix*

   DEFINITION: _____

8. retinopathy

prefix	*root*	*combining vowel*	*suffix*

   DEFINITION: _____

9. sclerokeratitis

prefix	*root*	*combining vowel*	*suffix*

   DEFINITION: _____

EXERCISE 13

Replace the italicized phrase with the correct medical term.

1. *Involuntary eye movements* might not be apparent to the patient.

   _____

2. Excessive ultraviolet light exposure can cause *irregular growth of the conjunctiva*.

   _____

3. During Shawna's well-baby visit, the pediatrician noted *an inability of the eyes to gaze in the same direction*.

   _____

4. *Conjunctivitis with hypertrophy of the conjunctiva* is prevalent in third-world countries.

   _____

5. Linda's *sty* was resolved without medical intervention.

   _____

6. *Nearsightedness* is a vision problem that requires corrective lenses.

   _____

7. Because of his *night blindness*, Wade seldom drove his car after dusk.

   _____

8. A decreased field of vision is often the result of *a degenerative disease of the retina*.

   _____

Diagnostic and Treatment Terms Related to the Eye

Review the pronunciation and definition of the diagnostic and treatment terms in Table 15-6. Complete the exercises for each set of terms.

TABLE 15-6 DIAGNOSTIC AND TREATMENT TERMS RELATED TO THE EYE

Term with Pronunciation	Definition
blepharoplasty (**BLEFF**-ah-roh-**plass**-tee) blephar/o = eyelid -plasty = surgical repair	surgical repair or plastic surgery of the eyelid
corneal transplant (**KOR**-nee-al) corne/o = cornea -al = pertaining to	surgical transplantation of a donor cornea into the eye of a recipient
cryoextraction of the lens (**krigh**-oh-ecks-**TRAK**-shun)	removal of the crystalline lens with a cooling probe
enucleation of the eye (ee-**noo**-klee-**AY**-shun)	removal of the eye from the orbit

(continues)

TABLE 15-6 DIAGNOSTIC AND TREATMENT TERMS RELATED TO THE EYE (continued)

Term with Pronunciation	Definition
extracapsular cataract extraction (ECCE) (**eks**-trah-**KAP**-syoo-lar **KAT**-ah-rakt)	removal of the crystalline lens and the anterior segment of the lens capsule
funduscopy (fun-**DOSS**-koh-pee) fund/o = fundus; base -scopy = examination with a scope	examination of the posterior inner part of the eye, known as the *fundus*, using an ophthalmoscope
intraocular lens implant (**in**-trah-**OK**-yoo-lar) intra- = within ocul/o = eye -ar = pertaining to	surgical implantation of a crystalline lens; usually done at the same time as cataract extraction
iridectomy (ir-id-**EK**-toh-mee) irid/o = iris -ectomy = surgical removal	excision of a section of the iris
keratoplasty (**KAIR**-ah-toh-**plass**-tee) kerat/o = cornea -plasty = surgical repair	surgical repair of the cornea characterized by the excision of an opaque section of the cornea
laser in situ keratomileusis (LASIK) (**kair**-ah-toh-mill-**YOO**-sis)	procedure to correct vision problems, especially myopia, by removing corneal tissue and permanently changing the shape of the cornea
ophthalmoscope (off-**THAL**-moh-skohp) ophthalm/o = eye -scope = instrument for viewing	instrument for viewing the interior of the eye
ophthalmoscopy (**off**-thal-**MOSS**-koh-pee) ophthalm/o = eye -scopy = visualization with a scope	examination of the interior of the eye
phacoemulsification (**fak**-oh-ee-**MULL**-sih-fih-**kay**-shun)	breaking the crystalline lens or its cataract into tiny particles that can be removed by suction or aspiration
photo-refractive keratectomy (PRK) (**FOH**-toh ree-**FRAK**-tiv kair-ah-**TEK**-toh-mee) kerat/o = cornea -ectomy = surgical removal	surgical removal of corneal surface cells to correct or reduce myopia

(continues)

TABLE 15-6 DIAGNOSTIC AND TREATMENT TERMS RELATED TO THE EYE
(continued)

Term with Pronunciation	Definition
radial keratotomy (RK) (**RAY**-dee-al **kair**-ah-**TOT**-oh-mee) kerat/o = cornea -(o)tomy = incision into	spoke-like incisions into the cornea to correct nearsightedness
retinal photocoagulation (**REH**-tin-al foh-toh-koh-**ag**-yoo-**LAY**-shun) retin/o = retina -al = pertaining to	laser surgery of the retina to correct retinal detachment and prevent hemorrhage of retinal blood vessels
scleral buckling (**SKLAIR**-al **BUK**-ling) scler/o = sclera -al = pertaining to	repair of retinal detachment by resecting or folding in of the sclera
trabeculectomy (trah-**bek**-yoo-**LEK**-toh-mee)	surgical excision of a portion of corneal and scleral tissue to decrease intraocular pressure
trabeculoplasty (trah-**BEK**-yoo-loh-**plass**-tee)	surgical creation of a permanent fistula to drain excess aqueous humor from the anterior chamber of the eye in order to relieve the intraocular pressure associated with glaucoma
vitrectomy (vih-**TREK**-toh-mee) vitre/o = glassy; jelly-like -ectomy = surgical removal	surgical removal of all or part of the vitreous humor

EXERCISE 14

Analyze each term by writing the prefix, root, combining vowel, and suffix separated by vertical slashes. Based on the meaning of the word parts, write a definition for each term. Check the definition in a medical dictionary.

1. blepharoplasty

prefix	*root*	*combining vowel*	*suffix*

DEFINITION: _____

2. funduscopy

prefix	*root*	*combining vowel*	*suffix*

DEFINITION: _____

3. iridectomy

prefix	root	combining vowel	suffix

DEFINITION: _____

4. keratoplasty

prefix	root	combining vowel	suffix

DEFINITION: _____

5. ophthalmoscope

prefix	root	combining vowel	suffix

DEFINITION: _____

6. ophthalmoscopy

prefix	root	combining vowel	suffix

DEFINITION: _____

7. vitrectomy

prefix	root	combining vowel	suffix

DEFINITION: _____

EXERCISE 15

Match each medical term in Column 1 with the correct definition in Column 2.

COLUMN 1

_____ 1. corneal transplant

_____ 2. cryoextraction of the lens

_____ 3. ECCE

_____ 4. enucleation of the eye

_____ 5. intraocular lens implant

_____ 6. phacoemulsification

_____ 7. photo-refractive keratectomy

_____ 8. radial keratotomy

_____ 9. retinal photocoagulation

_____ 10. scleral buckling

_____ 11. trabeculectomy

_____ 12. vitrectomy

COLUMN 2

a. breaking the lens into tiny particles

b. extracapsular cataract extraction

c. excision of corneal and scleral tissue

d. folding in of the sclera to repair a
   detached retina

e. laser surgery of the retina

f. removal of corneal surface cells

g. removal of the eye from the orbit

h. removal of the lens with a
   cooling probe

i. spoke-like incisions into the cornea

j. surgical implantation of a lens

k. surgical removal of vitreous humor

l. surgical transplantation of a donor
   cornea

Abbreviations

Review the abbreviations related to the eye in Table 15-7. Practice writing out the meaning of each abbreviation.

TABLE 15-7   ABBREVIATIONS

Abbreviation	Meaning
ECCE	extracapsular cataract extraction
EOM	extraocular movement
ICCE	intracapsular cataract extraction
IOL	intraocular lens
IOP	intraocular pressure
LASIK	laser in situ keratomileusis
OD	right eye (oculus dexter)
OS	left eye (oculus sinister)
OU	each eye (oculus uterque)
PERRLA	pupils equal, round, reactive to light and accommodation
PRK	photo-refractive keratectomy
REM	rapid eye movement
RK	radial keratotomy
VA	visual acuity
VF	visual field

The Ear

The visible parts of our ears, located on either side of the head, are called the *external ear*. The internal ear structures, called the *middle* and *inner* ear, are buried in the bony framework of the cranium. The structures of the ear function to provide our sense of hearing, balance, and equilibrium. Sound waves enter the ear, travel through the structures of the middle and inner ear, and are converted to electrical impulses that are transmitted to the cerebral cortex. In the cerebral cortex, the impulses are interpreted into the sounds that we hear. Our sense of hearing is dependent on the health of our ears, our hearing-related nerves, and our brain.

Word Roots Related to Hearing

To understand and use medical terms related to hearing, it is necessary to acquire a thorough knowledge of the associated word roots. Review the word roots in Table 15-8 and complete the exercises.

TABLE 15-8   WORD ROOTS: EAR

Word Root/Combining Form	Meaning
acoust/o	hearing
audi/o	hearing; sound
cochle/o	cochlea
labyrinth/o	inner ear; labyrinth

(continues)

TABLE 15-8 WORD ROOTS: EAR (continued)

Word Root/Combining Form	Meaning
myring/o	eardrum
ot/o	ear
staped/o	stapes; middle ear bone
tympan/o	eardrum

EXERCISE 16

Write the word root and its meaning on the spaces provided.

1. audiologist

   ROOT: _____ MEANING: _____

2. labyrinthitis

   ROOT: _____ MEANING: _____

3. myringotomy

   ROOT: _____ MEANING: _____

4. tympanoplasty

   ROOT: _____ MEANING: _____

5. otitis media

   ROOT: _____ MEANING: _____

6. stapedectomy

   ROOT: _____ MEANING: _____

7. cochleoma

   ROOT: _____ MEANING: _____

8. acoustic nerve

   ROOT: _____ MEANING: _____

EXERCISE 17

Write the correct word root(s) for the following definitions.

1. ear _____
2. eardrum _____
3. hearing _____
4. inner ear _____
5. middle ear bone _____

Structures of the Ear

The major structures of the ear are organized as the external, middle, and internal ear. Figure 15-11 illustrates these structures. Refer to the figure as you learn about the parts of the ear.

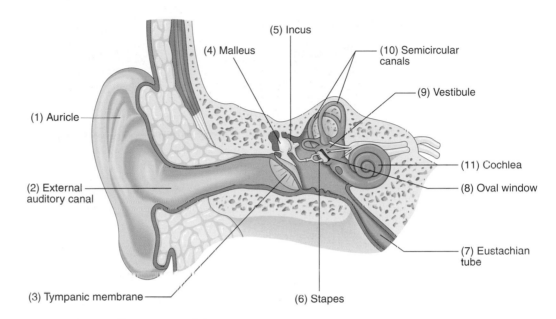

Figure 15-11   Structures of the ear

The external ear includes the (1) **auricle** (**OR**-ih-kal), or **pinna** (**PIN**-ah), which is a cartilaginous flap that directs sound waves into the (2) **external auditory canal**. The auditory canal is lined with hairs called **cilia** (**SILL**-ee-ah) and **ceruminous** (seh-**ROOM**-ih-nus) **glands**. Cilia help direct sound waves through the canal, and the ceruminous glands produce **cerumen** (seh-**ROO**-men), a substance commonly called *earwax* that protects and lubricates the ear. The external ear is separated from the middle ear by the (3) **tympanic** (tim-**PAN**-ik) **membrane**, or eardrum. The tympanic membrane transmits sound waves to the middle ear.

The middle ear includes three small bones called the **ossicles** (**OSS**-ih-kuhlz). The bone closest to the tympanic membrane is the (4) **malleus** (**MAL**-ee-us), commonly known as the *hammer;* the next bone is the (5) **incus** (**INK**-us), commonly known as the *anvil*; and the third bone is the (6) **stapes** (**STAY**-peez), commonly known as the *stirrup*. The middle ear also includes the (7) **eustachian** (yoo-**STAY**-shun) **tube** that connects the middle ear to the pharynx. Yawning and swallowing cause the eustachian tube to open and equalize the pressure between the middle ear and the outside atmosphere.

Vibrations of the tympanic membrane, which are caused by sound waves, set the ossicles in motion. The malleus transmits sound waves to the incus, which in turn transmits sound waves to the stapes. The stapes vibrate against the (8) **oval window**, which separates the middle ear from the inner ear.

The inner ear, called the **labyrinth** (**LAB**-ih-rinth), includes the (9) **vestibule** (**VESS**-tih-byool), the (10) **semicircular canals**, and the (11) **cochlea** (**KOK**-lee-ah). The cochlea is a spiral or snail-shaped structure that contains auditory fluids and the **organ of Corti**. The organ of Corti receives sound wave vibrations and converts them into nerve impulses. The impulses are carried to the brain by the **acoustic** (ah-**KOO**-stik) **nerve** and are then recognized as specific sounds. The semicircular canals are continuous with the vestibule and are filled with fluid necessary for balance and equilibrium. The process of converting sound waves into hearing is illustrated in Figure 15-12.

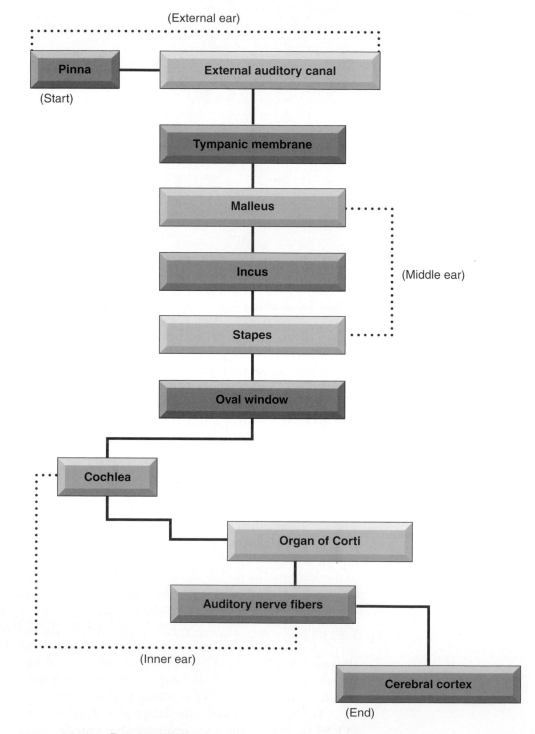

Figure 15-12 Process of hearing

EXERCISE 18

Identify the names of the structures shown in Figure 15-13. Write your answers on the spaces provided.

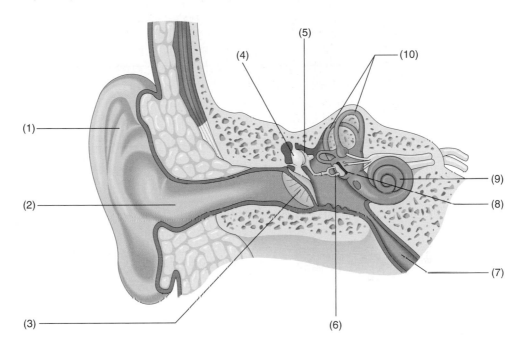

Figure 15-13 Labeling exercise

1. _____
2. _____
3. _____
4. _____
5. _____
6. _____
7. _____
8. _____
9. _____
10. _____

EXERCISE 19

Write the name of each defined structure of the ear.

1. anvil _____

2. converts sound waves into nerve impulses _____

3. eardrum _____

4. flap of the outer ear _____

5. hammer _____

6. inner ear _____

7. middle ear bones (one word) _____

8. secretes earwax _____

9. snail-shaped structure _____

10. stirrup _____

Medical Terminology Related to the Ear

Medical terms related to the ear are organized into three main categories: (1) general medical terms; (2) disease and condition terms; and (3) diagnostic procedure, surgery, and laboratory test terms. Table 15-9 lists roots, prefixes, and suffixes associated with these terms. Review the word parts in the table and complete the exercises.

TABLE 15-9 ROOTS, PREFIXES, AND SUFFIXES

Root	Meaning	Suffix	Meaning	Prefix	Meaning
laryng/o	larynx	-algia	pain	presby-	old
myc/o	fungus	-cusis; cusia	hearing		
rhin/o	nose	-gram	graphic record		
		-metry	to measure		
		-oma	tumor; mass		
		-plasty	surgical repair		
		-(r)rhea	flow; discharge		
		-(o)tomy	incision into		

EXERCISE 20

Write the root(s), suffix, and their meanings on the spaces provided. Based on the meaning of the word parts, write a definition for each term. Check the definition in a medical dictionary. Note that some terms might have more than one root.

1. otomycosis

   ROOT: _____ MEANING: _____

   ROOT: _____ MEANING: _____

   PREFIX: _____ MEANING: _____

   SUFFIX: _____ MEANING: _____

   DEFINITION: _____

2. otalgia

   ROOT: _____ MEANING: _____

   PREFIX: _____ MEANING: _____

   SUFFIX: _____ MEANING: _____

   DEFINITION: _____

3. otorrhea

    ROOT: _____   MEANING: _____

    PREFIX: _____   MEANING: _____

    SUFFIX: _____   MEANING: _____

    DEFINITION: _____

4. audiogram

    ROOT: _____   MEANING: _____

    PREFIX: _____   MEANING: _____

    SUFFIX: _____   MEANING: _____

    DEFINITION: _____

5. myringoplasty

    ROOT: _____   MEANING: _____

    PREFIX: _____   MEANING: _____

    SUFFIX: _____   MEANING: _____

    DEFINITION: _____

6. myringotomy

    ROOT: _____   MEANING: _____

    PREFIX: _____   MEANING: _____

    SUFFIX: _____   MEANING: _____

    DEFINITION: _____

7. presbycusis

    ROOT: _____   MEANING: _____

    PREFIX: _____   MEANING: _____

    SUFFIX: _____   MEANING: _____

    DEFINITION: _____

8. audiometry

    ROOT: _____   MEANING: _____

    PREFIX: _____   MEANING: _____

    SUFFIX: _____   MEANING: _____

    DEFINITION: _____

9. audiologist

    ROOT: _____   MEANING: _____

    PREFIX: _____   MEANING: _____

    SUFFIX: _____   MEANING: _____

    DEFINITION: _____

TABLE 15-13 ABBREVIATIONS (continued)

Abbreviation	Meaning
BOM	bilateral otitis media
EENT	eyes, ears, nose, throat
ENT	ears, nose, throat
TM	tympanic membrane

CHAPTER REVIEW

The Chapter Review can be used as a self-test. Go through each exercise and answer as many questions as you can without referring to previous exercises or earlier discussions within this chapter. Check your answers and fill in any blanks. Practice writing any terms you might have misspelled.

EXERCISE 26

Write the medical term for each definition.

1. within the eye   _____

2. physician who specializes in diseases and
   treatment of the eye   _____

3. inflammation of the eyelids   _____

4. inflammation of the conjunctiva   _____

5. abnormal protrusion of the eyeballs   _____

6. farsightedness   _____

7. nearsightedness   _____

8. impaired vision related to aging   _____

9. surgical repair of the eyelid   _____

10. abnormal sensitivity to light   _____

11. pertaining to hearing   _____

12. specialist who evaluates hearing loss   _____

13. ear, nose, and throat physician specialist   _____

14. excessive accumulation of earwax   _____

15. inflammation of the eardrum   _____

16. fungal infection of the ear   _____

17. AS   _____

18. ringing sensation in the ears   _____

19. dizziness   _____

20. incision into the eardrum   _____

EXERCISE 27

Write a brief definition for each medical term.

1. nasolacrimal _____
2. ophthalmology _____
3. blepharoptosis _____
4. diplopia _____
5. glaucoma _____
6. keratitis _____
7. nyctalopia _____
8. retinopathy _____
9. ophthalmoscope _____
10. cochlear _____
11. labyrinthitis _____
12. otalgia _____
13. otorrhea _____
14. presbycusis _____
15. audiometry _____
16. tympanoplasty _____

EXERCISE 28

Circle the medical term that best fits the definition.

DEFINITION	CIRCLE ONE TERM
1. agent that constricts the pupil	*mydriatic* OR *miotic*
2. cyst caused by an obstructed meibomian gland	*hordeolum* OR *chalazion*
3. divergent strabismus	*ectropion* OR *exotropia*
4. turning inward of the eyelash margin	*esotropia* OR *entropion*
5. increased intraocular pressure	*glaucoma* OR *cataract*
6. agent that dilates the pupil	*miotic* OR *mydriatic*
7. convergent strabismus	*esotropia* OR *entropion*
8. bacterial infection of an eyelash follicle	*pterygium* OR *hordeolum*
9. progressive cloudiness of the lens	*glaucoma* OR *cataract*
10. turning outward of the eyelash margins	*pterygium* OR *ectropion*
11. chronic, contagious conjunctivitis	*trachoma* OR *hordeolum*
12. inability of the eyes to gaze in the same direction	*nystagmus* OR *strabismus*
13. irregular thickening of the conjunctiva	*chalazion* OR *pterygium*
14. involuntary movement of the eyes	*nystagmus* OR *strabismus*

EXERCISE 29

Match the term or abbreviation in Column 1 with the description in Column 2

COLUMN 1	COLUMN 2
_____ 1. astigmatism	a. bilateral otitis media
_____ 2. audiogram	b. chronic inner ear disorder with fluid
_____ 3. audiology	accumulation
_____ 4. BOM	c. swimmer's ear
_____ 5. chalazion	d. surgical repair of the ear
_____ 6. cholesteatoma	e. graphic record of hearing
_____ 7. hordeolum	f. infection of the middle ear
_____ 8. Meniere's disease	g. mass of cellular debris and cholesterol
_____ 9. otitis externa	h. specialist of the ear, nose, and throat
_____ 10. otitis media	i. study of diseases and treatments of
_____ 11. otology	the ear
_____ 12. otoplasty	j. study of hearing
_____ 13. otorhinolaryngologist	k. inflammation of the iris, ciliary body,
_____ 14. retinoblastoma	and choroid
_____ 15. uveitis	l. irregularly focused light rays, abnormally
	shaped cornea
	m. sty
	n. cyst due to obstructed meibomian gland
	o. malignant tumor of the retina

EXERCISE 30

Read the following operative report. Write out the abbreviations and provide a brief definition of the italicized medical terms. Use a medical dictionary to look up the meaning of the terms.

PREOPERATIVE DIAGNOSIS: Nuclear (1) *cataract* with cortical spoking, (2) *OD*.

POSTOPERATIVE DIAGNOSIS: Nuclear cataract with cortical spoking, OD.

OPERATION PERFORMED: (3) *ECCE* with a posterior chamber (4) *intraocular* lens implant, OD.

DESCRIPTION OF PROCEDURE: The patient was placed in the supine position, and (5) *periorbital* anesthesia was achieved. The patient's periorbital areas were prepped and the right eye draped in the usual fashion for an (6) *ophthalmic* surgical procedure. The lids of the right eye were retracted, an 8-0 black silk bridle suture was passed under the superior rectus tendon, and the globe was retracted downward. A (7) *conjunctival* peritomy was then performed for 180 degrees. A (8) *corneoscleral* groove was then formed. Two preplaced 8-0 black silk sutures were then passed through the groove. The (9) *anterior chamber* was then entered with a razor blade incision through the groove and filled with Healon. The anterior (10) *capsulotomy* was then performed. The nucleus was then expressed without difficulty. The patient tolerated the procedure well and was transferred to the recovery room in excellent condition.

1. _____
2. _____
3. _____
4. _____
5. _____
6. _____
7. _____
8. _____
9. _____
10. _____

EXERCISE 31

Read the progress note and write a brief definition for each italicized medical term, abbreviation, or phrase.

PROGRESS NOTE

The patient is a nine-month-old infant who presents with tenderness, (1) *AU*. His mother states that he has been "fussy during feeding and does not have a fever." (2) *Otoscopic* examination reveals (3) *suppurative otitis media*, more pronounced in the left ear. The (4) *tympanic membrane* is edematous and bulging. I explained to mom due to recurring episodes of (5) *serous otitis media* and today's problem, she should consider bilateral (6) *myringotomy* and (7) *tympanostomy* with placement of tubes. We briefly discussed the pros and cons of this procedure and mom understands my concern related to (8) *labyrinthitis*. I prescribed (9) *otic* drops to be administered three times per day. A two-week follow-up visit will be scheduled.

1. _____
2. _____
3. _____
4. _____
5. _____
6. _____
7. _____
8. _____
9. _____

EXERCISE 32

Select the best answer for each question or statement.

1. Select the term for involuntary movements of the eyes.
   a. astigmatism
   b. nystagmus
   c. hordeolum
   d. pterygium

2. Which term means impaired vision related to aging?
   a. myopia
   b. hyperopia
   c. presbyopia
   d. esotropia

3. Select the term for abnormal cloudiness of the lens.
   a. cataract
   b. hordeolum
   c. glaucoma
   d. pterygium

4. Select the medical term for the condition commonly known as *cross-eyed*.
   a. ectropion
   b. entropion
   c. exotropia
   d. esotropia

5. Which medical term describes an irregular thickening of the conjunctiva?
   a. conjunctivitis
   b. pterygium
   c. hordeolum
   d. nystagmus

6. Choose the medical term for nearsightedness.
   a. myopia
   b. hyperopia
   c. nyctalopia
   d. exotropia

7. Select the medical term for the condition commonly known as a *sty*.
   a. pterygium
   b. hordeolum
   c. entropion
   d. dacryocystitis

8. Which medical term describes an abnormal protrusion of the eyeballs?
   a. exotropia
   b. hyperopia
   c. esotropia
   d. exophthalmia

9. Select the medical term for a drooping eyelid.
   a. blepharoptosis
   b. ectropion
   c. entropion
   d. hordeolum

10. Which term best describes the condition commonly known as *walleyed*?
    a. exophthalmia
    b. exotropia
    c. hyperopia
    d. esotropia

11. The structures of the inner ear are collectively known as which term?
    a. ossicles
    b. semicircular canals
    c. vestibule
    d. labyrinth

12. Which term describes the structure(s) of the ear that play a role in balance and equilibrium?
    a. labyrinth
    b. ossicles
    c. semicircular canals
    d. eustachian tube

13. Select the term for the structure(s) of the ear that house the organ of Corti.
    a. cochlea
    b. ossicles
    c. labyrinth
    d. eustachian tube

14. Collectively, what term describes the bones of the middle ear?
    a. ossicles
    b. labyrinth
    c. cochlea
    d. semicircular canals

15. Which term describes the ear structure(s) that help equalize the pressure between the ear and the atmosphere?
    a. cochlea
    b. labyrinth
    c. semicircular canals
    d. eustachian tube

16. Which abbreviation means left ear?
    a. AS
    b. AD
    c. LE
    d. AU

17. Which term names the structure that separates the middle ear from the inner ear?
    a. cochlea
    b. labyrinth
    c. oval window
    d. tympanic membrane

18. Select the term for a ringing sensation in the ears.
    a. tympanitis
    b. vertigo
    c. otosclerosis
    d. tinnitus

19. Select the correct abbreviation for right ear.
    a. AS
    b. AD
    c. RE
    d. AU

20. Which term is the test that uses a tuning fork to measure the conduction of sound waves?
    a. otoscopy
    b. Weber test
    c. sensorineural test
    d. Rinne test

CHALLENGE EXERCISES

1. *Laser surgery to correct various vision problems has been widely publicized. Visit a local ophthalmologist and gather information about the types of surgery being performed, the vision problems that can be corrected with each type of surgery, and the risks and benefits of the surgery. If you do not have access to a local ophthalmologist, search the Internet for the information, using the keywords "laser surgery" and "eye."*

2. *Interview a local audiologist or search the Internet using the keywords "audiology" or "audiologist" for specific information about the profession. What are the educational requirements? Is there a national or state certification or licensing examination? What type of equipment does an audiologist use? Are there many employment opportunities in the field?*

Pronunciation Review

Review the terms in the chapter. Pronounce each term using the following phonetic pronunciations. Check off the term when you are comfortable saying it.

TERM	PRONUNCIATION
☐ acoustic neuroma	ah-**KOO**-stik noo-**ROH**-mah
☐ aqueous humor	**AY**-kwee-us humor
☐ astigmatism	ah-**STIG**-mah-tizm
☐ audiogram	**AW**-dee-oh-gram
☐ audiologist	aw-dee-**ALL**-oh-jist

☐ audiology	**aw**-dee-**ALL**-oh-jee
☐ audiometry	**aw**-dee-**OM**-eh-tree
☐ auditory	**AW**-dih-tor-ee
☐ auricle	**OR**-ih-kal
☐ blepharitis	**bleh**-fah-**RIGH**-tis
☐ blepharoplasty	**BLEFF**-ah-roh-**plass**-tee
☐ blepharoptosis	**bleh**-fah-roh-**TOH**-sis
☐ cataract	**KAT**-ah-rakt
☐ cerumen	seh-**ROO**-men
☐ ceruminous gland	seh-**ROOM**-ih-nus gland
☐ chalazion	kah-**LAY**-zee-on
☐ cholesteatoma	**koh**-lee-**stee**-ah-**TOH**-mah
☐ choroid	**KOH**-royd
☐ cilia	**SILL**-ee-ah
☐ ciliary body	**SILL**-ee-air-ee body
☐ cochlea	**KOK**-lee-ah
☐ cochlear	**KOK**-lee-ar
☐ conductive deafness	kon-**DUK**-tiv deafness
☐ conjunctiva	kon-junk-**TIGH**-vah
☐ conjunctivitis	kon-**junk**-tih-**VIGH**-tis
☐ cornea	**KOR**-nee-ah
☐ corneal transplant	**KOR**-nee-al transplant
☐ cryoextraction of the lens	**krigh**-oh-eks-**TRAK**-shun of the lens
☐ crystalline lens	**KRIS**-tah-lin lens
☐ dacryocystitis	**dak**-ree-oh-sis-**TIGH**-tis
☐ diabetic retinopathy	**digh**-ah-**BET**-ik **reh**-tin-**OP**-ah-thee
☐ diplopia	dih-**PLOH**-pee-ah
☐ ectropion	ek-**TROH**-pee-on
☐ entropion	en-**TROH**-pee-on
☐ enucleation of the eye	ee-**noo**-klee-**AY**-shun of the eye
☐ esotropia	es-oh-**TROH**-pee-ah
☐ eustachian tube	yoo-**STAY**-shun tube
☐ exophthalmia	**eks**-off-**THAL**-mee-ah
☐ exotropia	**eks**-oh-**TROH**-pee-ah
☐ extracapsular cataract extraction	**eks**-trah-**KAPS**-yoo-lar **KAT**-ah-rakt extraction
☐ funduscopy	fun-**DOSS**-koh-pee
☐ glaucoma	glaw-**KOH**-mah
☐ hordeolum	hor-**DEE**-oh-lum
☐ hyperopia	**high**-per-**OH**-pee-ah
☐ impacted cerumen	impacted seh-**ROO**-men
☐ incus	**INK**-us
☐ intraocular	**in**-trah-**OK**-yoo-lar
☐ intraocular lens implant	**in**-trah-**OK**-yoo-lar lens implant
☐ iridectomy	ir-id-**EK**-toh-mee
☐ iris	**EYE**-ris
☐ iritis	ir-**EYE**-tis
☐ keratitis	**kair**-ah-**TIGH**-tis
☐ keratoplasty	**KAIR**-ah-toh-**plass**-tee
☐ labyrinth	**LAB**-ih-rinth
☐ labyrinthitis	**lab**-ih-rin-**THRIGH**-tis

☐ lacrimal	**LAK**-rih-mal
☐ lacrimal duct	**LAK**-rih-mal duct
☐ lacrimal fluid	**LAK**-rih-mal fluid
☐ lacrimal gland	**LAK**-rih-mal gland
☐ lacrimal sac	**LAK**-rih-mal sac
☐ malleus	**MAL**-lee-us
☐ meibomian glands	migh-**BOH**-mee-an glands
☐ Meniere's disease	man-ee-**AYRZ** disease
☐ miotic	migh-**OT**-ik
☐ mydriatic	mid-ree-**AT**-ik
☐ myopia	migh-**OH**-pee-ah
☐ myringitis	mir-in-**JIGH**-tis
☐ myringoplasty	mir-**IN**-goh-**plass**-tee
☐ myringotomy	mir-in-**GOT**-oh-mee
☐ nasolacrimal	**nay**-zoh-**LAK**-ree-mal
☐ nyctalopia	**nik**-toh-**LOH**-pee-ah
☐ nystagmus	nih-**STAG**-mus
☐ ophthalmologist	**off**-thall-**MALL**-oh-jist
☐ ophthalmology	**off**-thall-**MALL**-oh-jee
☐ ophthalmoscope	off-**THAL**-moh-skohp
☐ ophthalmoscopy	**off**-thal-**MOSS**-koh-pee
☐ optician	op-**TIH**-shun
☐ optometrist	op-**TOM**-eh-trist
☐ optometry	op-**TOM**-eh-tree
☐ organ of Corti	organ of **KOR**-tee
☐ ossicles	**OSS**-ih-kulz
☐ otalgia	oh-**TAL**-jee-ah
☐ otitis externa	oh-**TIGH**-tis eks-**TER**-nah
☐ otitis media	oh-**TIGH**-tis **MEE**-dee-ah
☐ otologist	oh-**TALL**-oh-jist
☐ otology	oh-**TALL**-oh-jee
☐ otomycosis	**oh**-toh-migh-**KOH**-sis
☐ otoplasty	**OH**-toh-**plass**-tee
☐ otorhinolaryngologist	**oh**-toh-**righ**-noh-**lair**-in-**GALL**-oh-jist
☐ otorhinolaryngology	**oh**-toh-**righ**-noh-**lair**-in-**GALL**-oh-jee
☐ otorrhea	oh-toh-**REE**-ah
☐ otosclerosis	**oh**-toh-sklair-**OH**-sis
☐ otoscope	**OH**-toh-skohp
☐ otoscopy	oh-**TOSS**-koh-pee
☐ phacoemulsification	**fak**-oh-ee-**MULL**-sih-fih-**kay**-shun
☐ photo-refractive keratectomy	**FOH**-toh ree-**FRAK**-tiv **kair**-ah-**TEK**-toh-mee
☐ photophobia	foh-toh-**FOH**-bee-ah
☐ photoretinitis	**foh**-toh-reh-tih-**NIGH-tis**
☐ presbycusis	prez-bee-**KOO**-sis
☐ presbyopia	prez-bee-**OH**-pee-ah
☐ pterygium	ter-**IJ**-ee-um
☐ radial keratotomy	**RAY**-dee-al **kair**-ah-**TOT**-oh-mee
☐ retina	**RET**-ih-nah
☐ retinal photocoagulation	**REH**-tin-al **foh**-toh-koh-**ag**-yoo-**LAY**-shun

☐ retinitis pigmentosa   **reh**-tih-**NIGH**-tis **pig**-men-**TOH**-sah
☐ retinoblastoma   **reh**-tin-oh-blass-**TOH**-mah
☐ retinopathy   **reh**-tin-**OP**-ah-thee
☐ Rinne test   **RIN**-nee test
☐ sensorineural deafness   **sen**-soh-ree-**NOO**-ral deafness
☐ serous otitis media   **SEER**-us oh-**TIGH**-tis media
☐ sclera   **SKLAIR**-ah
☐ scleral buckling   **SKLAIR**-al buckling
☐ stapedectomy   **stay**-pee-**DEK**-doh-mee
☐ stapes   **STAY**-peez
☐ strabismus   strah-**BIZ**-mus
☐ suppurative otitis media   **SOO**-per-ah-tiv oh-**TIGH**-tis media
☐ suspensatory ligaments   suh-**SPEN**-sah-tor-ee ligaments
☐ tinnitus   tin-**NIGH**-tus
☐ trabeculectomy   trah-**bek**-yoo-**LEK**-toh-mee
☐ trachoma   tray-**KOH**-mah
☐ tympanic membrane   tim-**PAN**-ik membrane
☐ tympanitis   **tim**-pah-**NIGH**-tis
☐ tympanoplasty   **tim**-pan-oh-**PLASS**-tee
☐ tympanotomy   **tim**-pan-**OT**-toh-mee
☐ uveitis   yoo-vee-**EYE**-tis
☐ vertigo   **VER**-tih-goh
☐ vestibule   **VESS**-tih-byool
☐ vitrectomy   vih-**TREK**-toh-mee
☐ vitreous humor   **VIH**-tree-us humor

Chapter 16
Specialty Terminology

OBJECTIVES

At the completion of this chapter, the student should be able to:

1. Define and spell medical terms related to oncology, pharmacology, and surgery.
2. Describe the difference between benign and malignant tumors.
3. Discuss four cancer treatment methods.
4. Compare five diagnostic methods related to cancer.
5. Interpret commonly used prescription medication abbreviations.
6. Differentiate between medication actions and medication effects.
7. Compare four types of anesthesia.
8. Describe six surgical positions.

OVERVIEW

This chapter introduces you to frequently used medical terminology related to the following: (1) **oncology** (on-**KALL**-oh-jee), the medical specialty for the study, diagnosis, and treatment of cancer; (2) **pharmacology** (**farm**-ah-**KALL**-oh-jee), the study of the nature, uses, and effects of drugs used for medicinal purposes; and (3) surgery. Some of the body system terms related to these topics have been presented in previous chapters. The terms presented in this chapter are more general and add to your knowledge of the language of the health-care industry.

Oncology

As stated in the overview, oncology is the medical specialty dedicated for the study, diagnosis, and treatment of cancer. Physicians who specialize in this field are called **oncologists** (on-**KALL**-oh-jists). A **radiation oncologist** is a physician who specializes in using radiation to treat cancer. A **radiation therapist** is an individual, usually a radiation technician (x-ray technician), with specialized training focused on working with equipment associated with radiation therapy.

Some texts define oncology as the sum of knowledge regarding tumors. Tumors, described as abnormal masses of tissue due to excessive cell growth, are generally classified as **benign** (bee-**NIGHN**) or **malignant** (mah-**LIG**-nant). Benign tumors are seldom life-threatening and do not spread to other parts of the body. Malignant tumors are referred to as cancer because they can be life-threatening, and are characterized by uncontrollable growth and **metastasis** (meh-**TASS**-tah-sis). According to the American Cancer Society (ACS), metastasis is the spread of cancer cells to other parts of the body.

Cancer

Cancer develops when cells in the body begin growing in an uncontrolled manner and continue to grow and form new abnormal cells. Cancer cells develop when the **DNA** (deoxyribonucleic acid) of our normal cells becomes damaged. DNA is in every cell and is responsible for directing all cellular activities, including cellular reproduction. Under normal conditions, the body is able to repair damaged DNA. In cancer cells, the DNA is not repairable, resulting in abnormal, uncontrolled cell growth and reproduction.

Damaged DNA can be inherited from genetic mutations in maternal or paternal chromosomes. About 5% of cancers in the United States are the result of inherited genetic mutations. According to the ACS, an individual's DNA becomes damaged by exposure to **carcinogens** (**kar-SIN**-oh-jenz), which are any substances that cause cancer or help cancer grow, such as the substances in tobacco products. Other environmental carcinogens include prolonged exposure to sunlight, exhaust fumes from vehicles, insecticides, and other chemicals. Regardless of the origin, cancer is the second leading cause of death in the United States.

Types of Cancer

There are two main categories of cancer that are classified according to the type of tissue where the tumor arises, or begins. The categories are **carcinomas** (**kar**-sin-**OH**-mahz) and **sarcomas** (sar-**KOH**-mahz).

Carcinomas are made up of epithelial cells and often infiltrate surrounding tissue. This is the largest group of malignant tumors and 80–90% of all cancers are carcinomas. In the early stages, this type of cancer might present as **carcinoma in situ** (**kar**-sin-**OH**-mah in **SIGH**-too), which means the tumor is confined to the organ where it first developed. The cancer has not metastasized and often is highly curable. Two types of carcinoma are **squamous** (**SKWAY**-mus) **cell carcinoma** and **adenocarcinoma** (**add**-in-noh-**kar**-sin-**OH**-mah). Squamous cell carcinoma begins in nonglandular cells such as the skin, as illustrated in Figure 16-1.

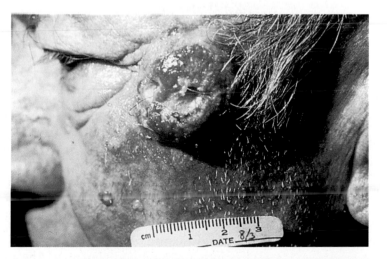

Figure 16-1   Squamous cell carcinoma (Courtesy of Robert A. Silverman, MD, Pediatric Dermatology, Georgetown University)

Adenocarcinoma begins in glandular tissue such as the ducts or lobules of the breast. Adenocarcinomas can also arise from the tissue of organs such as the stomach, colon, pancreas, and kidneys. Figure 16-2 illustrates adenocarcinoma of the colon.

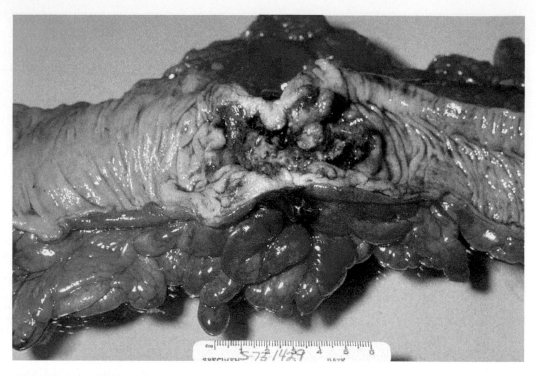

Figure 16-2 Adenocarcinoma of the colon (Centers for Disease Control/Dr. Edwin P. Ewing, Jr.)

Sarcomas begin in connective tissue such as bone, cartilage, and muscles. Recall that smooth muscle cancer is called leiomyosarcoma, and skeletal muscle cancer is called rhabdomyosarcoma. The five-year survival rate associated with sarcomas ranges from 60–75%, depending on the primary site.

Diagnostic Methods

Several **biopsy** methods are available to confirm a cancer diagnosis. All methods involve removing or withdrawing a sample of the suspicious tissue or tumor. The sample is then examined under a microscope to asses the type of cellular growth associated with the tumor. Diagnostic methods include:

- **Fine needle aspiration biopsy** (FNB)—A very thin needle attached to a syringe is used to withdraw a small amount of tissue from the suspected tumor.
- **Needle core biopsy**—A slightly larger needle is used in this type of biopsy. The larger needle allows the physician to withdraw a larger sample of tissue.
- **Excisional** or **incisional biopsy**—A surgeon cuts through the skin and removes the entire tumor, which is known as an excisional biopsy; or the surgeon removes a small part of a large tumor, which is known as an incisional biopsy. These biopsies are often done with local or regional anesthesia.
- **Endoscopic biopsy**—During an endoscopic biopsy, a flexible tube is inserted into a natural body opening. The tube contains a viewing lens or camera, a fiber-optic light, and small instruments for removing samples of the tumor or suspicious tissue.
- **Laparoscopy**, **thoracoscopy**, or **mediastinoscopy**—These methods are similar to an endoscopic biopsy, but each requires a small incision to introduce the endoscope into the body. When the sample is taken from tumors or tissue in the abdominal or pelvic cavities, the procedure is called *laparoscopy*. If the procedure involves the chest, it is called a *thoracoscopy* or *mediastinoscopy*.

- **Open surgical exploration**—When a needle or endoscopic biopsy method does not or will not provide enough information about a suspected malignancy, a *laparotomy* might be necessary. Laparotomy requires general anesthesia and often involves an incision from the lower end of the sternum to the lower part of the abdomen. With this method, the physician can visually examine the site of the tumor as well as take biopsies. If this procedure involves the chest, it is called *thoracotomy* or *mediastinotomy*.

Grading and Staging Malignant Tumors

To determine the best course of treatment, oncologists must know the characteristics of malignant tumors or cancers. This information is obtained through gross and microscopic examinations of the tumor and its cells. After these examinations are completed, the tumor is assigned a **grade** on a scale from 1 to 4, which measures the extent to which malignant cells and tissue resemble the "normal," or parent cells. Grade 1 tumors have cells that are very much like normal cells; grade 4 tumors have cells that are the least like normal cells. The term **differentiation** (**diff**-er-en-shee-**AY**-shun), which means the cells have developed into what they are supposed to be, is also used when tumors are graded. Therefore, a tumor that is categorized as *grade 1* is composed of cells that are very close to normal. Table 16-1 lists tumor grades and their definitions.

TABLE 16-1   TUMOR GRADES

Grade	Description
GX	grade cannot be assessed
G1	well-differentiated cells; tumor cells look very much like parent cells
G2	moderately differentiated; tumor cells resemble parent cells
G3	poorly differentiated; tumor cells barely resemble parent cells
G4	undifferentiated; tumor cells are unlike parent cells

Staging is used in conjunction with grading to further identify the characteristics of malignant tumors. Staging tells the oncologist the relative size of the tumor and the extent to which the tumor has metastasized. The **TNM staging system** is an internationally recognized method for staging malignant tumors. In this system, *T* refers to the size of the primary tumor, *N* refers to the involvement of regional lymph nodes, and *M* refers to how far the tumor has metastasized. Numerical values for staging range from 0 to 4, with 0 indicating the least involvement or size, and 4 indicating the highest degree of size and metastasis. Table 16-2 lists tumor stages and their definitions.

TABLE 16-2   TNM STAGING SYSTEM

Tumor	Description
T_0	no evidence of a primary tumor
T_{IS}	carcinoma in situ
T_1, T_2, T_3, T_4	progressive size of the tumor: T_1 is the smallest; T_4 is the largest
T_x	tumor cannot be assessed

(continues)

TABLE 16-2 TNM STAGING SYSTEM (continued)

Node	Description
N_0	regional lymph nodes not abnormal or not involved
N_1, N_2, N_3, N_4	increasing lymph node involvement: regional or distant; N_1 is the least number of involved lymph nodes; N_4 is the highest lymph node involvement
N_x	regional lymph nodes cannot be clinically assessed

Metastasis	Description
M_0	no evidence of metastasis
M_1, M_2, M_3	ascending degrees of metastasis: M_1 indicates less metastasis than M_2, which indicates less metastasis than M_3

EXERCISE 1

Write a brief definition for each term.

1. benign _____
2. biopsy _____
3. carcinogen _____
4. carcinoma in situ _____
5. differentiation _____
6. fine needle aspiration biopsy _____
7. malignant _____
8. metastasis _____
9. oncology _____
10. radiation oncologist _____
11. sarcoma _____
12. undifferentiated _____

EXERCISE 2

Read the following statements and write the meaning of the grade and stage for each malignant tumor.

1. adenocarcinoma of the stomach; G3, T_2, N_0, M_0

   _____

2. osteosarcoma; G4, T_3, N_2, M_1

   _____

3. adenocarcinoma of the lung; G4, T_4, N_4, M_4

   _____

Treating Cancer   Surgery is the most common way to treat cancer and offers the greatest chance for curing cancers that have not metastasized. **Curative** surgery is described as a primary cancer treatment when the tumor is *in situ* and can be removed in total. **Debulking** surgery means the surgeon removes as much of the tumor as possible, but total removal would cause significant damage to organs or tissue near the tumor. The remainder of the tumor or cancer is then treated with chemotherapy or radiation therapy, and sometimes with both.

Radiation therapy is defined as treating cancer with high-energy rays (such as x-rays) to kill or shrink cancer cells. There are two general categories of radiation therapy: external and internal. **External beam radiation** is the most widely used type of radiation therapy. As the name implies, the radiation is delivered from a source outside the body and the beams are focused on the area affected by cancer. The equipment that delivers the beams is called a **linear accelerator**. External beam radiation provides treatment for large areas of the body such as the area of the main tumor and nearby lymph nodes.

Internal radiation therapy is also called **brachytherapy (brack-ee-THEH-rah-pee)**, which means short-distance therapy. With this treatment method, the radiation source is placed directly into the tumor or cavity close to the tumor. There are two main types of internal radiation: (1) **interstitial (in-ter-STISH-al) radiation**, during which small pellets, wires, tubes, or containers of radioactive material are placed directly into or close to the tumor; and (2) **intracavity radiation**, during which a container of radioactive material is placed in a body cavity such as the vagina. Radioactive material is intended to destroy cancer cells, but also affects normal body tissue and cells such as bone marrow, the gastrointestinal tract, and reproductive organs.

Chemotherapy involves using anticancer drugs either alone or in combinations to treat cancer. This type of treatment has been available since the early 1950s. As with all cancer treatments, the objective of chemotherapy is to destroy cancer cells and tissue. The medications used in chemotherapy also have an effect on bone marrow, the gastrointestinal tract, reproductive organs, and hair follicles. Chemotherapy medications are given in the following ways:

- **Intravenous (IV)**—Medication is injected directly into a vein via a small catheter.
- **Vascular access device (VAD)**—A catheter is surgically placed under the skin into a blood vessel usually in the chest area; medications are injected into the VAD.
- **Orally**—Medications in the form of a pill, capsule, or liquid are taken by mouth.

Chemotherapy is usually given over the course of several weeks. The time between treatments allows the body's normal tissue, specifically the bone marrow, a recovery period. The chemotherapy medications travel throughout the bloodstream and can destroy cancer cells that have metastasized. Side effects of chemotherapy include nausea, vomiting, hair loss, and **neutropenia (noo-troh-PEE-nee-ah)**, which is a decrease in the number of neutrophils (white blood cells). The action of chemotherapeutic agents on bone marrow is responsible for neutropenia.

EXERCISE 3

Write the medical term for each definition or abbreviation.

1. treatment method to totally remove an
   in situ tumor _____

2. surgical removal of as much of the tumor as
   possible _____

3. most commonly used type of radiation therapy _____

4. another term for internal radiation therapy _____

5. radioactive material is placed directly into or near
   the tumor _____

6. using medications to treat cancer _____

7. VAD

Pharmacology

Pharmacology is the study of the nature, uses, and effects of drugs for medicinal purposes. A **pharmacist** is a specialist who is licensed to formulate and dispense medications. A basic understanding of the special terms related to pharmacology will add to your knowledge of the language of the health-care industry. This section covers the following topics:

- The difference between prescription and over-the-counter medications
- Routes of medication administration
- Medical terms related to medication action and effects
- Abbreviations related to medications

Some health-care professionals refer to medications as drugs. To differentiate between legal and illegal drugs, this text refers to all substances taken to treat or relieve the signs or symptoms of illness as **medications**.

Medications are dispensed under one of two names: the **generic name** or the **brand name**. The federal government assigns the generic name, which can be used by any manufacturer. Levothyroxine is the generic name for a medication prescribed to replace certain thyroid hormones. The brand name, also called the trade or private name, indicates ownership by a specific manufacturer. Synthroid is a brand name for levothyroxine; both medications are used to replace the same thyroid hormone.

Prescription and Over-the-Counter Medications

A **prescription** (**Rx**) is an order for medication, therapy, or other intervention that must be authorized by a licensed health-care professional. Prescriptions are usually given in writing by a physician. In some states, health-care professionals such as nurse practitioners or physician assistants can write prescriptions. Some prescriptions can be refilled by telephone.

A **prescription medication** is a medication that may be dispensed only with a prescription from an appropriately licensed health-care professional. A pharmacist or **pharmacy technician**, an individual who works under the direct supervision of a pharmacist, must dispense the medication. Erythromycin is an example of a familiar prescription medication.

An **over-the-counter medication (OTC)** is a medication that may be dispensed without a written prescription. Aspirin is an example of a familiar OTC medication. Many prescription medications are available in a less potent form as an OTC. Motrin is an example of a medication that is available as both an OTC and a prescription medication.

All medications must be taken as directed by the prescription or according to the product directions. Abbreviations are often used to note the time and frequency for administering or taking prescription medications. However, health-care professionals and various health-care organizations have identified abbreviations and other symbols that contribute to medication errors. Therefore, the Joint Commission, an agency that accredits health-care organizations, has issued an official "do not use" list of abbreviations and symbols. The Institute for Safe Medication Practices (ISMP) has published the ISMP List of Error-Prone Abbreviations, Symbols, and Dosage Designations. Table 16-3, which lists some of the commonly used abbreviations related to the time and frequency of administration for prescription medications, includes the "do not use" and error-prone abbreviations. Abbreviations from the Joint Commission's "do not use" list are flagged with an asterisk. Abbreviations from the ISMP's list are flagged with two asterisks. Even though these abbreviations should not be in current use, they are present in medical reports that were generated before the lists were published. Note that the abbreviations are taken from the Latin phrases that describe time and frequency.

TABLE 16-3 TIME AND FREQUENCY OF ADMINISTRATION

Abbreviation	Meaning	Latin Phrase
ac	before meals	*ante cibum*
ad lib	as desired	*ad libitum*
bid.	twice a day	*bis in die*
h, hr	hour	(none)
pc	after meals	*post cibum*
**hs	at bedtime	*hor somni*
po	by mouth	*per os*
prn	as needed	*pro re nata*
q	every	*quaque*
qam	every morning	(none)
*qd	every day	*quaque die*
qh	every hour	*quaque hora*
q2h, q3h, etc.	every 2 hours, etc.	(none)
qid	four times a day	*quarter in die*
*qod	every other day	(none)
sos	if necessary	(none)
stat	immediately	(none)
tid	three times a day	*ter in die*

* Joint Commission - Do Not Use
** ISMP - Error-Prone Abbreviations

The **dosage**, which is the amount taken, of the medication is also written as an abbreviation. Some of these abbreviations are familiar, such as **cc** to indicate cubic centimeter; others are less familiar, such as **dr** to indicate dram. Table 16-4 lists some of the commonly used abbreviations related to dosage. As in Table 16-3, abbreviations from the Joint Commission's "do not use" list are flagged with an asterisk. Abbreviations from the ISMP's list are flagged with two asterisks.

TABLE 16-4   ABBREVIATIONS FOR MEDICATION DOSAGE

Abbreviation	Meaning
¨cc	cubic centimeter
cm	centimeter
dr	dram
Gm, g, gm	gram
gr	grain
gtt	drops
kg	kilogram
L	liter
mg	milligram
mEq	millequivalent
mL	milliliter
oz	ounce
**ss̄	one-half
T, Tbsp	tablespoon
t, tsp	teaspoon

* Joint Commission - Do Not Use
** ISMP - Error-Prone Abbreviations

EXERCISE 4

Write the abbreviation for each definition.

1. after meals   _____

2. as desired   _____

3. as needed   _____

4. at bedtime   _____

5. before meals   _____

6. by mouth   _____

7. every   _____

8. four times a day   _____

9. three times a day   _____

10. twice a day   _____

EXERCISE 5

Write the meaning for each abbreviation.

1. cc   _____

2. cm   _____

3. dr   _____

4. Gm, g, gm   _____

5. gr   _____

6. gtt   _____

7. kg   _____

8. L   _____

9. mg   _____

10. mEq   _____

11. mL   _____

12. oz   _____

13. T, Tbsp   _____

14. t, tsp   _____

Routes of Administration

For a medication to be effective, it must be introduced into the body. Medications can be delivered through the digestive tract or bypassing the digestive tract. Table 16-5 lists the most common digestive tract routes of administration.

TABLE 16-5   DIGESTIVE TRACT ROUTES OF ADMINISTRATION

Route	Description	Advantages/Disadvantages
oral	given by mouth, swallowed	+ easy, safe, economical – slow absorption; might be destroyed by digestive juices
rectal	inserted into the rectum	+ patient does not have to swallow – slow irregular absorption
nasogastric	delivered through a tube placed through the nose and into the stomach	+ patient does not have to swallow – slow absorption; might be destroyed by digestive juices

Parenteral (pah-**REN**-ter-al) **routes** of administration bypass the digestive tract. These routes deliver medication through mucous membranes, the skin, muscle tissue, and veins. **Intravenous** (**IV**) administration delivers the medication directly into the bloodstream. Table 16-6 lists commonly used parenteral routes of medication administration. Three types of injections are illustrated in Figure 16-3.

TABLE 16-6 PARENTAL ROUTES OF ADMINISTRATION

Route	Description	Examples
inhalation	taken through the nose or mouth; absorbed into the bloodstream through the lungs	asthma and anesthesia medications
intradermal (ID)	injection into the dermis of the skin	vaccinations, tuberculosis and allergy tests
intramuscular (IM)	injection into muscle tissue	antibiotics
intravenous (IV)	injection directly into a vein	antibiotics, blood
sublingual	under the tongue; absorbed through the mucous membranes of the mouth	nitroglycerin
*subcutaneous (SC, SQ, SubQ)	injection into the fatty layer of the skin, just below the dermis	insulin, hormones, local anesthetics
topical	on the skin or mucous membrane	ointments, sprays, powders
transdermal	through the skin; continuous administration via a patch or disk	hormones, nitroglycerin

* Joint Commission - Do Not Use
** ISMP - Error-Prone Abbreviations

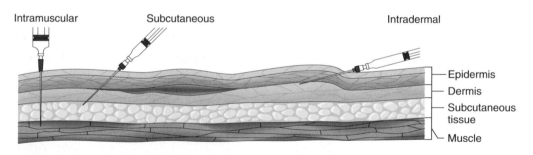

Intramuscular   Subcutaneous   Intradermal

Epidermis
Dermis
Subcutaneous tissue
Muscle

Figure 16-3 Types of injections

EXERCISE 6

With the exception of pharmac/o, *which means drug, the roots, prefixes, and suffixes associated with pharmacology were covered in previous chapters. Using your knowledge of these word parts, analyze the listed terms by separating the prefix, root, combining vowel, and suffix with vertical slashes. Write a brief definition for each term. Some terms have more than one root.*

1. intradermal

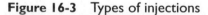

prefix   *root*   *combining vowel*   *suffix*

2. intramuscular

prefix   *root*   *combining vowel*   *suffix*

3. intravenous

prefix	root	combining vowel	suffix

4. nasogastric

prefix	root	combining vowel	suffix

5. oral

prefix	root	combining vowel	suffix

6. rectal

prefix	root	combining vowel	suffix

7. sublingual

prefix	root	combining vowel	suffix

8. subcutaneous

prefix	root	combining vowel	suffix

9. transdermal

prefix	root	combining vowel	suffix

Medication Actions and Effects

Once taken, all medications have an effect on the body. Of course, we want the medication to have the **desired effect**, to act as it was intended to act. For example, antibiotics should reduce or eliminate disease-causing bacteria; sedatives should induce a state of relaxation; anticoagulants should prevent abnormal blood clotting.

There are times, however, when medications produce an undesired or unanticipated effect. Table 16-7 lists both desirable and undesirable effects of medications.

TABLE 16-7 MEDICATION EFFECTS

Effect	Description
addiction	compulsive, uncontrollable dependence on a medication
adverse reaction	an unexpected effect of taking a medication
anaphylactic (**an**-ah-fih-**LAK**-tik) shock	serious and profound state of shock caused by an adverse reaction to a medication
cumulation (**KYOOM**-yoo-**lay**-shun)	medication levels accumulate in body tissues because the medication is not completely excreted before the next dose is given
local effect	response to a medication is confined to a specific body area, organ, or part

(continues)

☐ curette, curet   **KOO**-ret

☐ differentiation   **diff**-er-en-shee-**AY**-shun

☐ dilator   **DIGH**-lay-tor

☐ dorsal   **DOOR**-sall

☐ dorsal recumbent   **DOOR**-sall ree-**KUM**-bent

☐ endobronchial   **en**-doh-**BRONG**-kee-al

☐ endotracheal   **en**-doh-**TRAY**-kee-al

☐ epidural   ep-ih-**DOO**-ral

☐ forceps   **FOR**-seps

☐ hemostat   **HEE**-moh-stat

☐ inhalation   **in**-hah-**LAY**-shun

☐ insufflation   in-soo-**FLAY**-shun

☐ interstitial   in-ter-**STISH**-al

☐ intradermal   **in**-trah-**DERM**-al

☐ intramuscular   **in**-trah-**MUSS**-kyoo-lar

☐ intravenous   **in**-trah-**VEE**-nus

☐ malignant   mah-**LIG**-nant

☐ metastasis   meh-**TASS**-tah-sis

☐ neutropenia   noo-troh-**PEE**-nee-ah

☐ oncologist   on-**KALL**-oh-jist

☐ oncology   on-**KALL**-oh-jee

☐ palliative   **PAL**-ee-ah-tiv

☐ parenteral   pah-**REN**-ter-al

☐ pharmacist   **FARM**-ah-sist

☐ pharmacologist   **far**-mah-**KALL**-oh-jist

☐ pharmacology   **far**-mah-**KALL**-oh-jee

☐ placebo   plah-**SEE**-boh

☐ potentiation   poh-**ten**-she-**AY**-shun

☐ prophylactic   proh-fih-**LAK**-tik

☐ retractor   ree-**TRAK**-tor

☐ scalpel   **SKAL**-pal

☐ squamous   **SKWAY**-mus

☐ subcutaneous   **sub**-kyoo-**TAY**-nee-us

☐ sublingual   sub-**LING**-wall

☐ tenaculum   teh-**NAK**-yoo-lum

☐ therapeutic   **thair**-ah-**PYOO**-tik

☐ Trendelenberg   tren-**DELL**-en-burg

Appendix A
Part 1: Word Element to Meaning

WORD ROOTS

Root	Meaning
abdomin/o	abdomen
acid/o	sour; bitter
acoust/o	hearing
acr/o	extremities
aden/o	gland
adenoid/o	adenoid
adip/o	fat
adren/o	adrenal glands
adrenal/o	adrenal glands
agglutin/o	to clump
alveol/o	alveolus
amni/o	amnion
amnion/o	amnion
an/o	anus
andr/o	male; man
aneurysm/o	aneurysm
angi/o	vessel
ankyl/o	stiff
anthrac/o	coal
append/o	appendix
appendic/o	appendix
aque/o	watery
arachn/o	spider
arter/o	artery
arteri/o	artery
arteriol/o	arteriole
arthr/o	joint
articul/o	joint
atel/o	incomplete
ather/o	fat; fatty plaque; fatty, yellowish plaque

Root	Meaning
audi/o	hearing; sound
balan/o	glans penis
bas/o	base
bil/i	bile; gall
blast/o	immature
blephar/o	eyelid
bronch/o; bronch/i	bronchus
bronchiol/o	bronchiole
bucc/o	cheek
burs/o	bursa; sac
calc/i	calcium
cardi/o	heart
carp/o	wrist bones
cec/o	cecum
celi/o	abdomen
cephal/o	head
cerebell/o	cerebellum
cerebr/o	cerebrum
cervic/o	cervix
cheil/o	lips
chol/e	bile; gall
cholangi/o	bile duct
cholecyst/o	gallbladder
choledoch/o	common bile duct
chondr/o	cartilage
chori/o	chorion
clavicul/o	clavicle; collarbone
coagul/o	clotting
coccyg/o	coccyx; tailbone
cochle/o	cochlea
col/o	colon
colon/o	colon

Root	Meaning	Root	Meaning
colp/o	vagina	glomerul/o	glomerulus
coni/o	dust	gloss/o	tongue
conjunctiv/o	conjunctiva	gluc/o	glucose; sugar; sweet
cor/o	heart		
corne/o	cornea	glyc/o	glucose; sugar; sweet
coron/o	heart		
cortic/o	cortex	gonad/o	sex glands
cost/o	rib	granul/o	granules
crani/o	cranium; skull	gravid/o	pregnancy
cry/o	cold	gyn/o	woman
crypt/o	hidden	gynec/o	woman
cut/o	skin	hem/o	blood
cutane/o	skin	hemat/o	blood
cyan/o	blue; bluish	hepat/o	liver
cyst/o	bladder; sac; urinary bladder	hidr/o	sweat
		humer/o	humerus; upper arm bone
dacry/o	tears		
dacryocyst/o	tear sac	hydr/o	water; fluid
dendr/o	branching	hyster/o	uterus
derm/o	skin	ile/o	ileum
dermat/o	skin	ili/o	ilium; pelvic bone
dipl/o	two; double	immun/o	protection
dips/o	thirst	ir/o	iris
duoden/o	duodenum	irid/o	iris
electr/o	electricity	is/o	equal
embry/o	embryo	ischi/o	ischium; pelvic bone
encephal/o	brain		
endocrin/o	endocrine	jejun/o	jejunum
enter/o	intestines	kal/i	potassium
eosin/o	rosy red; rosy	kary/o	nucleus
epididym/o	epididymis	kerat/o	cornea; horny tissue; hard
epiglott/o	epiglottis		
epis/o	vulva	ket/o	ketone bodies
esophag/o	esophagus	kyph/o	humpback
fasci/o	fascia; fibrous tissue	labyrinth/o	inner ear; labyrinth
		lacrim/o	tears
femor/o	femur; thigh bone	lact/o	milk
fet/o; fet/i	fetus	lamin/o	lamina; thin flat plate or layer
fibr/o	fiber; fibrous tissue		
fibul/o	fibula; outer lower leg bone	lapar/o	abdominal wall
		laryng/o	larynx
fund/o	fundus	leiomy/o	smooth muscle
gastr/o	stomach	leuk/o	white
gingiv/o	gums	ligament/o	ligament
glauc/o	silver; gray	lingu/o	tongue
gli/o	neuroglia; nerve cell	lip/o	fat

Root	Meaning	Root	Meaning
lith/o	stone	ot/o	ear
lord/o	swayback	ovari/o	ovary
lumb/o	lower back	ox/i	oxygen
lymph/o	lymph	pachy/o	thick
lymphaden/o	lymph gland	palpebr/o	eyelid
lymphangi/o	lymph vessel	pancreat/o	pancreas
mamm/o	breast	par/o	bear; give birth to; labor; childbirth
mandibul/o	mandible; lower jawbone	part/o	bear; give birth to; labor; childbirth
mast/o	breast	patell/o	patella; kneecap
maxill/o	maxilla; upper jaw bone	pector/o	chest
meat/o	meatus; opening	pelv/i	pelvis
melan/o	black	perine/o	perineum
men/o	menses; menstruation	peritone/o	peritoneum
		phac/o	lens
mening/o	meninges	phag/o	to eat
metacarp/o	hand bones	phak/o	lens
metatars/o	foot bones	phalang/o	finger and toe bones
metr/i; metr/o	uterus		
morph/o	form; shape	pharyng/o	pharynx
muc/o	mucus	phleb/o	vein
my/o	muscle	phot/o	light
myc/o	fungus	phren/o	diaphragm
myel/o	bone marrow; spinal cord	pil/o	hair
		pleur/o	pleura
myring/o	eardrum	pneum/o	lung; air
nas/o	nose	poikil/o	varied; irregular
nat/o	birth	polyp/o	polyp
natr/o	sodium	proct/o	rectum
nephr/o	kidney	prostat/o	prostate gland
neur/o	nerve	pub/o	pubis; pelvic bone
noct/o	night	pubi/o	pubis; pelvic bone
nucle/o	nucleus	puerper/o	childbirth
nyctal/o	night	pulmon/o	lungs
ocul/o	eye	pupill/o	pupil
olig/o	few; diminished	py/o	pus
onych/o	nail	pyel/o	renal pelvis
oophor/o	ovary	quadr/i	four
ophthalm/o	eye	radi/o	radius; outer lower arm bone
opt/o	vision; eye		
or/o	mouth	rect/o	rectum
orch/o	testis; testicle	ren/o	kidney
orchi/o	testis; testicle	retin/o	retina
orchid/o	testis; testicle	rhabdomy/o	skeletal muscle; striated muscle
orth/o	straight		
oste/o	bone	rhin/o	nose

Root	Meaning	Root	Meaning
rhytid/o	wrinkles	tend/o	tendon
salping/o	fallopian tubes; oviducts	tendin/o	tendon
		tenosynov/o	tendon sheath
sarc/o	flesh	test/o	testis; testicle
scapula/o	scapula; shoulder blade	testicul/o	testis; testicle
		thec/o	sheath
scler/o	sclera; hard	thorac/o	chest
scoli/o	crooked; bent	thromb/o	clot; thrombus
seb/o	sebum	thym/o	thymus gland
semin/i	semen	thyr/o	thyroid gland
sial/o	salivary gland; saliva	thyroid/o	thyroid gland
		tonsill/o	tonsils
sigmoid/o	sigmoid colon	toxic/o	poison
sinus/o	sinus	trache/o	trachea
somat/o	body	trich/o	hair
sperm/o	sperm; spermatic cord	tympan/o	eardrum
		ungu/o	nail
spermat/o	sperm; spermatic cord	ur/o	urine; urinary system
spher/o	sphere; round	ureter/o	ureter
sphygm/o	pulse	urethr/o	urethra
spir/o	breathe; breath	uter/o	uterus
splen/o	spleen	uve/o	uvea
spondyl/o	vertebra; vertebral column	vagin/o	vagina
		vas/o	vessel; vas deferens
squam/o	scale		
staped/o	stapes; middle ear bone	ven/o	vein
		ventricul/o	ventricle
stern/o	sternum; breastbone	vertebr/o	vertebra; vertebral column
steth/o	chest	vesic/o	urinary bladder
stomat/o	mouth	vitre/o	glassy; jelly-like
sud/o	sweat	vulv/o	vulva
sudor/o	sweat	xanth/o	yellow
tars/o	ankle bones	xer/o	dry
ten/o	tendon		

PREFIXES

Prefix	Meaning	Prefix	Meaning
a-	no; not; without	astr-	star
ab-	away from	auto-	self
an-	no; not; without	bi-	two; double; both
ana-	no; not; without	brady-	slow
ante-	before; forward	carcin-	cancer; malignant
anti-	against	contra-	against; opposite

Prefix	Meaning	Prefix	Meaning
dura-	hard	non-	not
dys-	abnormal; painful; difficult	nulli-	none
echo-	sound	oxy-	sharp; quick
ect-	outside; out	pan-	all
en-	within; in; inward	para-	beside; around
endo-	within; inner	per-	through
epi-	above; upon	peri-	around; surrounding
eso-	within; in; inward	poly-	many; excessive
eu-	same; normal	post-	after
ex-	out; outward	pre-	before; in front of
hemi-	half	presby-	old
hyper-	above; excessive	primi-	first; one
hypo-	deficient; below	retro-	backward; behind; upward
infra-	below; inferior		
inter-	between	semi-	half
intra-	within	sub-	under; below; beneath
iso-	same; equal		
macro-	large	super-	above; over; excess
mal-	bad; poor; abnormal		
		supra-	above; on top of
meta-	change; after; beyond	sym-	with; association
		syn-	together; with; union
micro-	small		
mono-	one	tachy-	fast
multi-	many	tri-	three
neo-	new	uni-	one

SUFFIXES

Suffix	Meaning	Suffix	Meaning
-ac	pertaining to	-crit	to separate
-al	pertaining to	-cusia	hearing
-algia	pain	-cusis	hearing
-ary	pertaining to	-cytosis	condition of cells
-asthenia	without feeling or sensation	-desis	binding; fixation
		-dynia	pain
-blast	immature; embryonic	-ectasis	stretching; dilatation
-capnia	carbon dioxide	-ectomy	surgical removal; excision
-cele	hernia; protrusion		
-centesis	surgical puncture to remove fluid	-emesis	vomiting
		-emia	blood condition
-clasia	surgical breaking	-gen	producing; forming
-clasis	surgical breaking	-genesis	producing; forming
-crine	to secrete	-genic	producing; forming

Suffix	Meaning	Suffix	Meaning
-globin	protein	-phonia	sound; voice
-globulin	protein	-phoresis	carrying;
-gram	record; picture;		transmission
	x-ray film	-phoria	feeling; mental
-graph	instrument for		state
	recording	-plasty	surgical repair
-graphy	process of	-plegia	paralysis
	recording	-pnea	breathing
-ia	condition;	-poiesis	formation;
	abnormal condition		production of
-iac	pertaining to	-ptosis	drooping; sagging
-iasis	condition;	-ptysis	spitting up
	abnormal condition	-(r)rhagia	hemorrhage
-ic	pertaining to	-(r)rhaphy	suture of
-itis	inflammation	-(r)rhea	discharge; flow
-kinesia	movement	-(r)rhexis	rupture
-(o)logist	specialist	-sclerosis	hardening
-(o)logy	study of	-scope	instrument for
-lysis	destruction;		viewing
	breakdown	-scopy	visualization with a
-lytic	destruction;		scope
	breakdown	-somnia	sleep
-malacia	softening	-stasis	control; stop;
-megaly	enlarged;		stopping or
	enlargement		controlling
-meter	instrument to	-stenosis	narrowing
	measure	-(o)stomy	creating a new or
-metry	measuring; to		artificial opening
	measure	-therapy	treatment
-oid	like; resembling	-thorax	chest; pleural
-oma	tumor		cavity
-opia	vision	-tocia	labor; birth
-osis	condition;	-(o)tomy	incision into
	abnormal condition	-tonia	muscle tone
-ous	pertaining to	-tresia	opening
-paresis	partial paralysis	-tripsy	crushing
-pathy	disease; illness	-trophy	growth;
-penia	deficiency;		development
	decreased number	-tropia	to turn; turning
		-tropin	stimulating effect
			of a hormone
-pepsia	digestion	-tropion	to turn; turning
-pexy	surgical fixation	-uria	urine; urination
-phagia	eating; swallowing	-version	to turn
-philia	attraction to		

Appendix A
Part 2: Meaning to Word Element

WORD ROOTS

Meaning	Root
abdomen	abdomin/o; celi/o
abdominal wall	lapar/o
adenoid	adenoid/o
adrenal glands	adren/o; adrenal/o
air	pneum/o
alveolus	alveol/o
amnion	amni/o; amnion/o
aneurysm	aneurysm/o
ankle bones	tars/o
anus	an/o
appendix	append/o; appendic/o
arteriole	arteriol/o
artery	arter/o; arteri/o
base	bas/o
bear	par/o; part/o
bent	scoli/o
bile	bil/i; chol/e
bile duct	cholangi/o
birth	nat/o
bitter	acid/o
black	melan/o
bladder	cyst/o
blood	hem/o; hemat/o
blue	cyan/o
bluish	cyan/o
body	somat/o
bone	oste/o
bone marrow	myel/o
brain	encephal/o
branching	dendr/o
breast	mamm/o; mast/o
breastbone	stern/o

Meaning	Root
breath	spir/o
breathe	spir/o
bronchiole	bronchiol/o
bronchus	bronch/o; bronch/i
bursa	burs/o
calcium	calc/i
cartilage	chondr/o
cecum	cec/o
cerebellum	cerebell/o
cerebrum	cerebr/o
cervix	cervic/o
cheek	bucc/o
chest	pector/o; steth/o; thorac/o
childbirth	par/o; part/o; puerper/o
chorion	chori/o
clavicle	clavicul/o
clot	thromb/o
clotting	coagul/o
to clump	agglutin/o
coal	anthrac/o
coccyx	coccyg/o
cochlea	cochle/o
cold	cry/o
collarbone	clavicul/o
colon	col/o; colon/o
common bile duct	choledoch/o
conjunctiva	conjunctiv/o
cornea	corne/o; kerat/o
cortex	cortic/o
cranium	crani/o
crooked	scoli/o

Meaning	Root	Meaning	Root
diaphragm	phren/o	glassy	vitre/o
diminished	olig/o	glomerulus	glomerul/o
double	dipl/o	glucose	gluc/o; glyc/o
dry	xer/o	granules	granul/o
duodenum	duoden/o	gray	glauc/o
dust	coni/o	gums	gingiv/o
ear	ot/o	hair	pil/o; trich/o
eardrum	myring/o; tympan/o	hand bones	metacarp/o
to eat	phag/o	hard	kerat/o; scler/o
electricity	electr/o	head	cephal/o
embryo	embry/o	hearing	acoust/o; audi/o
endocrine	endocrin/o	heart	cardi/o; cor/o;
epididymis	epididym/o		coron/o
epiglottis	epiglott/o	hidden	crypt/o
equal	is/o	horny tissue	kerat/o
esophagus	esophag/o	humerus	humer/o
extremities	acr/o	humpback	kyph/o
eye	ocul/o; ophthalm/o;	ileum	ile/o
	opt/o	ilium	ili/o
eyelid	blephar/o;	immature	blast/o
	palpebr/o	incomplete	atel/o
fallopian tubes	salping/o	inner ear	labyrinth/o
fascia	fasci/o	intestines	enter/o
fat	adip/o; lip/o	iris	ir/o; irid/o
fatty, yellowish	ather/o	irregular	poikil/o
plaque		ischium	ischi/o
femur	femor/o	jejunum	jejun/o
fetus	fet/o; fet/i	jelly-like	vitre/o
few	olig/o	joint	arthr/o; articul/o
fiber	fibr/o	ketone bodies	ket/o
fibrous tissue	fasci/o; fibr/o	kidney	ren/o; nephr/o
fibula	fibul/o	kneecap	patell/o
finger and toe	phalang/o	labor	par/o; part/o
bones		labyrinth	labyrinth/o
flesh	sarc/o	lamina	lamin/o
fluid	hydr/o	larynx	laryng/o
foot bones	metatars/o	lens	phac/o; phak/o
form	morph/o	ligament	ligament/o
four	quadr/i	light	phot/o
fundus	fund/o	lips	cheil/o
fungus	myc/o	liver	hepat/o
gall	bil/i; chol/e	lower back	lumb/o
gallbladder	cholecyst/o	lower jawbone	mandibul/o
give birth to	par/o; part/o	lung	pneum/o
gland	aden/o	lungs	pulmon/o
glans penis	balan/o	lymph	lymph/o

Meaning	Root
lymph gland	lymphaden/o
lymph vessel	lymphangi/o
male	andr/o
man	andr/o
mandible	mandibul/o
maxilla	maxill/o
meatus	meat/o
meninges	mening/o
menses	men/o
menstruation	men/o
middle ear bone	staped/o
milk	lact/o
mouth	or/o; stomat/o
mucus	muc/o
muscle	my/o
nail	onych/o; ungu/o
nerve	neur/o
nerve cell	gli/o
neuroglia	gli/o
night	noct/o; nyctal/o
nose	nas/o; rhin/o
nucleus	kary/o; nucle/o
opening	meat/o
outer lower arm bone	radi/o
outer lower leg bone	fibul/o
ovary	oophor/o; ovari/o
oviducts	salping/o
oxygen	ox/i
pancreas	pancreat/o
patella	patell/o
pelvic bone	ili/o; ischi/o; pubi/o; pub/o
pelvis	pelv/i
perineum	perine/o
peritoneum	peritone/o
pharynx	pharyng/o
pleura	pleur/o
poison	toxic/o
polyp	polyp/o
potassium	kal/i
pregnancy	gravid/o
prostate gland	prostat/o
protection	immun/o
pubis	pubi/o; pub/o
pulse	sphygm/o

Meaning	Root
pupil	pupill/o
pus	py/o
radius	radi/o
rectum	proct/o; rect/o
renal pelvis	pyel/o
retina	retin/o
rib	cost/o
rosy	eosin/o
rosy red	eosin/o
round	spher/o
sac	cyst/o; burs/o
saliva	sial/o
salivary gland	sial/o
scale	squam/o
scapula	scapula/o
sclera	scler/o
sebum	seb/o
semen	semin/i
sex glands	gonad/o
shape	morph/o
sheath	thec/o
shoulder blade	scapula/o
sigmoid colon	sigmoid/o
silver	glauc/o
sinus	sinus/o
skeletal muscle	rhabdomy/o
skin	cut/o; cutane/o; derm/o; dermat/o
skull	crani/o
smooth muscle	leiomy/o
sodium	natr/o
sound	acoust/o; audi/o; ech/o
sour	acid/o
sperm	sperm/o; spermat/o
spermatic cord	sperm/o; spermat/o
sphere	spher/o
spider	arachn/o
spinal cord	myel/o
spleen	splen/o
stapes	staped/o
sternum	stern/o
stiff	ankyl/o
stomach	gastr/o
stone	lith/o
straight	orth/o

Meaning	Root
striated muscle	rhabdomy/o
sugar	gluc/o; glyc/o
swayback	lord/o
sweat	hidr/o; sud/o; sudor/o
sweet	gluc/o; glyc/o
tailbone	coccyg/o
tear sac	dacryocyst/o
tears	dacry/o; lacrim/o
tendon	ten/o; tend/o; tendin/o
tendon sheath	tenosynov/o
testicle	orch/o; orchi/o; orchid/o; test/o; testicul/o
testis	orch/o; orchi/o; orchid/o; test/o; testicul/o
thick	pachy/o
thigh bone	femor/o
thin flat plate or layer	lamin/o
thirst	dips/o
thrombus	thromb/o
thymus gland	thym/o
thyroid gland	thyr/o; thyroid/o
tongue	gloss/o; lingu/o
tonsils	tonsill/o
trachea	trache/o
two	dipl/o

Meaning	Root
upper arm bone	humer/o
upper jawbone	maxill/o
ureter	ureter/o
urethra	urethr/o
urinary bladder	vesic/o; cyst/o
urinary system	ur/o
urine	ur/o
uterus	hyster/o; metr/i; metr/o; uter/o
uvea	uve/o
vagina	colp/o; vagin/o
varied	poikil/o
vas deferens	vas/o
vein	phleb/o; ven/o
ventricle	ventricul/o
vertebra	spondyl/o; vertebr/o
vertebral column	spondyl/o; vertebr/o
vessel	angi/o; vas/o
vision	opt/o
vulva	epis/o; vulv/o
water	hydr/o
watery	aque/o
white	leuk/o
woman	gyn/o; gynec/o
wrinkles	rhytid/o
wrist bones	carp/o
yellow	xanth/o

PREFIXES

Meaning	Prefix
abnormal	dys-; mal-
above; on top of; upon	supra-; epi-
above; over; excess; excessive	super-; hyper-
after	post-; meta-
against	anti-; contra-
all	pan-
around	para-; peri-
association	sym-
away from	ab-
backward	retro-

Meaning	Prefix
bad	mal-
before	ante-; pre-
behind	retro-
below	infra-; hypo-; sub-
beneath	sub-
beside	para-
between	inter-
beyond	meta-
both	bi-
cancer	carcin-
change	meta-
deficient	hypo-

Meaning	Prefix
difficult	dys-
double	bi-
equal	iso-
excessive	poly-; hyper-; super-
fast	tachy-
first	primi-
forward	ante-
half	hemi-; semi-
hard	dura-
in	en-; eso-
in front of	pre-
inferior	infra-
inner	endo-
inward	en-; eso-
large	macro-
malignant	carcin-
many	multi-; poly-
new	neo-
no	a-; an-; ana-
none	nulli-
normal	eu-
not	a-; an-; ana-; non-
old	presby-
one	mono-; primi-; uni-
opposite	contra-

Meaning	Prefix
out	ect-; ex-
outside	ect-
outward	ex-
painful	dys-
poor	mal-
quick	oxy-
same	eu-; iso-
self	auto-
sharp	oxy-
slow	brady-
small	micro-
sound	echo-
star	astr-
surrounding	peri-
three	tri-
through	per-
together	syn-
two	bi-
under	sub-
union	syn-
upward	retro-
with	syn-; sym-
within	en-; eso-; endo-; intra-
without	a-; an-; ana-

SUFFIXES

Meaning	Suffix
abnormal condition	-ia; -iasis; -osis
attraction to	-philia
binding	-desis
birth	-tocia
blood condition	-emia
breakdown	-lysis; -lytic
breathing	-pnea
carbon dioxide	-capnia
carrying	-phoresis
chest	-thorax
condition	-ia; -iasis; -osis
condition of cells	-cytosis
control; controlling	-stasis
creating a new or artificial opening	-(o)stomy

crushing	-tripsy
decreased number	-penia
deficiency	-penia
destruction	-lysis; -lytic
development	-trophy
digestion	-pepsia
dilatation	-ectasis
discharge	-(r)rhea
disease	-pathy
drooping	-ptosis
eating	-phagia
embryonic	-blast
enlarged	-megaly
excision	-ectomy
feeling	-phoria
fixation	-desis
flow	-(r)rhea
formation	-poiesis

Meaning	Suffix
forming	-genesis; -genic; -gen
growth	-trophy
hardening	-sclerosis
hearing	-cusis; cusia
hemorrhage	-(r)rhagia
hernia	-cele
illness	-pathy
immature	-blast
incision into	-(o)tomy
inflammation	-itis
instrument for recording	-graph
instrument for viewing	-scope
instrument to measure	-meter
labor	-tocia
like	-oid
to measure; measuring	-metry
mental state	-phoria
movement	-kinesia
muscle tone	-tonia
narrowing	-stenosis
opening	-tresia
pain	-algia; -dynia
paralysis	-plegia
partial paralysis	-paresis
pertaining to	-ac; -al; -ary; -iac; -ic; -ous
picture	-gram
pleural cavity	-thorax
process of recording	-graphy
producing	-genesis; -genic; -gen
production of	-poiesis
protein	-globin; -globulin

Meaning	Suffix
protrusion	-cele
record	-gram
resembling	-oid
rupture	-(r)rhexis
sagging	-ptosis
to secrete	-crine
to separate	-crit
sleep	-somnia
softening	-malacia
sound	-phonia
specialist	-(o)logist
spitting up	-ptysis
stimulating effect of a hormone	-tropin
stop; stopping	-stasis
stretching	-ectasis
study of	-(o)logy
surgical breaking	-clasis; -clasia
surgical fixation	-pexy
surgical puncture to remove fluid	-centesis
surgical removal	-ectomy
surgical repair	-plasty
suture of	-(r)rhaphy
swallowing	-phagia
transmission	-phoresis
treatment	-therapy
tumor	-oma
to turn; turning	-tropia; -tropion; -version
urine; urination	-uria
vision	-opia
visualization with a scope	-scopy
voice	-phonia
vomiting	-emesis
without feeling or sensation	-asthenia
x-ray film	-gram

Appendix B
Abbreviation List

Abbreviation	Meaning
ac	before meals
ABG	arterial blood gases
AC	air conduction
ACTH	adrenocorticotropic hormone
ad lib	as desired
AD	right ear (auris dextra)
ADH	antidiuretic hormone
AIDS	acquired immune deficiency syndrome
ALS	amyotrophic lateral sclerosis
ANS	autonomic nervous system
ARD	acute respiratory distress
ARDS	adult respiratory distress syndrome
ARF	acute respiratory failure
AS	left ear (auris sinistra)
ASHD	arteriosclerotic heart disease
AU	each ear (auris unitas)
AV node	atrioventricular node
BBB	bundle branch block
bid	twice a day
BC	bone conduction
BE	barium enema
BOM	bilateral otitis media
BP	blood pressure
BPH	benign prostatic hypertrophy
BUN	blood urea nitrogen
Bx, Bx	biopsy
c̄	with
CABG	coronary artery bypass graft
CAD	coronary artery disease
CAPD	continuous ambulatory peritoneal dialysis
CAT	computed axial tomography
CBC	complete blood count
cc	cubic centimeter
CCPD	continuous cycler-assisted peritoneal dialysis

Abbreviation	Meaning
CF	cystic fibrosis
CHF	congestive heart failure
cm	centimeter
CNS	central nervous system
CO_2	carbon dioxide
COPD	chronic obstructive pulmonary disease
CP	cerebral palsy
CPR	cardiopulmonary resuscitation
C-section	cesarean section
CSF	cerebrospinal fluid
CST	contraction stimulation test
CVA	cerebrovascular accident
CVS	chorionic villus sampling
D&C	dilatation and curettage
DEXA	duel-energy x-ray absorptiometry
DIP	distal interphalangeal
dr	dram
DTR	deep tendon reflexes
DVT	deep vein thrombosis
ECCE	extracapsular cataract extraction
EDB	expected date of birth
EDC	expected or estimated date of confinement
EDD	expected date of delivery
EEG	electroencephalography
EENT	eyes, ears, nose, throat
EGD	esophagogastroduodenoscopy
EKG, ECG	electrocardiogram
EMG	electromyography
ENT	ears, nose, throat
EOM	extraocular movement
ERCP	endoscopic retrograde cholangiopancreatography
ESR	erythrocyte sedimentation rate
FBS	fasting blood sugar
FHR	fetal heart rate
FM	fibromyalgia
FSH	follicle-stimulating hormone
fx	fracture
GERD	gastroesophageal reflux disease
GH	growth hormone
GI	gastrointestinal
GI series	gastrointestinal series
Gm, g, gm	gram
gr	grain
gtt	drops
GTT	glucose tolerance test
GYN	gynecology

Abbreviation	Meaning
h, hr	hour
hs	at bedtime
HD	Huntington's disease
Hct	hematocrit
Hgb	hemoglobin
HHD	hypertensive heart disease
HIV	human immunodeficiency virus
HPV	human papillomavirus
HSV	herpes simplex virus
ICCE	intracapsular cataract extraction
ICP	intracranial pressure
ID	intradermal
IDDM	insulin-dependent diabetes mellitus
IM	intramuscular
inj	injection
IOL	intraocular lens
IOP	intraocular pressure
IU	international unit
IV	intravenous
IVP	intravenous pyelography
kg	kilogram
KUB	kidneys, ureters, and bladder
L	liter
LAGBP	laparoscopic adjustable gastric bypass
LASIK	laser in situ keratomileusis
L&D	labor and delivery
LH	luteinizing hormone
LLQ	left lower quadrant
LMP	last menstrual period
LP	lumbar puncture
LUQ	left upper quadrant
MCH	mean corpuscular hemoglobin
MCHC	mean corpuscular hemoglobin concentration
MCP	metacarpophalangeal
MCV	mean corpuscular volume
MD	muscular dystrophy
mEq	milliequivalent
mg	milligram
MI	myocardial infarction
mL	milliliter
MRI	magnetic resonance imaging
MS	multiple sclerosis
MSH	melanocyte-stimulating hormone
MTP	metatarsophalangeal
NG	nasogastric
NHL	non-Hodgkin's lymphoma
NIDDM	non–insulin-dependent diabetes mellitus

Abbreviation	Meaning
NIPD	nocturnal intermittent peritomeal dialysis
NPO, npo	nothing by mouth
NSD	normal spontaneous delivery
OB	obstetrics
OD	right eye (oculus dexter)
oint., ung	ointment
ORIF	open reduction internal fixation
OS	left eye (oculus sinister)
OTC	over-the-counter
OU	each eye (oculus uterque)
oz	ounce
pc	after meals
po	by mouth
prn	as needed
PAC	premature atrial contraction
PAP	prostatic acid phosphatase
Pap smear	Papanicolaou smear
PAT	paroxysmal atrial tachycardia
PCP	*Pneumocystis carinii* pneumonia
PEG	pneumoencephalogram
PERRLA	pupils equal, round, reactive to light and accommodation
PFTs	pulmonary function tests
PID	pelvic inflammatory disease
PIH	pregnancy-induced hypertension
PIP	proximal interphalangeal
PMS	premenstrual syndrome
PNS	peripheral nervous system
PPS	postpolio sydrome
PRK	photo-refractive keratectomy
PSA	prostate-specific antigen
PT	prothrombin time
PTCA	percutaneous transluminal coronary angioplasty
PTH	parathyroid hormone
PVC	premature ventricular contraction
q	every
q2h	every 2 hours
qam	every morning
qd	every day
qh	every hour
qid	four times a day
qod	every other day
RA	rheumatoid arthritis
RAIU	radioactive iodine uptake test
RBC	red blood cell
RDS	respiratory distress syndrome
REM	rapid eye movement

Abbreviation	Meaning
RF	rheumatoid factor
RHD	rheumatic heart disease
RK	radial keratotomy
RLQ	right lower quadrant
RUQ	right upper quadrant
Rx	treatment; prescription
RYGBP	Roux-en-y gastric bypass
$\bar{s}$	without
SA node	sinoatrial node
SBF	small bowel follow-through
SC	subcutaneous
sig	write on label
SNS	somatic nervous system
SOB	shortness of breath
sol	solution
sos	if necessary
$\overline{ss}$	one-half
stat	immediately
STH	somatotropin hormone
STI	sexually transmitted infection
subQ	subcutaneous
supp	suppository
SVD	spontaneous vaginal delivery
T, Tbsp	tablespoon
t, tsp	teaspoon
tid	three times a day
T_3	triiodothyronine
T_4	thyroxine
tab	tablet
TAH	total abdominal hysterectomy
TB	tuberculosis
TEE	transesophageal echocardiogram
TENS	transcutaneous electrical nerve stimulation
THR	total hip replacement
TIA	transient ischemic attack
tinct	tincture
TM	tympanic membrane
TO	telephone order
TPN	total parenteral nutrition
TSH	thyroid-stimulating hormone
TSS	toxic shock syndrome
TURP	transurethral resection of the prostate
TVH	total vaginal hysterectomy
U	unit
UA	urinalysis
UGI	upper gastrointestinal series

Abbreviation	Meaning
UPPP	uvulopalatopharyngoplasty
URI	upper respiratory tract infection
UTI	urinary tract infection
VA	visual acuity
VAD	vascular access device
VF	visual field
VO	verbal order
V/Q scan	ventilation/perfusion scan
WBC	white blood cell

Appendix C
Health-Related Web Sites

Name	Web Address	Brief Description
American Cancer Society	www.cancer.org	primary resource for information about cancer prevention, detection, and treatment
Center for Disease Control	www.cdc.gov	primary resource for information about current activities related to prevention and control of communicable diseases
Discovery Health	http://health.discovery.com	Discovery Channel's health Web site; user-friendly information about a wide variety of health issues
Mayo Clinic	www.mayohealth.org/home	Mayo Clinic home page; user friendly access to information from a highly respected leading institution in health care
Medical Dictionary	www.medicaldictionary.com	A comprehensive medical dictionary
Medline	www.medlineplus.gov	A subservice of the National Library of Medicine; information available by subject
Merck Manual Home Edition	www.merck.com/mmhe/index.html	consumer friendly, online version of the widely used medical reference *The Merck Manual*
WebMD	http://health.msn.com	MSN health Web site; user friendly alphabetic index of diseases, conditions, and more

INDEX